AF709995

中医科普系列—抑郁症

Depression

Help From Chinese Medicine

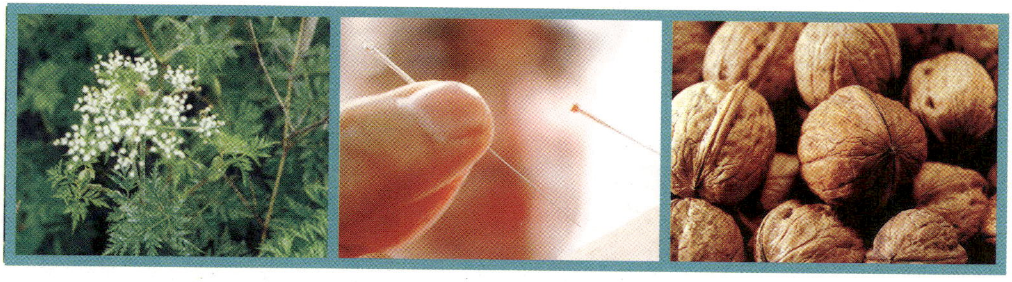

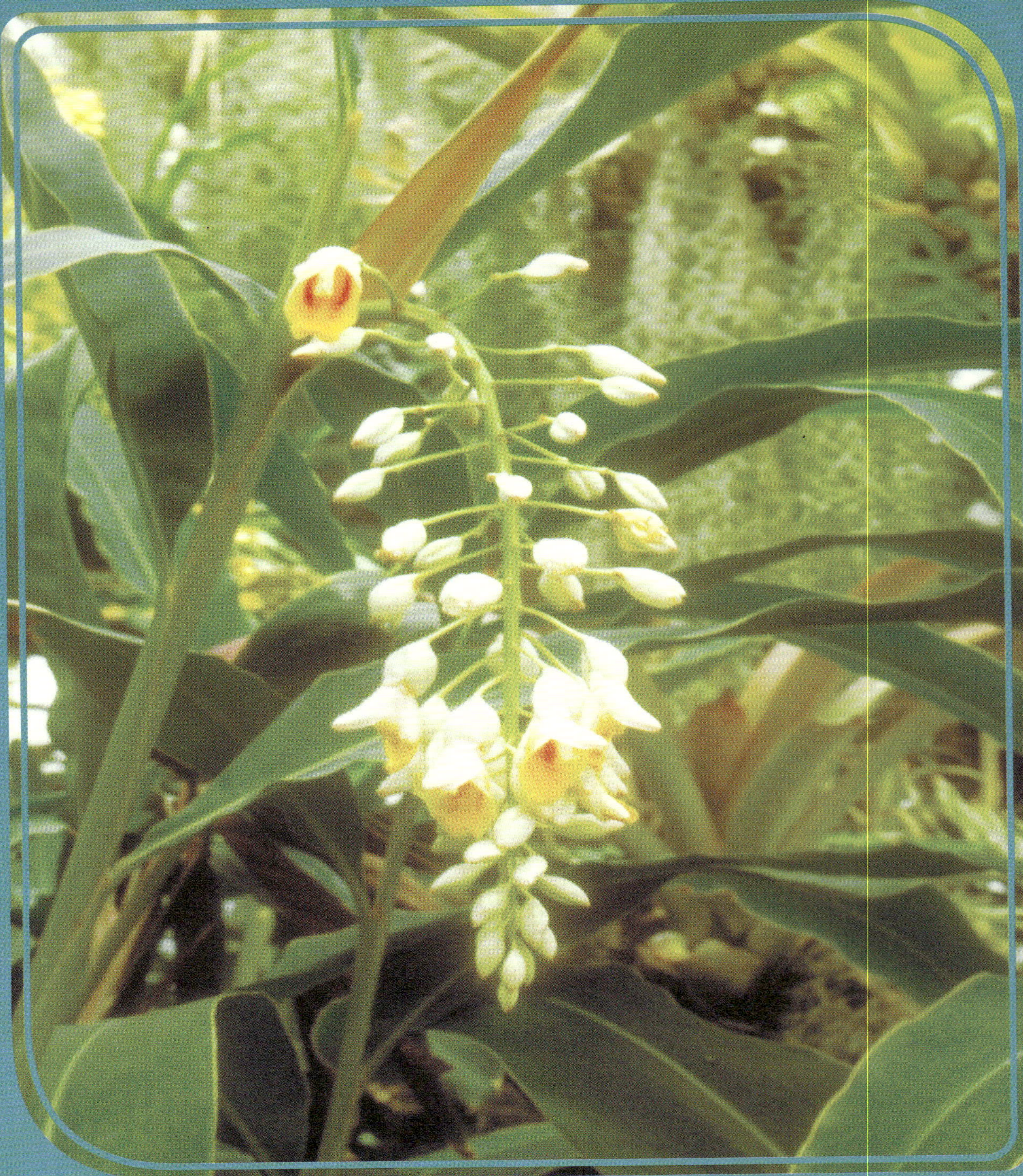

中医科普系列—抑郁症

Depression

Help From Chinese Medicine

Chen Yun-hui, Ph.D. TCM

Carl Stimson, L.Ac.

Edited by Mark Mondot, L.Ac.
Photographed and Designed by Beijing Sense Media Inc., Ltd.

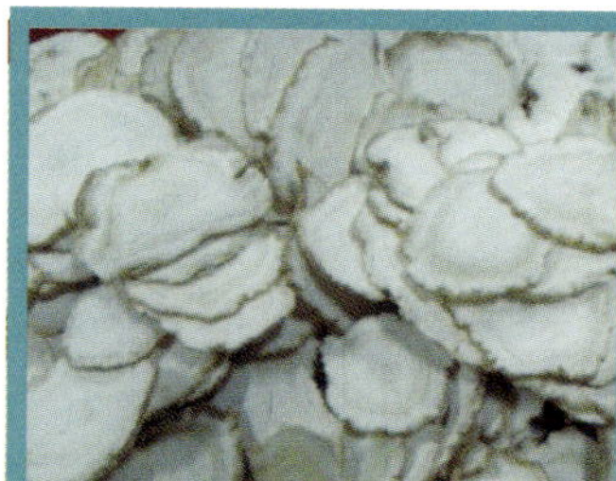
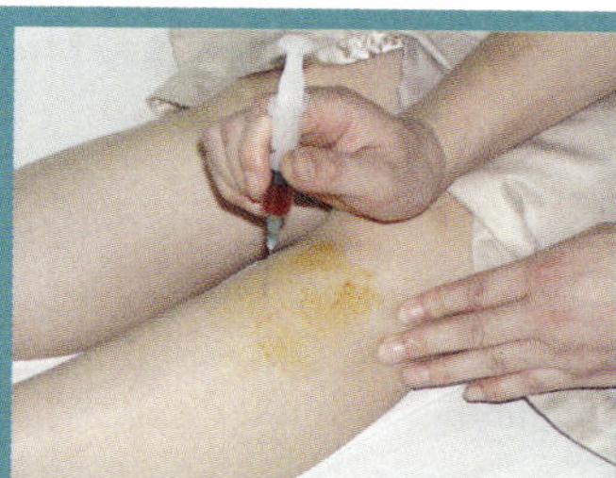
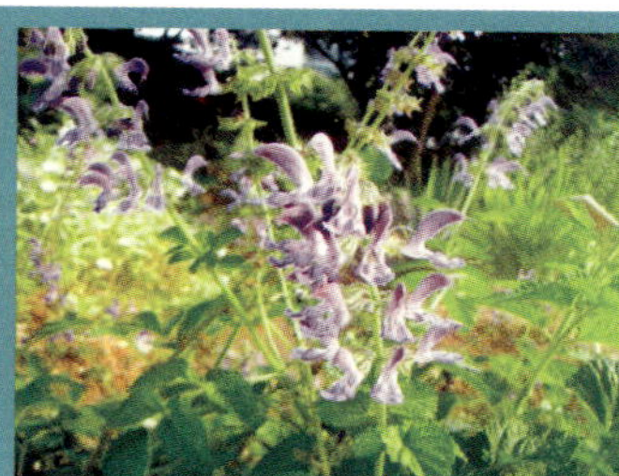

人民卫生出版社
PMPH
PEOPLE'S MEDICAL PUBLISHING HOUSE
BEIJING • LONDON • NEW YORK

人民卫生出版社
PMPH PEOPLE'S MEDICAL PUBLISHING HOUSE
Website: http://www.pmph.com

Book Title: Depression — Help From Chinese Medicine
中医科普系列—抑郁症

Contact address: Bldg 3, 3 Qu, Fangqunyuan, Fangzhuang, Beijing 100078, P.R. China
Phone/fax: 8610 6769 1034, E-mail: pmph@pmph.com

For text and trade sales, as well as review copy enquiries, please contact at pmphsales@gmail.com

Disclaimer

This book is for educational and reference purposes only. In view of the possibility of human error or changes in medical science, the author, editor, publisher or any other party involved in the publication of this work do not guarantee that the information contained herein is in any respect accurate or complete. The medicinal therapies and treatment techniques presented in this book are provided for the purpose of reference only. If readers wish to attempt any of the techniques or utilize any of the medicinal therapies contained in this book, the publisher assumes no responsibility for any such actions.

It is the responsibility of the readers to understand and adhere to local laws and regulations concerning the practice of these techniques and methods. The authors, editors, and publishers disclaim all responsibility for any liability, loss, injury, or damage incurred as a consequence, directly or indirectly, of the use and application of any of the content of this book.

Images in this book are from the Beijing Sense Media Inc., Ltd.
Phone: 8610 6403 7576, E-mail: sshg@sshg6688.com

First published: **2009**
ISBN: 978-7-117-11472-1/R·11473

Cataloguing in Publication Data:
A catalog record for this book is available from the CIP-Database China.

Printed in The People's Republic of China

ISBN 978-7-117-11472-1
9 787117 114721 >

Foreword

Depression is one of the major problems facing our society since our increasingly busy lifestyles have put tremendous pressure and stress on each one of us. Depression can also cause or coexist with a variety of illnesses such as cardiovascular diseases, gastrointestinal diseases, cancer, etc. It should be diagnosed and treated properly as other diseases, but ironically even if you are properly diagnosed and treated, you may still need to worry about the side effects and the remission associated with antidepressants.

During my visit to the U.S. in 2007, one of my friends asked, "How do people in China deal with depression?" Indeed, more and more people struggling with depression start to ask, "Are there any safe and effective treatments that I can use regularly? Is there any natural way to deal with depression?" Many popular antidepressants are not available in rural hospitals in China, but this does not necessarily mean that the Chinese experience less stress than people from other countries do, since it is very hard to avoid stress in today's world, no matter where you are. The difference is that people in China dealing with depression and emotional problems can get help from Chinese medicine instead of solely relying on biomedicine.

With a time-honored history, Chinese medicine has formed a unique system to diagnose and cure disease, which is fundamentally different from that of Western medicine. In Chinese medicine, the understanding of the human body is based on the holistic concept, and the treatment of disease is based primarily on syndrome differentiation. With Chinese medicine, you have at your disposal an arsenal of complementary therapeutic methods to manage depression. To name but just a few, acupuncture stimulates certain areas of the external body to relieve depression, and medicinals act on *zang-fu* organs internally. In case of slight and mild depression, these therapies may work as a stand-alone treatment. While for severe depression, please contact your physician and get immediate treatment, meanwhile look at the alternative therapies offered in this book and see whether you can use them as an approach to make the antidepressant more effective or to fight against the side effects. Due to potential interactions, please consult with your physician before you begin taking any medicinals.

Moreover, not everyone with an interest in Chinese medicine has depression or other health problems. You may simply want to remain happy and healthy, with a fresh daily supply of energy and vigor. No matter how you choose to use this book, I sincerely hope it will help you deal with depression and provide you with potent strategies that help you stay cheerful and vigorous for your whole life.

Chen Yun-hui
June 1, 2009

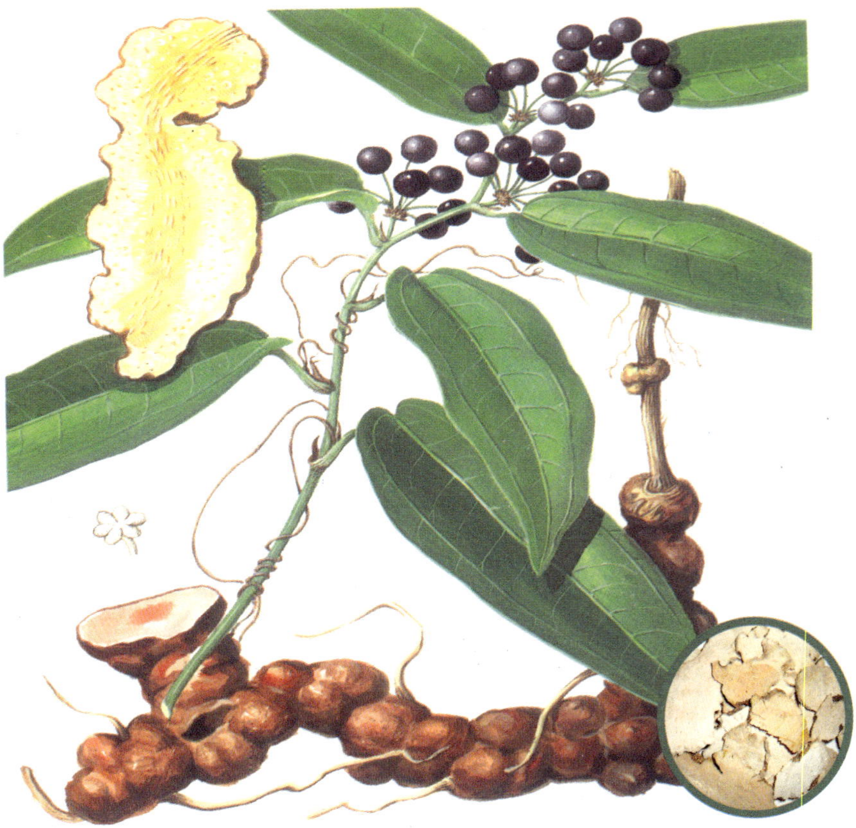

Smilacis Glabre

Guide to the Book

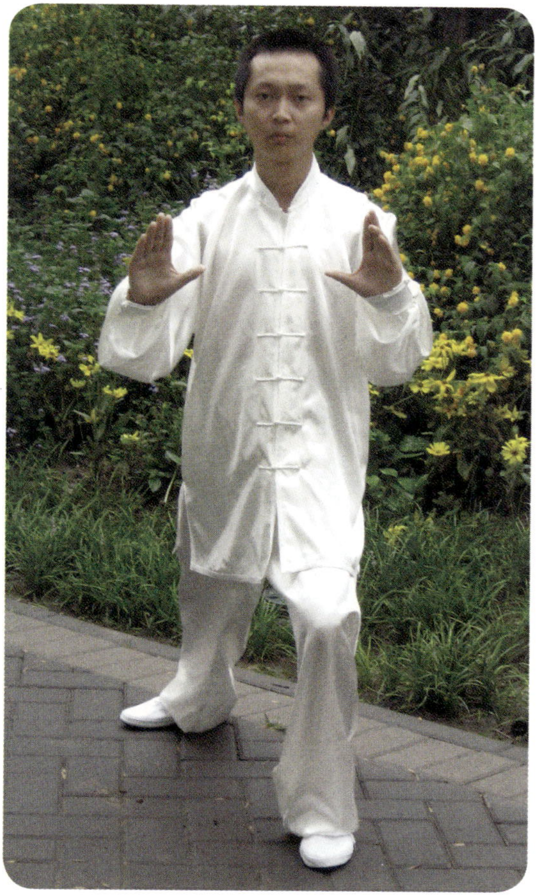

Explain

You may be considering getting help managing your depression with Chinese medicine but you have no idea what the treatment will be like. Or you may have already begun treatment and want to know more about the theories and methods used, and participate in the changes happening to you. If you find yourself in one of these situations, then this is the right book for you. It will help you to better understand what Chinese medicine is, how it can help, and what is involved in treatment. The basic theories will be introduced and the methods used by practitioners around the world will be explained in detail. Explanations of commonly known techniques such as acupuncture and medicinals, as well as lesser known modalities like moxibustion and tui na (massage) will help clear up any questions or misconceptions as well as prepare you for treatment. And lastly, where available, excerpts from modern research and clinical trials are included to inspire confidence in the ancient theories and methods.

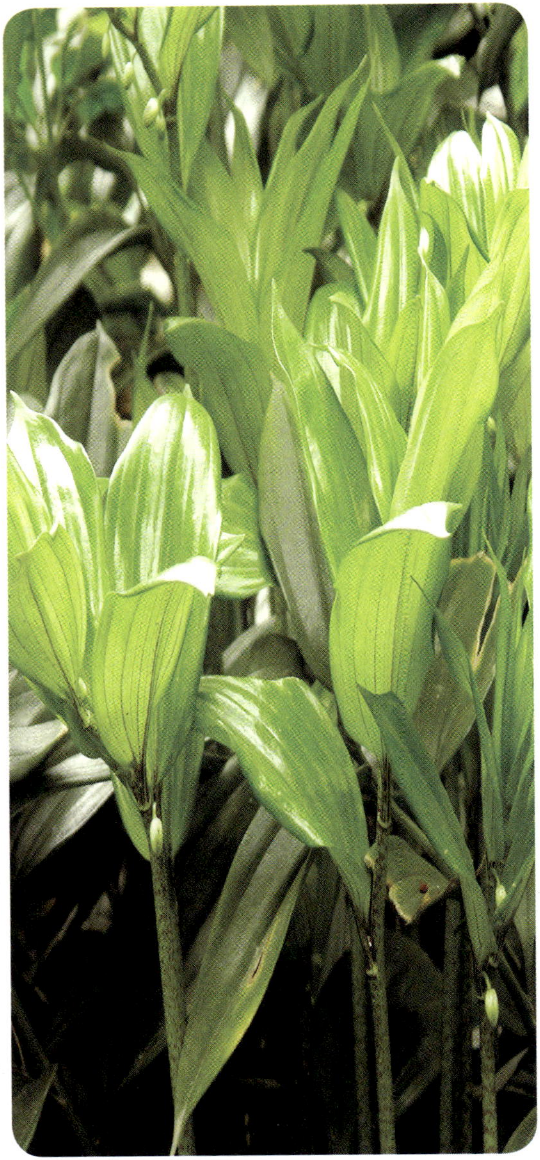

Solomonseal

Guide

The second purpose of this book is to provide you with a resource that can be used to help implement lifestyle changes that will alleviate symptoms as well as increase general health and prevent future illness. There is helpful information on eating habits, exercise programs, and a variety of at-home treatments that are both easy and affordable. From experience, doctors of Chinese medicine know that with proper treatment the amount and intensity of biomedical intervention necessary can be reduced or even eliminated. It is our hope that with the help of this book as a guide, all kinds of medical intervention can be reduced so that your time, energy, and money can be better spent doing the things you love.

While there is a lot of valuable information in the following chapters, this book is in no way intended to substitute for the care of a trained professional. Making a proper diagnosis and prescribing effective treatments are skills that take years to master and is especially difficult in complex problems such as depression. Chinese medicine is a highly individualized system, and the help of a proper guide, especially in the beginning stages of treatment, is essential. For suggestions on how to go about finding a qualified practitioner, please see the appendix.

Table of Contents

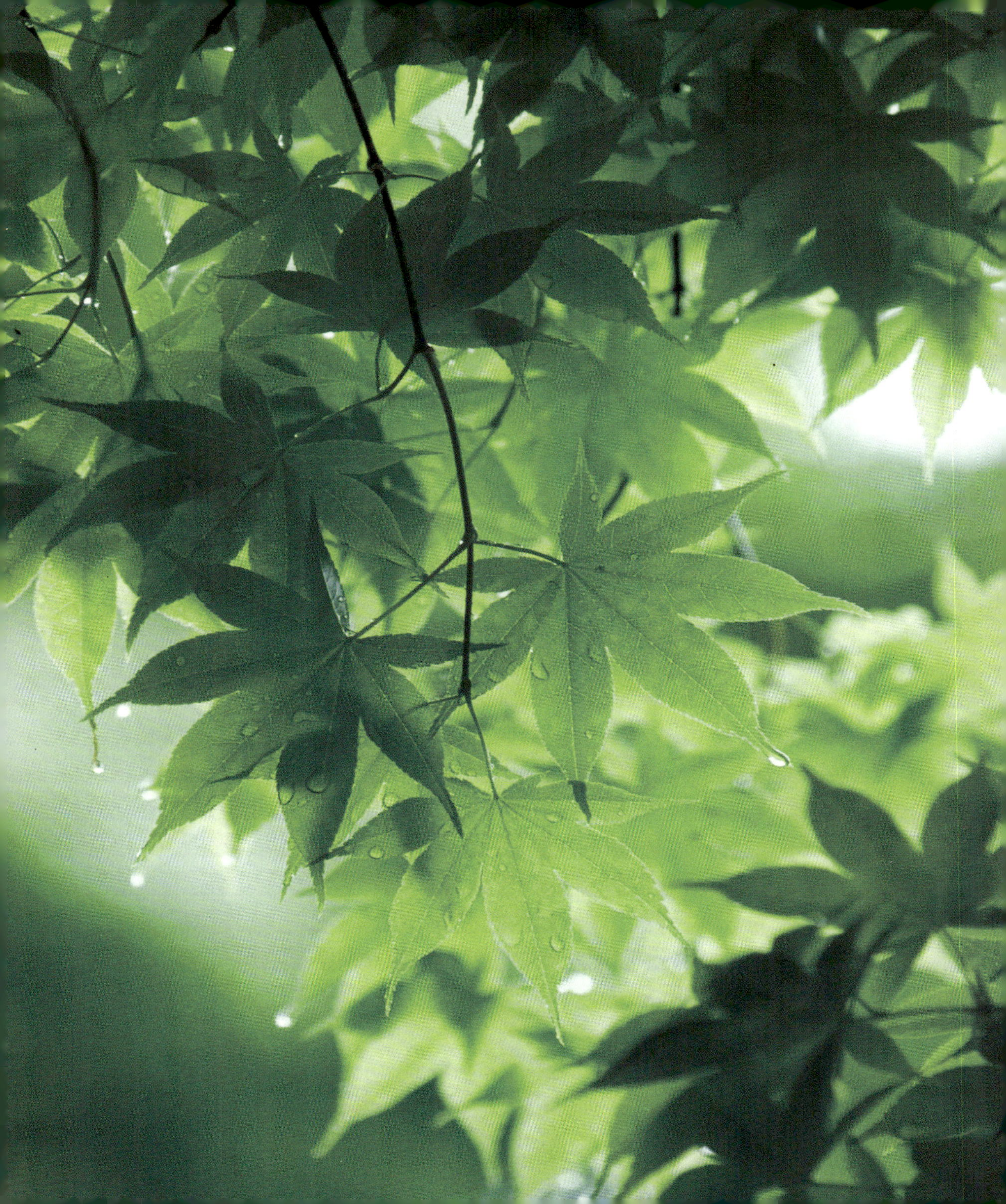

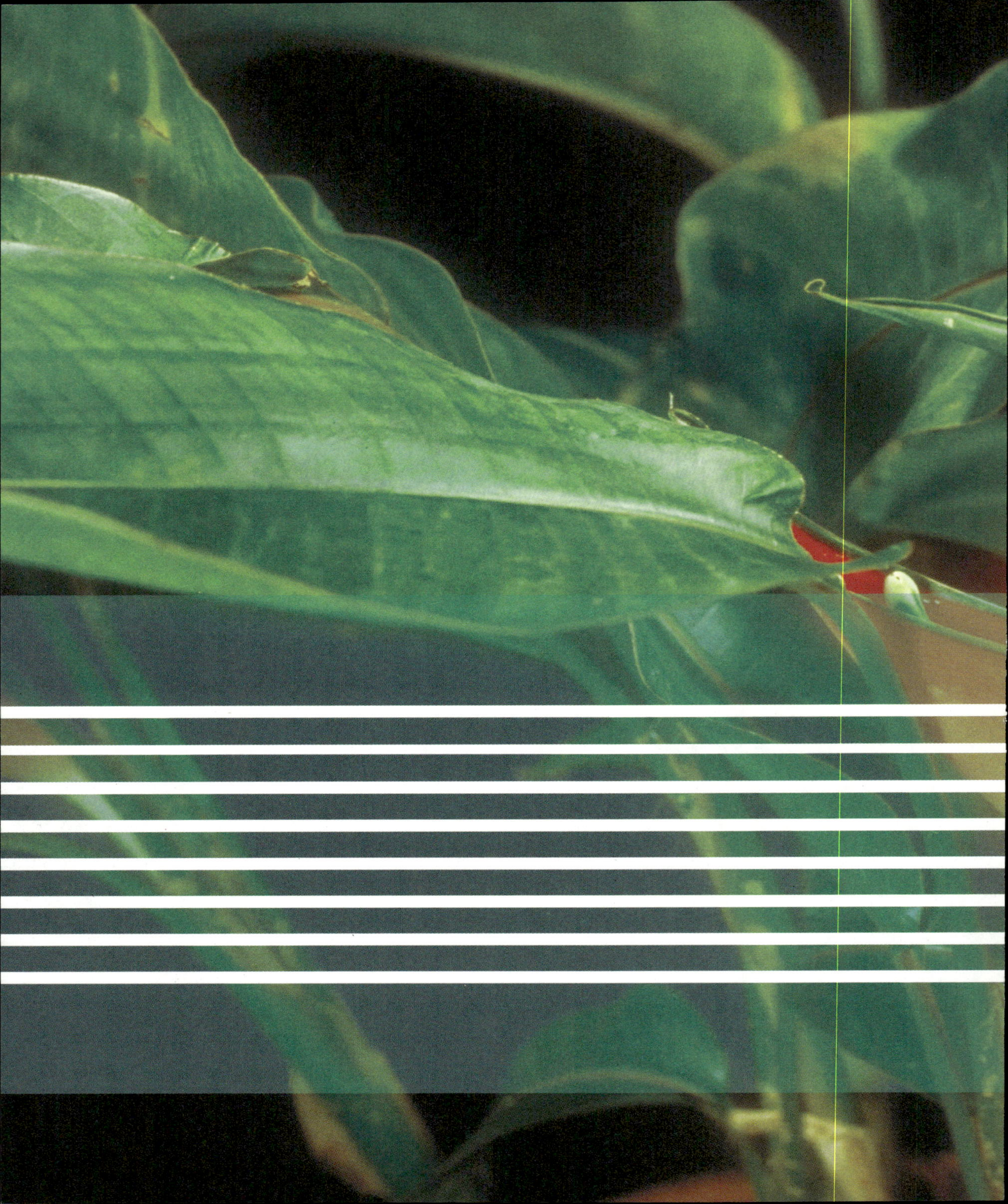

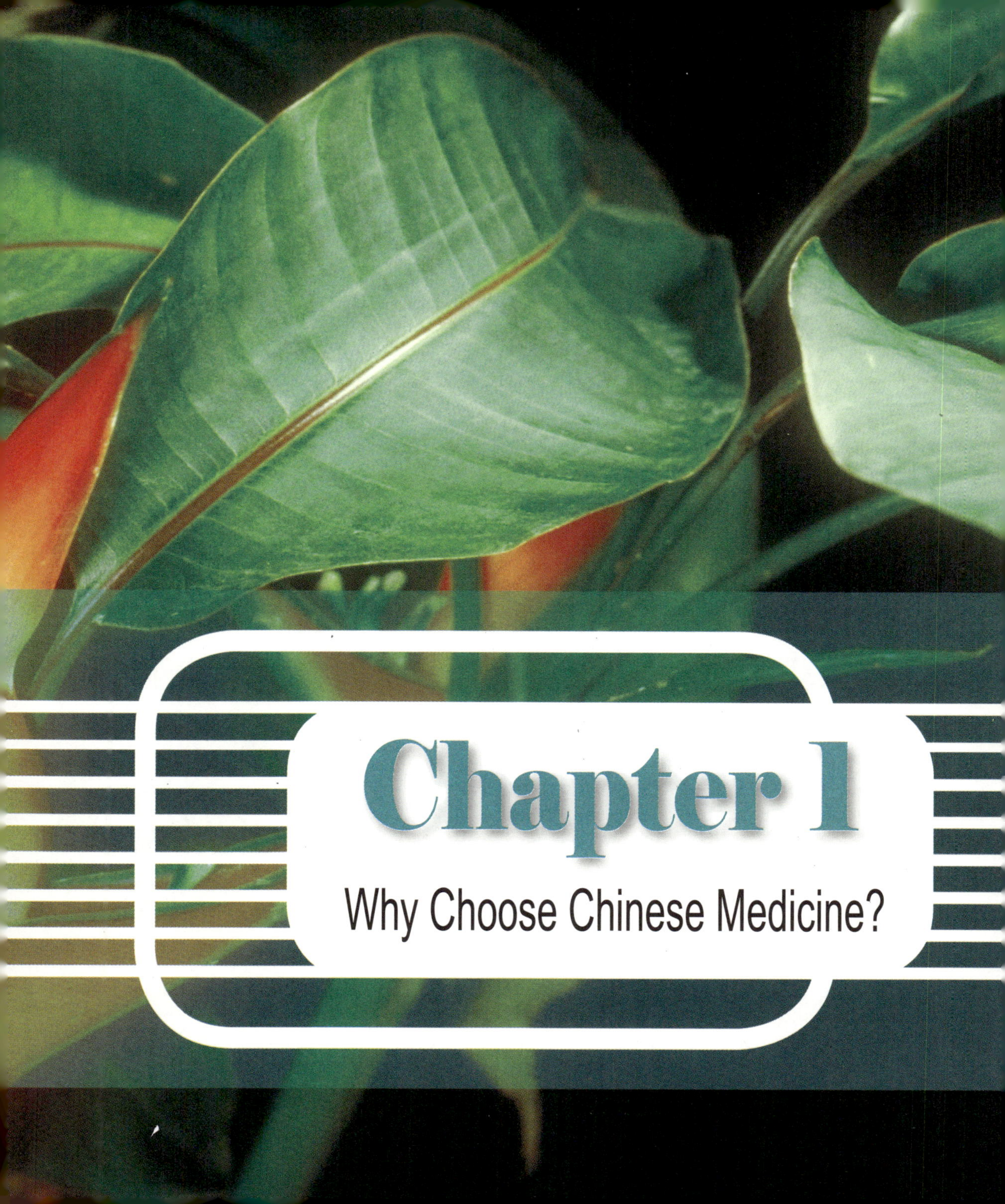

Chapter 1

Why Choose Chinese Medicine?

Chinese medicine includes a wide range of traditional medical practices originating in China that has developed over thousands of years. It is considered a complementary or alternative medical system in most parts of the world and has amazingly exploded in popularity over the past few decades. Techniques that have been used in Asia for thousands of years have finally found their way to the West and are being heartily embraced. Currently, it is an important part of the public health care system within China, and the efficacy of Chinese medicine is now being acknowledged by more and more people around the world.[1] Acupuncture, tui na, tai ji, five-phase theory, and yin-yang theory seem to be everywhere, most countries and regions worldwide have various kinds of Chinese medicine clinics and research centers. The medical community has taken notice, and government sponsored research on Chinese medicine and other natural medicines now reach nearly $300 million dollars every year in the USA alone.[2] The public is also interested, with acupuncture appearing in places from the Oprah Winfrey Show to hip-hop lyrics.

An ancient and mystical art, Chinese medicine has been rigorously practiced for thousands of years in China. So far, Chinese medicine has been exported to over 130 countries and regions, and over 10,000 doctors have been sent to other countries, especially developing countries, to provide services to the local people. Just by 1998, China conducted governmental level exchanges and cooperation on Chinese medicine with over 40 countries and regions including the USA, Japan, and France.[1] There are now well established schools all over North America and Europe as well as a growing field in South America, Africa, and the Middle East, not to mention its firm establishment in many other Asian countries. It is not unusual these days for hospitals in major cities to employ a Chinese medical practitioner and many insurance companies are choosing to cover treatments due to its efficacy, low cost, and safety.

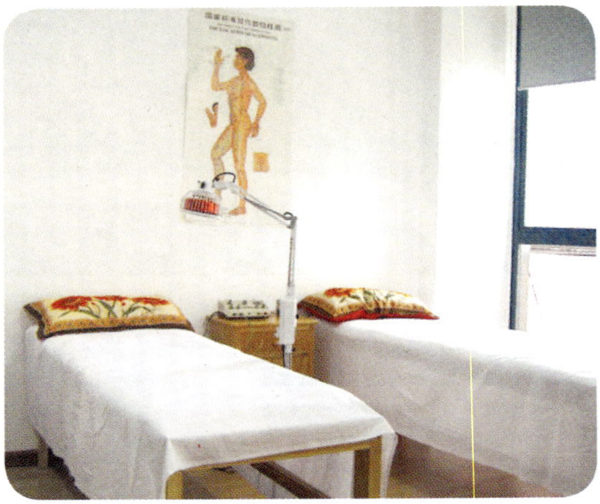

As most people grew up with conventional biomedical treatment, it is difficult to resist comparing Chinese medicine to biomedicine. Most people outside of Asia still do not consider it a scientific medical practice, so there is no shortage of critics and doubters in the biomedical community. Most theories of Chinese medicine are based upon meticulous observation of nature, the cosmos, and the human body, not research-based, and still waiting to be proven. However, ironically enough, most of these critics have had no significant training in Chinese medicine and are largely ignorant of its theories and techniques.

Despite the temptation and tendency to do so, Chinese medicine can not be compared across the board with modern biomedicine. To quote Judith Farquhar from her lecture in Beijing in 2005, the comparison "should engage with realities more than with ideals." Before comparisons are made, those making the comparisons should be familiar with each system. Thousands of years of empirical knowledge about Chinese medicine have been recorded using its own terminology system, while evaluation of the efficacy of Chinese medicine needs to be in line with modern research standards. The unique characteristics of diagnosis and treatment in Chinese medicine make it difficult to fit it into research methods that have been tailored for biomedical study. The fact is that the two systems are different in terms of many facets, such as philosophy, principles, and approach to treatment, and

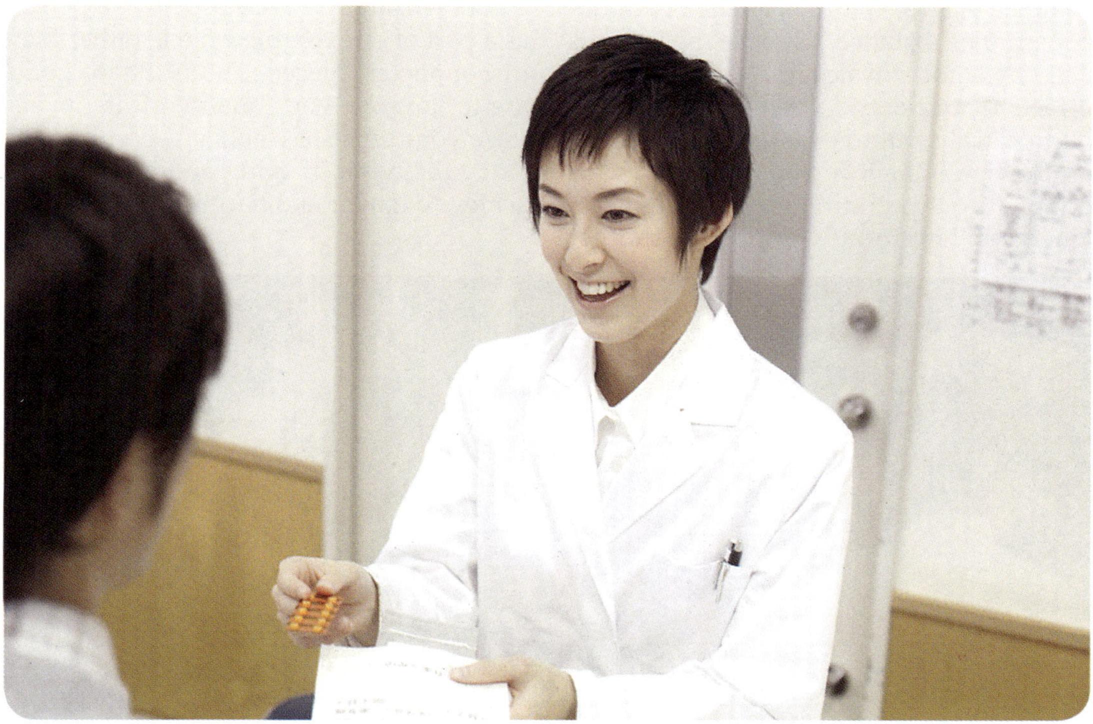

the differences are fundamental between Chinese medicine and biomedicine that lie outside the realm of lab tests and clinical trials. For instance, any two people with the same infection will be treated with a standard course of antibiotics in biomedical practice, whereas each person in Chinese medicine will receive a different treatment even for the same illness depending on their condition of pattern differentiation.

Furthermore, there is no necessity for comparison. Both types of medicine are valuable, using both medicines will provide a stronger and more viable form of healthcare, and offer the patient maximum benefit. For instance, Chinese medicine is used by some physicians to treat the side effects of radio and chemo-therapy, the withdrawal symptoms of antidepressants, antibiotic-resistant infections, and a variety of chronic conditions. Chinese medicine lays the groundwork for a stronger body and helps you prevent future illness, which will also benefit you when a traumatic accident happens, as the stronger and healthier body will fight infection and rebuild itself quicker and better. As you read this book, we hope you will begin to understand the power and subtlety the Chinese medicine system has to offer.

Chinese medicine can offer a transformational experience for those who suffer from depression or any other disease. It is more than relieving your depression. It is about recovering your natural ability to heal. Looking at the entire picture, Chinese medicine views spiritual, mental, emotional, and physical aspect of a person as a part of one complete circle rather than disconnected pieces. The ultimate goals are to improve your quality of life, maximize your sense of wellbeing, eliminate or delay the onset of aging and disease, and achieve a longer and happier life.

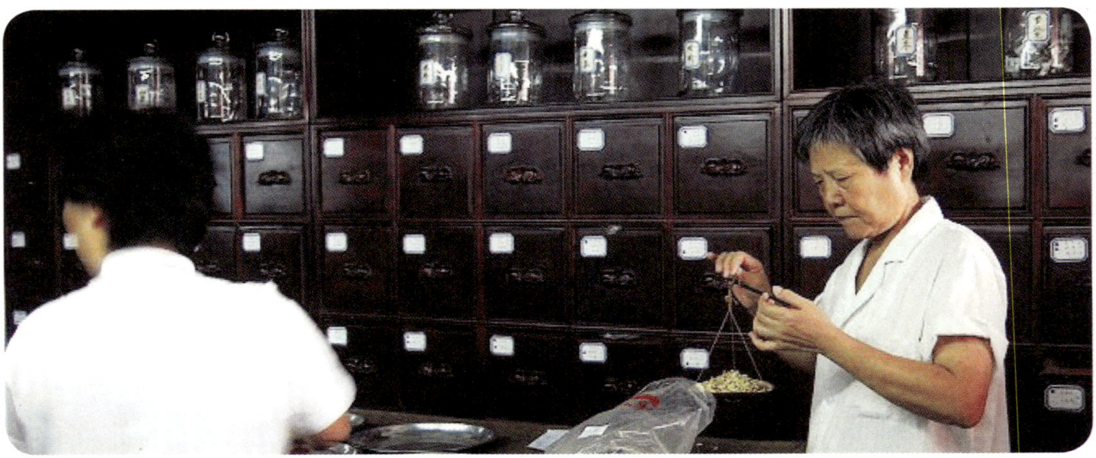

While biomedical treatment thrives in emergency rooms and during surgery, it seems to lose its power when faced with the many chronic diseases plaguing modern society, especially chronic diseases like heart disease, stroke, cancer, diabetes, and lung disorders, which are now labeled the world's leading killers by the World Health Organization. With depression specifically, biomedicine focuses principally on the physical body, relying on the pathologic lesions and discounting the patient's feelings about what may happen inside his body. Applying X-ray, CT, and MRI detection may allow the doctor to see inside the human body, but it may not give any clue to the emotional health of the patient. The problem lies primarily in a lack of a holistic view and correspondingly comprehensive treatment plan. Due to the increasing dissatisfaction of patients with their treatment regimens, one has to wonder if biomedicine is really capable of comprehensive treatment, or only claims to.

In 2007, the Centers for Disease Control and Prevention made the intriguing announcement that antidepressants were among the most-prescribed drugs. Its study reported 118 million out of a total of 2.4 billion drugs that doctors prescribed in visits to hospitals in 2005 were for antidepressants.[3] Those drugs, known as Selective Serotonin Reuptake Inhibitors (SSRI), can be very helpful for some people to ease the symptoms of depression; on the other hand, the side effects that associate with these drugs plus the withdrawal problems that result from stopping the medication are very terrible. Prozac, for instance, is currently used by more than five million Americans, but unfortunately, over the last seven years there have been 31,000 reports of adverse reactions to this powerful drug. An American review of spontaneous adverse drug reactions report found that "during a ten year period, Prozac was associated with more hospitalisations, deaths, or other serious adverse effects reported to the FDA than any other drug in America."[4] And, it is also worthwhile to note that according to the manufacturer's product information, this drug

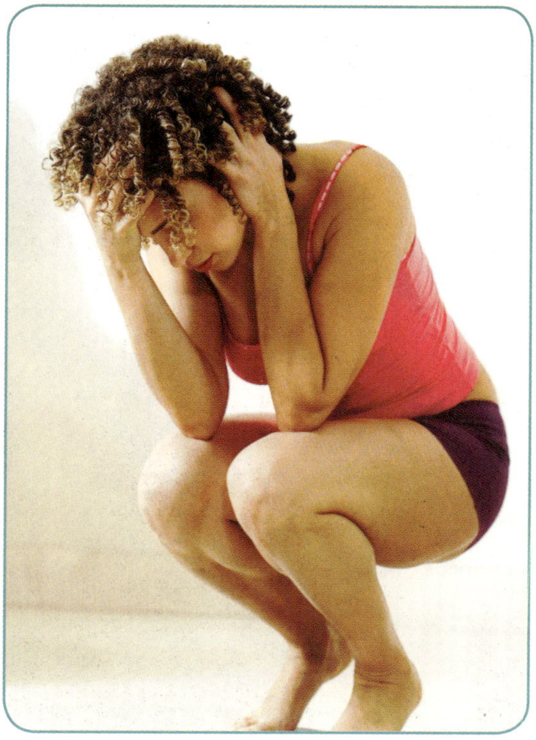

has many side effects. Up to 70 percent of patients on antidepressants report sexual side effects, yet the number of Americans who take the drugs (213 million prescriptions written by U.S. doctors in 2003) has ballooned since Prozac was introduced in the late 1980s.[5] In addition, people who hastily stop taking SSRI drugs are vulnerable to develop such withdrawal symptoms as dramatic changes in mood, insomnia, appetite changes, and agitation.

This is not to say that biomedicine does not have its merits. Many drugs produced by modern science do wonderful things with very few side-effects, especially if their dosage is low and administration period is short enough. Many patients still should seek care from a biomedical doctor even while getting treatment with Chinese medicine. But not attempting to restore the body's innate ability to maintain itself is contrary to the fundamental principles behind Chinese medicine. Great importance is given to the concept behind the cliché, "Use it or lose it." The analogy we wish to draw from this is that the use of drugs that substitute for a function or substance will help in the short term, but will lead to a decrease in function over the long run.

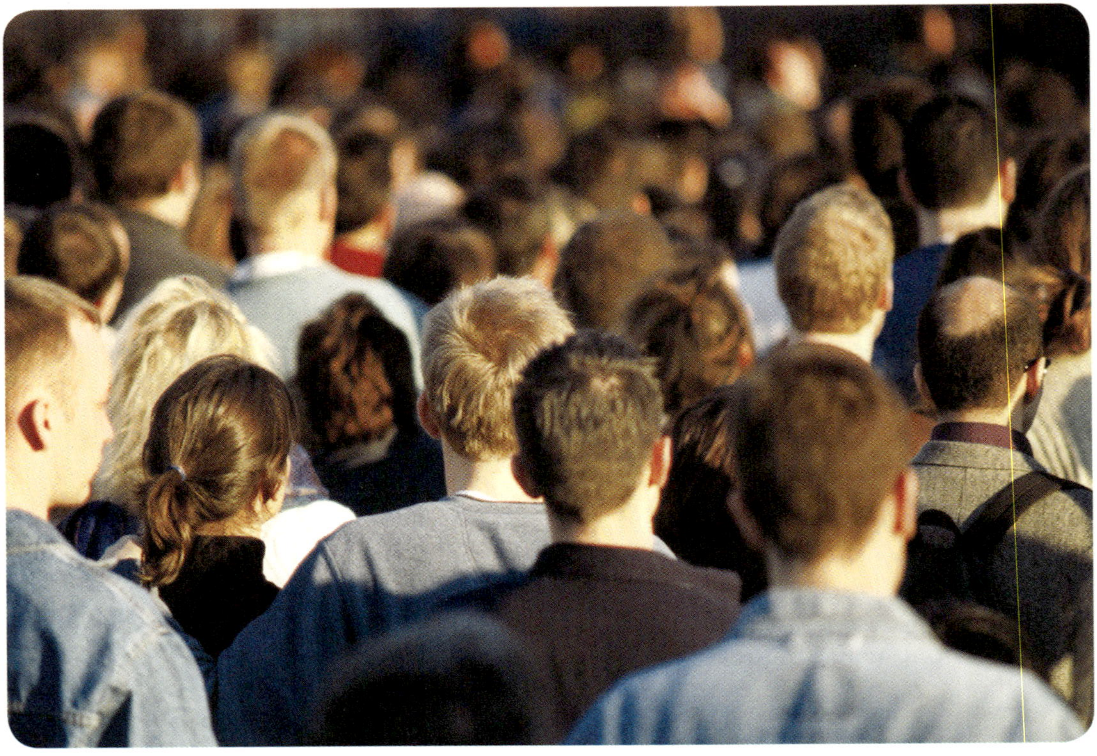

Chinese medicine focuses on treating the person who happens to be ill rather than concentrating on the disease mechanism which happens to be inside a person like is done in biomedicine. Chinese medicine treatment is primarily non-invasive and includes the use of Chinese medicinals, acupuncture, massage, meditation, mental and physical disciplines, and dietary therapy. The treatment methods of Chinese medicine, like other natural medical systems, are not intended to substitute for a bodily function or substance. The underlying mechanism of the treatment methods used is to help the body recover using natural substances and manual methods to stimulate the body's general function. They are intended to help the body do its job, help repair any damage, or aid in removing pathogens. Eventually, when the body has been "re-trained" to maintain balance on its own and is healthy enough to do the job itself, treatment is no longer necessary, which can be reduced and then eliminated. As an example, modern research has shown that the common medicinals used to treat infections can not be compared to the potent antibiotics used in hospitals. Many of these medicinals can only inhibit the growth of the bacteria, not destroy them. Yet experienced doctors of Chinese medicine will tell you that when properly prescribed, these medicinals are effective in the treatment of infectious disease, and in chronic cases they are often a better choice than the standard biomedical treatment. Let us take the disease of eczema as another example, there is no definitive cure for it in biomedicine, while Chinese medicine has long held that clearing heat, removing dampness in one's body, and strengthening the spleen are the effective therapeutic methods. In an article published in the August issue of the British Journal of Dermatology, doctors at the Chinese University of Hong Kong described how they ascertained the efficacy of the five Chinese medicinals which have long been used to treat eczema. The five medicinals are Flos Lonicerae, Medicinala Menthae, Cortex Moutan, Rhizoma Atractylodis, and Cortex Phellodendri.[6]

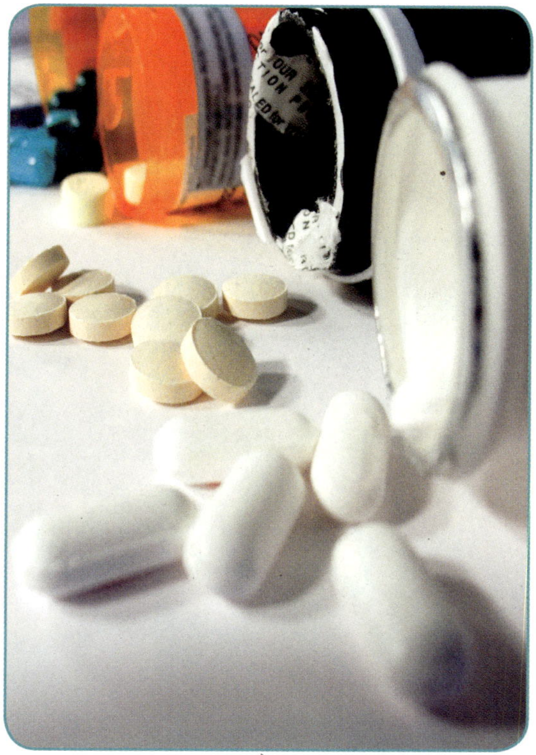

The language Chinese medicine uses (qi, yin-yang, five phases, etc.) is antique, but the idea it embraces is very advanced. Those insights were usually achieved through extensive experience and deep meditation. The knowledge has been passed down through generations.

If you are ready to take an active role in your health and in your life, Chinese medicine is right for you. But remember, achieving good health is not like climbing a mountain, with a visible goal, but like maintaining a garden, giving constant care and paying attention to changes in the environment. Chinese medicine has been helping make what is sometimes seen as an arduous task a rewarding joy for millions of people for thousands of years. If you also want your garden to thrive, come and join the community of natural medicine, learn more about Chinese medicine.

Let us start by reading about a real case before introducing the basic concepts of Chinese medicine.

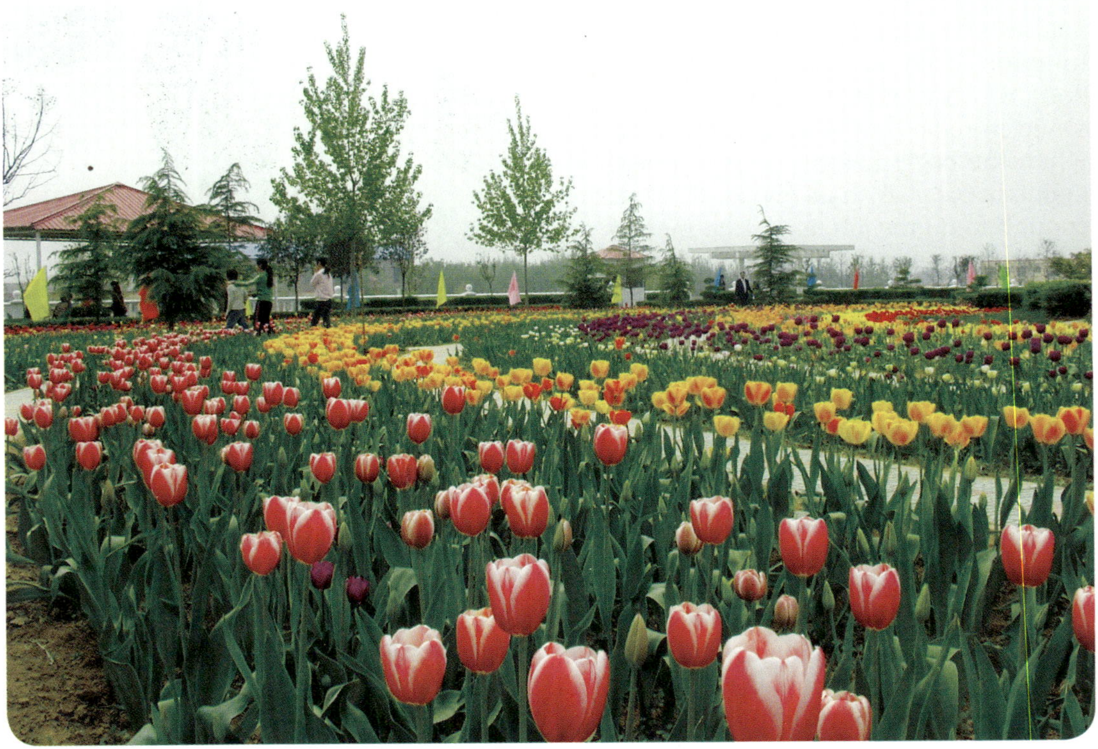

Case One

Mr. Yao is a 23-year-old medical graduate student who has had clinical depression for two years. Initially he wanted to be a resident physician, but lost interest, and felt that further study overseas was a good choice that could bring him to a higher level of understanding, more self-sufficiency, and greater respect. He worked really hard and then lost interest. Gradually, he found it difficult for him to concentrate on his academic work, particularly at times when he was feeling bad. He came to the clinic with a sad face, lassitude, fear and restlessness, shortness of breath, palpitation, chest oppression, lack of interest in most things, insomnia, poor appetite, dizziness, loose stool, normal urination, pale tongue with thin coating, and thin pulses. In Chinese medicine, this case was differentiated as deficiency pattern of spleen and heart. The corresponding therapeutic methods adopted were to strengthen the spleen, fortify the heart, tonify qi, and nourish blood. Selected acupoints included DU 20 (*bǎi huì*), *yìn táng*, ear *shén mén*, RN 12 (*zhōng wǎn*), BL 15 (*xīn shù*), BL 20 (*pí shù*), ST 36 (*zú sān lǐ*), SP 6 (*sān yīn jiāo*), the first three acupoints were manipulated with an even supplementing and draining manner, the remaining five were manipulated in a supplementing manner. The needles were left in place for 35 minutes. The treatment was conducted twice a week. A modified formula of *Guī Pí Tāng* (Spleen Restoring Decoction) was prescribed and the patient was asked to take a dose twice daily. After two months of treatment, the patient's condition was improved by a large margin, his sleep was better, lassitude was alleviated, palpation and chest oppression were relieved, but his shortness of breath and fear and restlessness were still problems. The treatment was continued for another two months and all the symptoms of depression were erased. Thereafter, to consolidate the therapeutic effect, acupuncture treatment was given for another six weeks, once a week. There were no side effects such as nausea and agitation and no withdrawal symptoms over the follow-up period of two years.

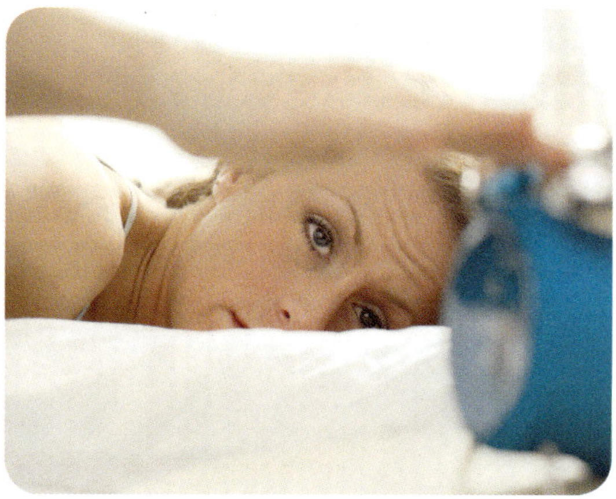

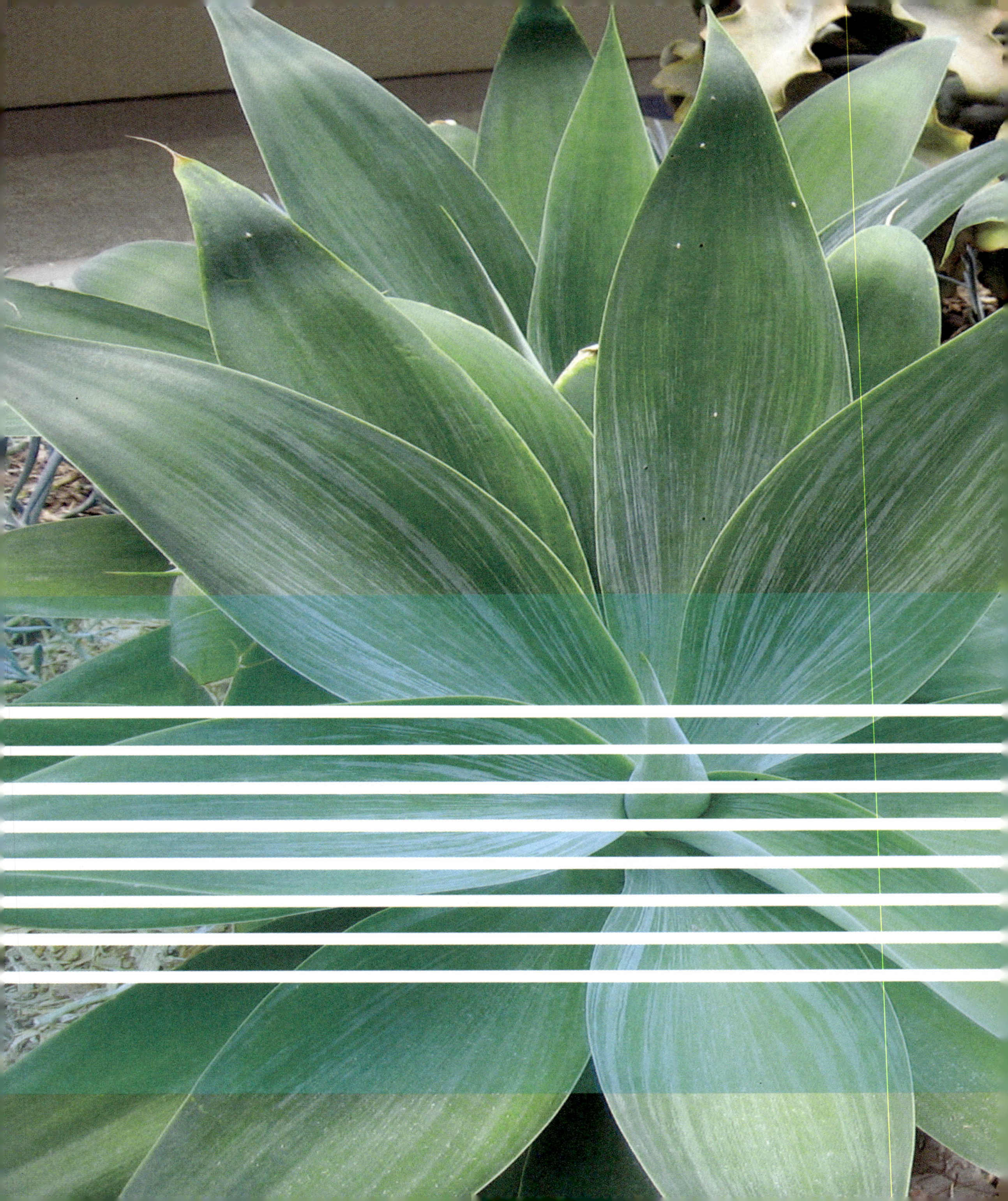

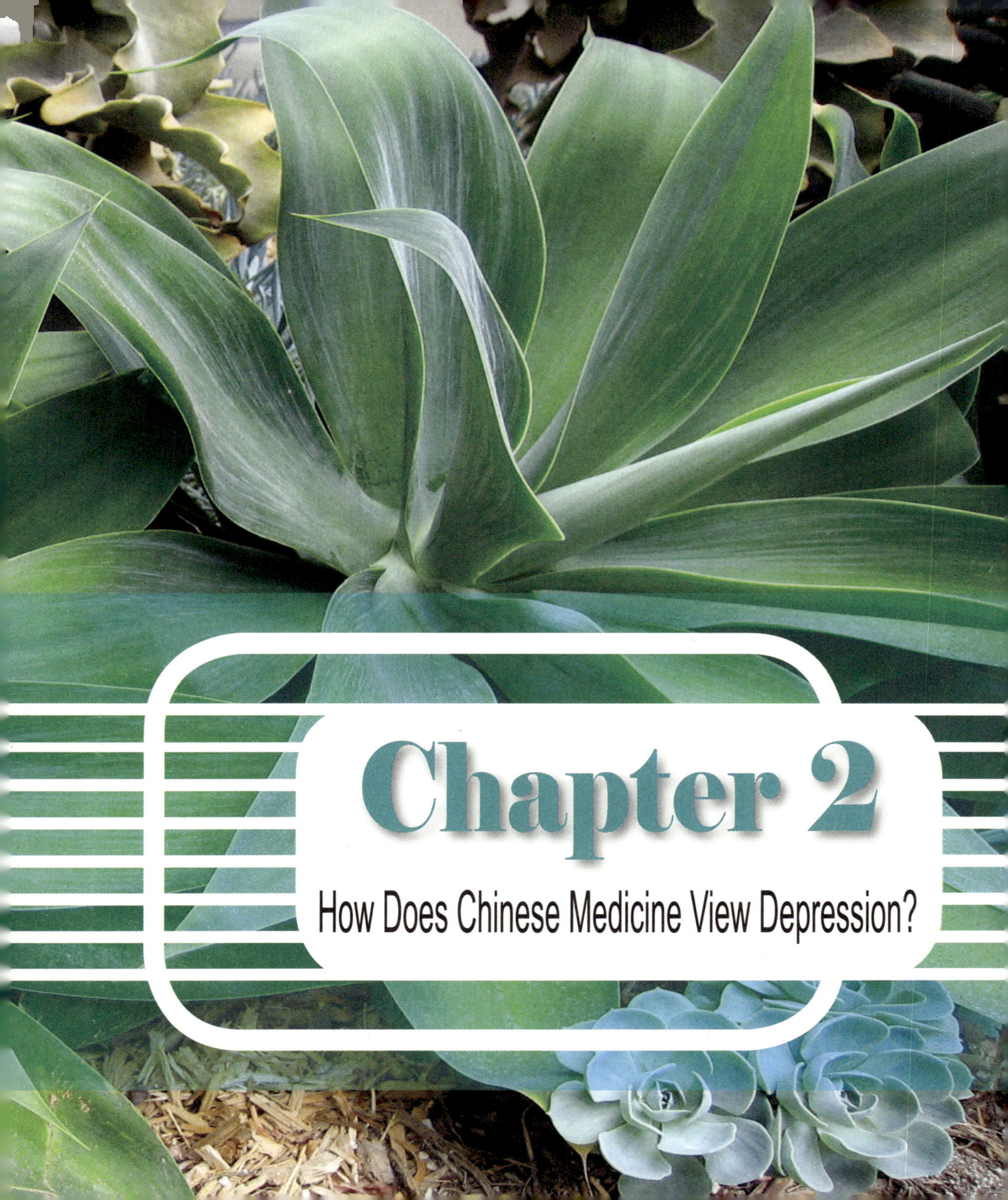

Chapter 2

How Does Chinese Medicine View Depression?

Many people in Western countries are under the impression that Chinese medicine involves some kind of sorcery with mysterious spirits. And indeed the ancient language of Chinese medicine can reinforce this view by referring to the "spirits" of the heart, lungs, liver, etc., or by insisting on the existence of the *jīng-luò*, which is the network that runs throughout the human body and is responsible for transporting qi and blood. People do often find it difficult to translate a Chinese medicine diagnosis into the biomedical words in which they are familiar. For instance, there is no direct and simple translation for how physicians of Chinese medicine diagnose patients' condition as "heat with dampness," "qi deficiency and blood stagnation," with a need to "strengthen the spleen." However, to wise doctors and open-minded patients, the words used matter little, what is important is if the underlying concepts are able to be applied and beneficial results obtained.

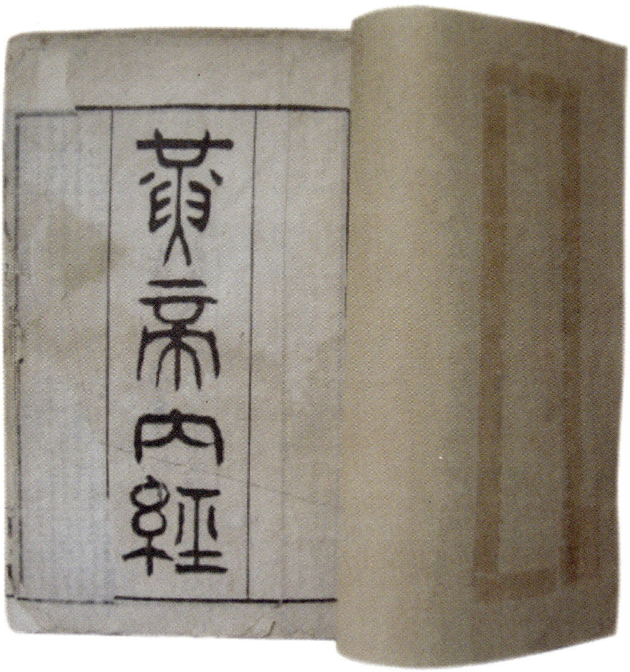

The Yellow Emperor's Inner Classic
(Huáng Dì Nèi Jīng)

Introduction to Chinese Medicine

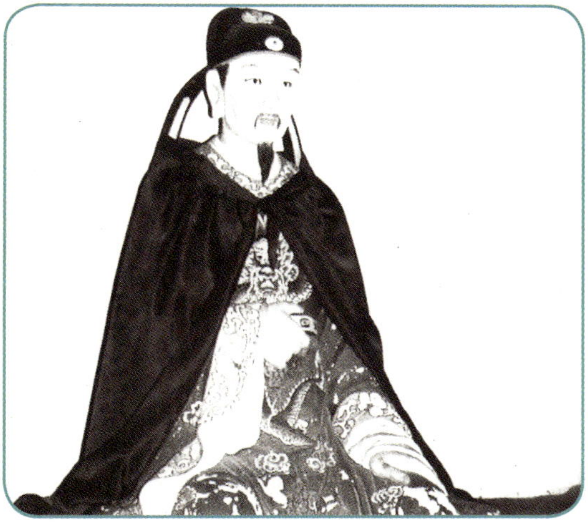

Zhang Zhong-jing

Chinese Medicine enjoys a rich tradition and the longest continuous history among the world's natural medicines. Its legends suggest a history of 5,000 years, while archeological evidence dates back to 1,700 B.C. The earliest existing literature dates from 2,000 B.C. and includes material from even earlier times.[7] Chinese medicine is remarkable in having not only survived, but thrived during thousands of years of political and social ups-and-downs, and in remaining relevant and continuing to grow despite the rise of biomedicine. It is presently providing safe and effective care at an increasing rate to people all over the globe.

Perhaps an illustrative example of how Chinese medicine has greatly benefited society at large will help you understand its potential value to the world. During the infamous flu epidemic of 1918 that swept over the world causing millions of deaths, the death rate in China was lower than in other countries.[8] It is estimated that over 2% of the world's population died during the flu with some countries suffering as much as a 20% loss of life. The statistics on China's southern province of Guangdong, however, say only 0.1% of the population died. During this time, biomedical treatment was largely unavailable to the vast majority of China's huge population. The people relied on the methods and theories of Chinese medicine to maintain health and treat disease. It is incredible to think that this natural system of health care was effective against one of the deadliest, most rapidly spreading diseases in the past century.[7]

Recently, people across the world have been drawn to Chinese medicine because it focuses on healing the person as a whole and seeking the root cause of illness. Chinese medicine is based on the traditional philosophy and culture of ancient China, the essence of which is the relationship between man, the universe, and the *dào* ("law" or "way") of nature. The *dào* of nature is a dynamic balance between yin and yang, and health is the balance between the body's yin and yang as well as its qi and blood, and between the body and the external environment. When this balance is disrupted, disease, pain, and suffering arise. The basic principle of treatment in Chinese medicine is to discover and act on the fundamental cause of the imbalance to restore harmony to yin, yang, qi, and blood, i.e. the ability of the body to heal itself. A qualified Chinese medicine practitioner should receive systematic and special training so as to view the body, mind, emotion, and spirit as one system.

August 12, 2008, The Times reported that for the first time in Olympic history, the athletes' village was equipped with a clinic offering traditional Chinese treatments and the initiative proved to be a success since Olympic athletes queued to try old Chinese remedies. Tony Smith, the coach of the Canadian gymnastics team, told the state newspaper China Daily that he was astonished when a niggling pain in his back vanished after a single acupuncture session. "It really does work," he said. "I will definitely recommend it to my athletes." Smith, who has long suffered from lower back pain, had just about given up hope after none of the various treatments he tried made any difference. "I thought I should give Chinese acupuncture a try, and found it really relieves the pain," he said. "I'll try it again this week. If it still works, I'll carry on with the treatment when I get back to Canada." Ola Ronsen, the head doctor for the Norwegian team, said: "I talked to one of the Chinese practitioners before we arrived, mostly focusing on sleep disturbances and other types of imbalances." When he arrived, he went for a full check-up. "The doctor discovered problems I didn't tell him of," he said.[9]

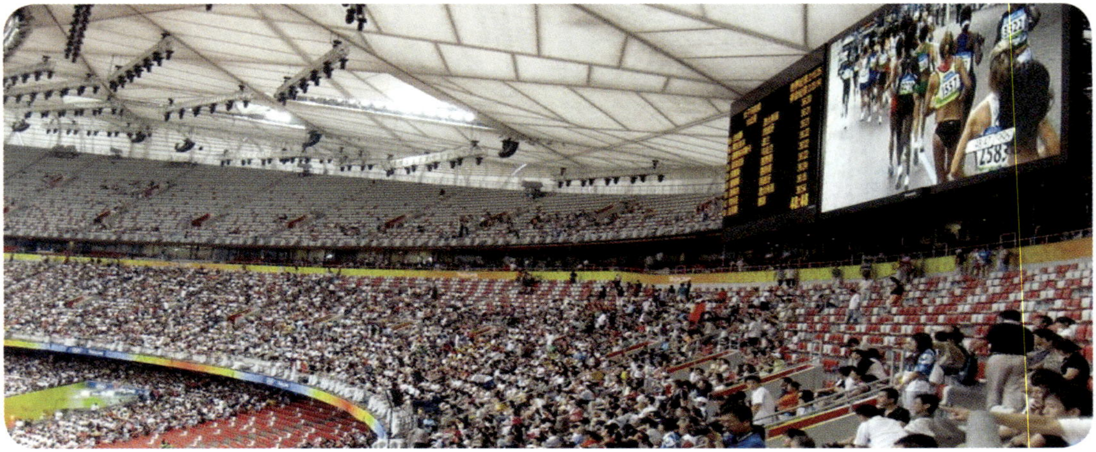

Key Concepts in Chinese Medicine

1. Qi

The concept of qi is much more than a medical term. Indeed, it is inseparable from ancient Chinese philosophy and is used by both fields to explain the forces that animate and control everything in the universe, from the cycle of seasons, to the origins and effects of emotions, to the inner workings of the human body. Originally, qi was not a philosophic concept but just referred to air, a substance which cannot be seen but the movement of which can be felt. Gradually, its meaning was extended to the philosophical field as a symbol for the primordial substance that was endowed with two properties: invisibility and motion. The ancient Chinese philosophy holds qi is invisible, moving and changing constantly, creating various kinds of things, giving rise to energy and activities, and making things in the

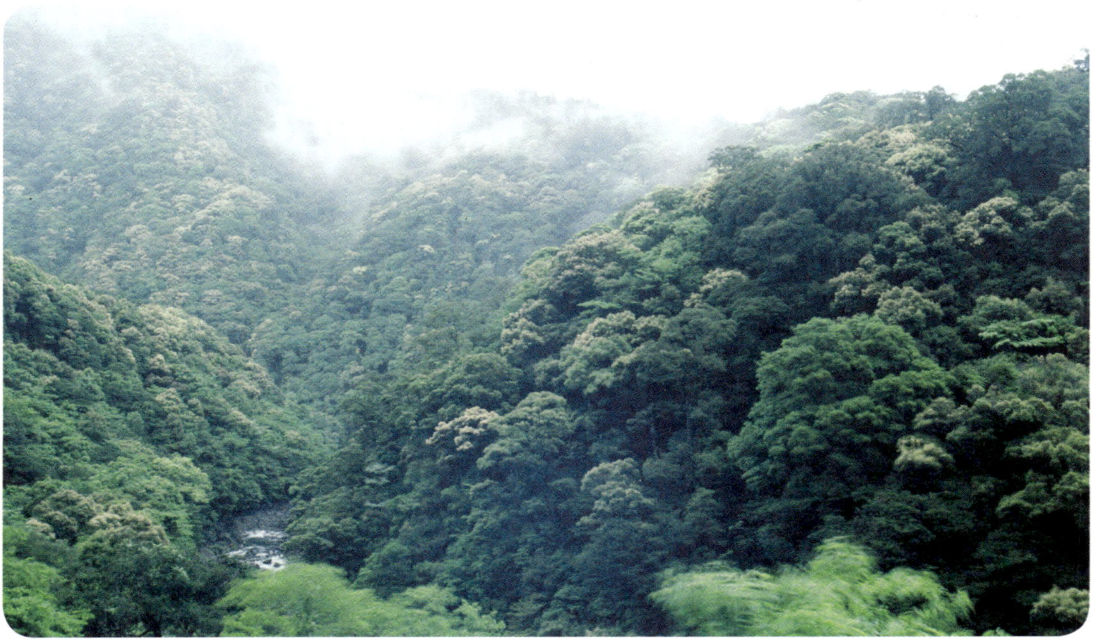

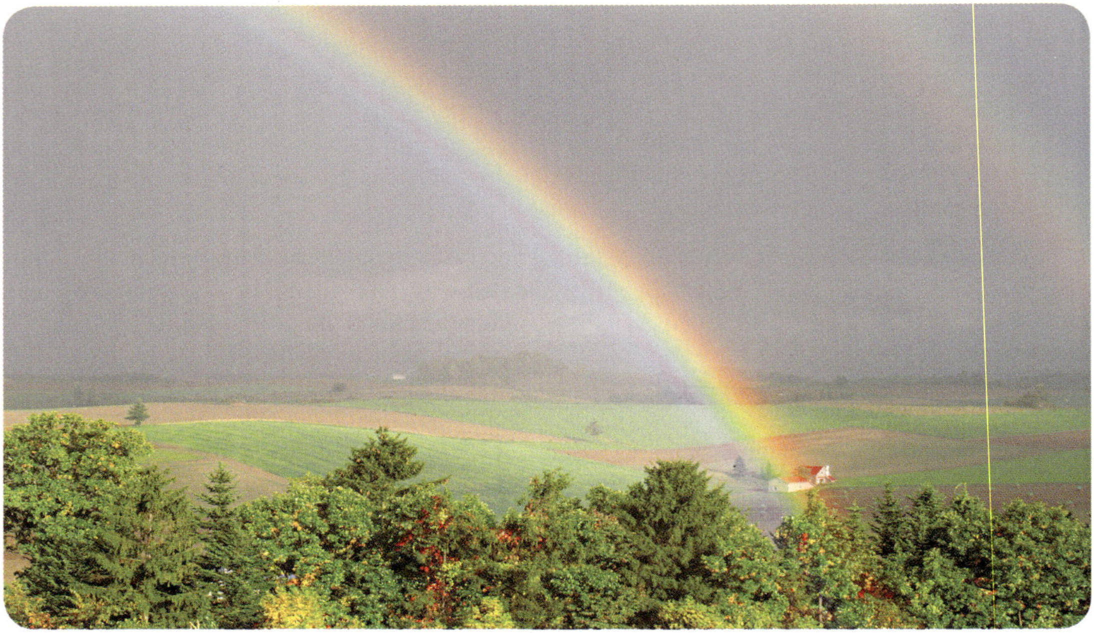

world transform from one to another. Qi was thought to be the most fundamental element making up the universe, and everything in this world is produced by the movement and change of qi. Accordingly, human life is also endowed with the nature of qi, which is the most fundamental substance in the construction of the human body and in the maintenance of its life activities. As *The Yellow Emperor's Inner Classic* (*Huáng Dì Nèi Jīng*,黄帝内经) stated: "Human life originates in the qi of Heaven and Earth, and develops according to the normal order of the four seasons." Various actions and changes of qi will bring the transformation of energy. In Chinese medicine, all life activities, including mental activities such as thought, will, and emotions, are based on the movements and changes of qi. There is no simple literal English translation of qi. Different translators have rendered it as air, vapor, or energy and all of these are partially, but not completely, accurate.

The concept of qi is somewhat similar to pneuma in ancient Greece or prana in India, which were used to describe an underlying life force that was seen as having a strong connection to air and breath. As the most basic and all-pervasive concept in Chinese medicine, qi in its most fundamental sense is energy in all its interpretations. Qi is the vital substance that constitutes the human body and maintains life activities: breathing, moving, thinking, working, and feeling. In Chinese medicine, qi is treated as the essential substance of the human body, and its movements explain various life processes. All substances in the body are transformed by constant motion and change of qi. The *zang-fu* organs, the channels and collaterals, the five sense organs, the nine orifices, and the body itself are formed by the motion, transformation, and accumulation of qi. A healthy body requires normal circulations of qi on all levels. When the flow of qi within the body is out of balance under physical, emotional, or environmental disturbance, illness may result. Some of qi's important characteristics are:

➡ Qi is indeed a kind of life force, but it is also a tangible vital substance that makes up everything in the cosmos, including humans.

➡ Qi is the medium for transformation that stimulates the process of change. Everything in the universe, organic or inorganic, is made of qi and defined by qi. Mountains, rivers, animals, plants, even human emotions all have qi.

➡ Qi cannot be defined as simply "energy", cannot be labeled a mere material substance, nor is it something in between. It is what connects humankind and the natural environment.

➡ Qi is the media that makes the relationships and interactions between things and lives possible.

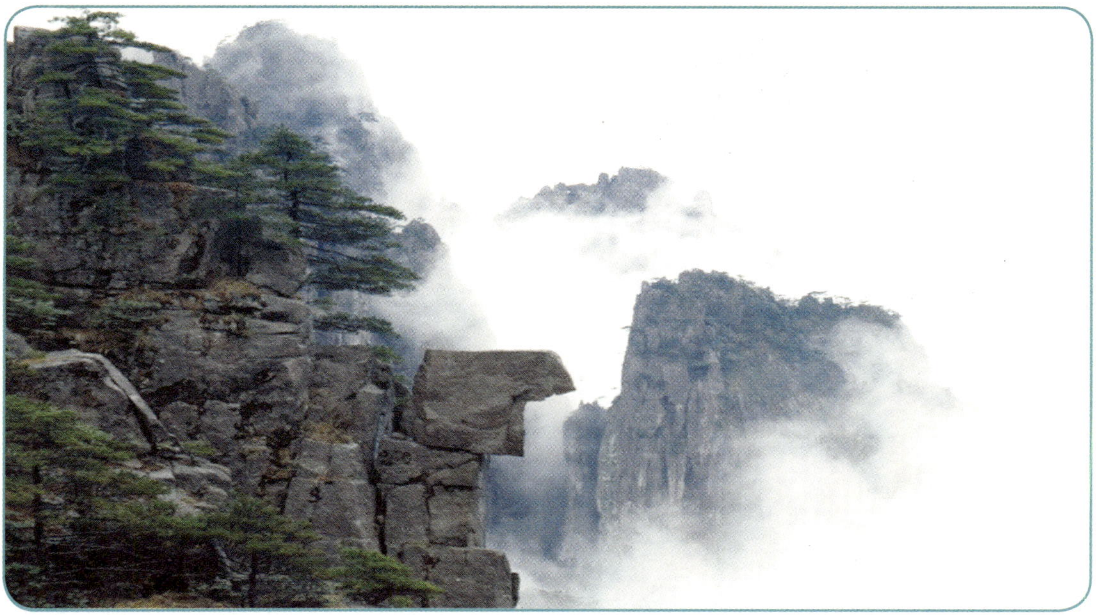

It can be difficult to understand the ancient Chinese claim that qi is both an ethereal life force as well as a material substance. To understand better, let us look at two very different categories of phenomena, human emotions and simple writing utensils, and see how qi exists in both of them.

First, take emotions. If a doctor of Chinese medicine was asked to describe the qi of the emotion of joy, he or she would probably say that its qi was light, rising, dispersing, and possibly warm. On the other hand, if asked to describe the qi of fear, the words used would be more along the lines of dark, sinking, or cold. These descriptions are not based on any lab tests or scientific evidence, but are based primarily on the practitioner's own experience of the resonance between the emotional state and his or her perception.

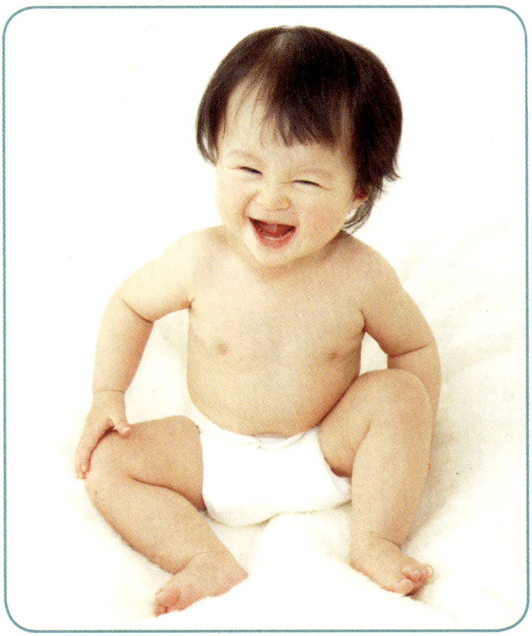

Now let us look at the other end of the spectrum, at two examples of solid, tangible writing utensils. One a well-worn wooden pencil and a cartoon character design, the kind a first grader might use to scratch out the ABC's; the other a sleek, expensive ink pen, probably black or silver that could be used to sign legal contracts. Similar to the description of joy above, the qi of the pencil could be described as light, familiar, or warm; and similar to the qi of fear above, the pen's qi would be described as dark, heavy, and cold.

We can see that qi is not merely energy, as the physical substance of the pencils was a crucial part of describing their qi. Likewise, we saw that qi cannot be limited to physical characteristics because the emotions described above, which have their distinct qi, have no tangible substance.

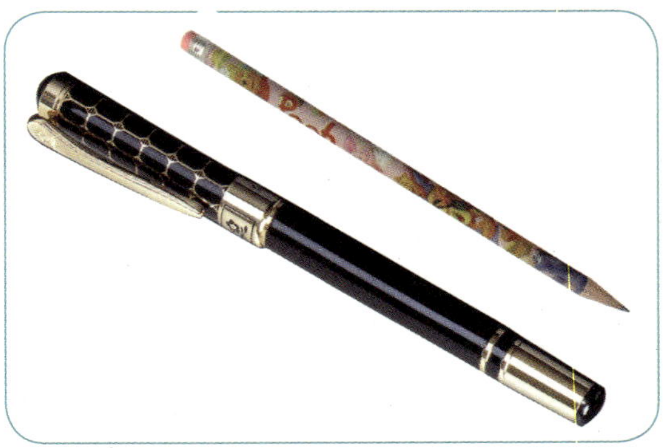

Chinese medicine, over thousands of years and with the help of countless doctors, patients, and philosophers has established a system in which the different phenomena of the universe can be described by qi and likewise the relationships between these phenomena can be described. Thus a Chinese doctor, when asked to describe the qi of something or the other, is not merely relying on his own experience and perceptions, but is using established theories to come up with an accurate description that anyone trained in qi will be able to agree with. In fact, it does not necessarily take training to understand qi. Most people would find the metaphorical descriptions of joy, fear, the pencil, and the pen easy to relate to. All people can think and talk in terms of qi, since it is based on the common sense of the natural world. The genius of Chinese medicine lies in its clear definitions and natural categorizations.

To understand what doctors of Chinese medicine aim to do in their treatments, we have to understand this well-used but rarely understood word, qi. Matter and energy are not independent of each other. As shown in Einstein's famous equation $E=mc^2$, there is an intrinsic relationship between matter and energy. Qi is a concept that bridges this relationship. It is the force that animates life. It is also the matter that constitutes life. Qi is shared by everything in the universe. It is the medium by which everything interacts. To quote one of the original textbooks of Chinese medicine in English *The Web that Has No Weaver*:

"The interaction, or resonance, is realized by qi. Health is the harmonious resonance while disease is the disharmony. Components of the universe, the qi of medicinals (plants, animal parts, and stones), acupoints (junctions of the human networks), lifestyle activities (movement

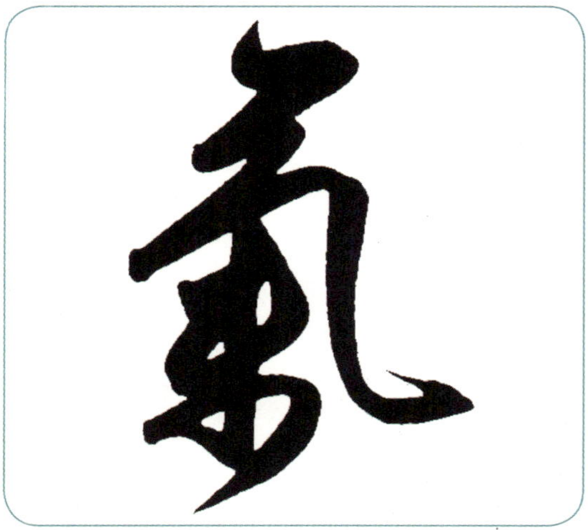

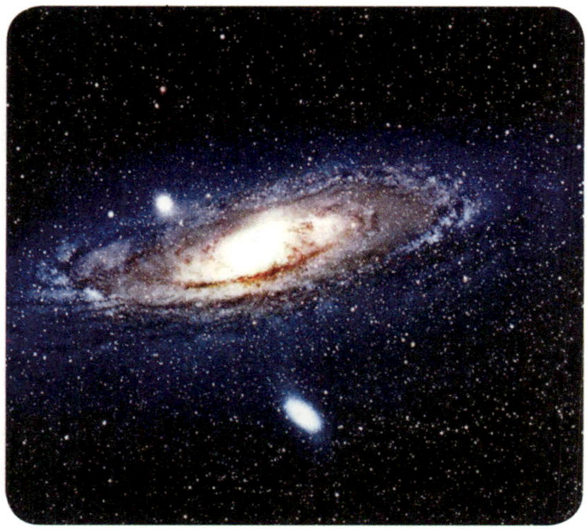

and rest, foods and relationships) or living environments (seasons, weather, or even air conditions) share a resonating frequency that already exists in a person. A medicine or a conscious shift in a person's behavior can resonate with the condition within a person (e.g. a pattern of a disharmony) and induce a person toward health."

In Chinese medicine, disease is defined as an outcome of struggle between vital qi (also known as normal qi and healthy qi) and evil qi (also known as pathogenic qi). Between these two kinds of qi, emphasis is often put on the former, as was stated in *The Yellow Emperor's Inner Classic* "If vital qi prevails, attack of evil qi never avails."

The vital qi covers all the substances and energy important for life activities and the body's resistance against disease. It primarily comes from three resources: primordial qi inherited from parents at conception, qi of food essence transformed by the spleen, and fresh air inhaled by the lungs. Primordial qi, as the basic building block of human beings, is derived from parents before birth and is stored in the kidney after birth to determine the growth, development, and reproductive activity of a human being. While qi of food essence and fresh air are acquired after birth, since the former is generated by what we eat and distributed all over the body to produce what we need through the interaction of multiple organs and the latter is inhaled by the lung. So eating a healthy diet and breathing fresh air are important steps towards creating a healthy balance in the body. Evil qi is harmful to health. It includes various

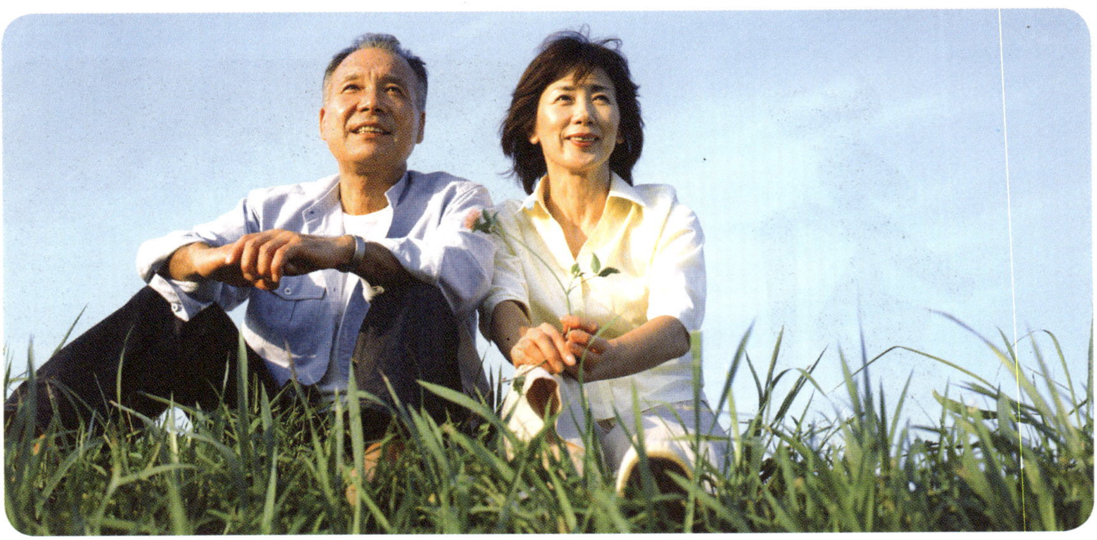

pathogenic factors, for example, emotional expressions such as anger, joy, fear, and sadness are all considered evil qi, if they happen in excess.

It is reasonable to say that in addition to congenital constitution, food and nutrients, and environment, the formation of qi in the human body is closely related to the function of such *zang-fu* organs as the kidney, spleen and stomach, and lung. Only when these organs run well can the qi of the body flourish. Otherwise, the formation of qi and the physiological function of qi will be impacted.

In terms of the human body and its various activities, Chinese medicine describes qi as having five major functions: promoting, warming, defending, securing, and transforming.

> Promoting

"Qi is the source of all movements."

Qi is a powerful substance that ignites and promotes all movements. Here 'movement' is in its broadest sense and includes all physiological and psychological activities: walking, dancing, breathing, the heart beating, the blood flowing, the distribution of body fluids, speaking, thinking, birth, growth, development, maturation, and aging. Just as wind provides energy to turn the turbine of a windmill, qi promotes all normal functions of the human body and the activities of qi can take place at any organ. The vigor and the movements of qi play a very important role in promoting the functional activities of *zang-fu* organs and channels and collaterals. It also promotes the formation and distribution of blood and body fluids, since the blood and body fluids pertain to be yin in property and rely on the activities of qi. Furthermore, qi is a vigorous

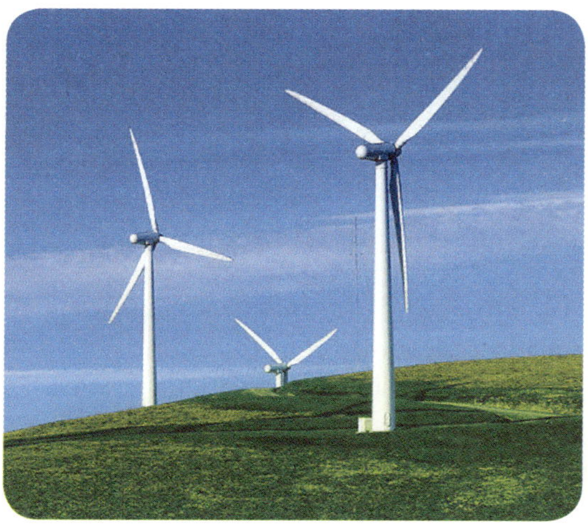

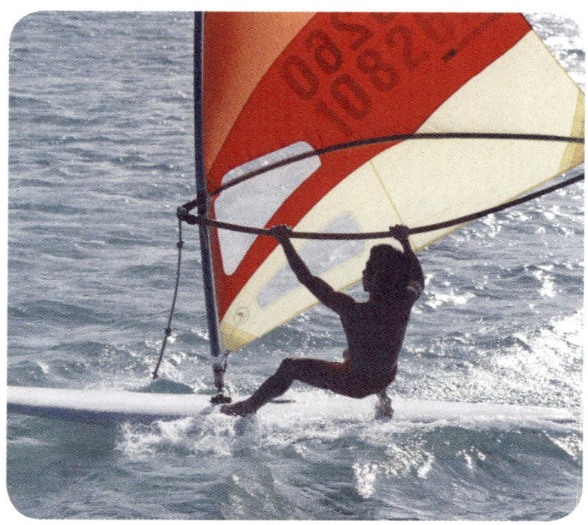

substance that flows fast in the human body and capable of activating the moving of blood and body fluids, and transforming them into various secretions and excretions.

If there is a deficiency of qi, its promoting functions are affected. Correspondingly, the growth and development of the human body are delayed, the organs and channels fail to function properly, the formation of blood and body fluid is hindered, and the flow of blood and body fluids is stagnated, which in turn leads to blood stagnation, phlegm, or edema.

> Warming

"Qi warms the body and is the source of the heat energy of the body."

As a yang substance in constant movement, qi is rich in heat. Maintenance of normal body temperature relies on the warming function of qi. This warming function also helps to smooth the flow and distribution of blood and body fluids, just like the water in a river flow in warm weather and freeze in cold weather. This warmth is also necessary for the internal organs to maintain normal function. The warmth can be manifested as the actual body temperature, in the normal function of the organs, or as the patient's subjective feeling of hot or cold. The difference between one person's qi and another person's can help to explain why some people tend to wear more clothes than others even though the temperature of the environment is the same.

Pathologically, disorders of qi in its warming function are mainly categorized into two kinds: when qi is deficient failing to produce adequate heat, internal cold might arise, with manifestation as aversion to cold and desire for warmth, cold limbs, lower body temperature, etc.; when qi is excessive or accumulated as a result of sluggish flow of qi in a local area, internal heat might appear.

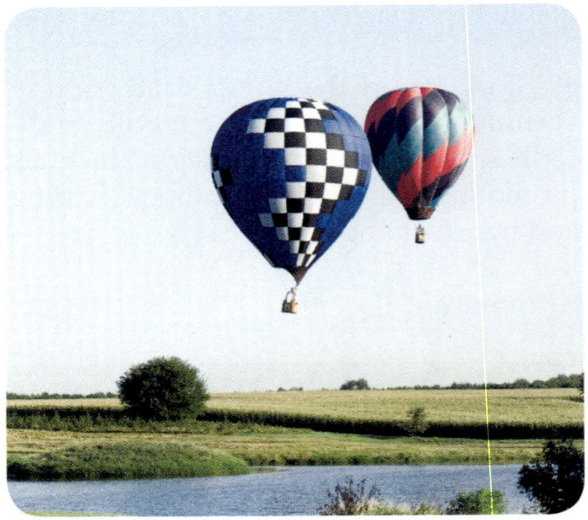

> Defending

"Qi protects the body, resisting the invasion of various external pathogens and preventing disease."

In Chinese medicine, one of the main causes of disease is the invasion of external pathogens through either the skin or the nose and mouth. By protecting the body surface, controlling the opening and closing of pores, as well as preventing and resisting the invasion of external pathogenic factors, qi is particularly important for defending against external attacks and maintaining good health. This function is often compared to immunity in biomedicine. Harmony of qi in the body is what protects us from pathogens in our environment. A quote from the most famous text of Chinese medicine, the *Yellow Emperor's Inner Classic* states: "If things from outside are able to harm the body, the qi must be weak." When qi is weak, we are vulnerable to disease. When qi is plentiful, we are less susceptible to illness. Qi can also help fight pathogens when they attack. The prognosis of disease is simply the dynamic balance sheet between the body's healthy qi, and the attacking qi of the pathogenic factors.

Pathologically, disorders of qi in its defensive function will weaken the resistance of the body against the invasion of these pathogenic factors, which will make people more susceptible to diseases such as the common cold.

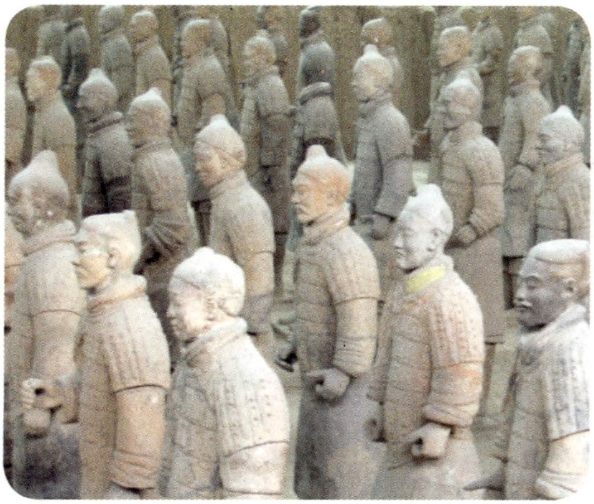

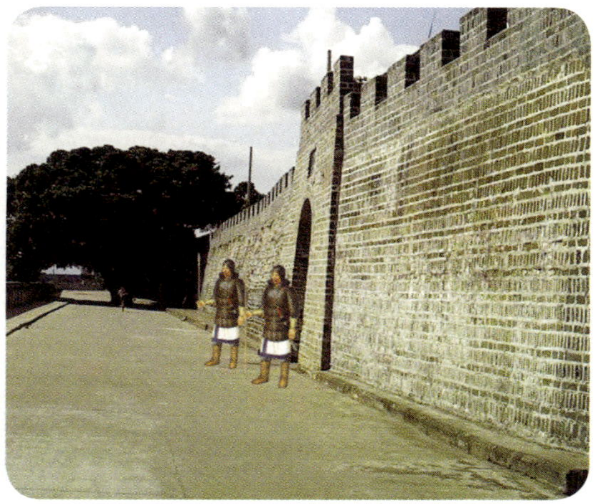

> Securing

"Qi keeps things in their proper place."

This means controlling bodily substances such as blood, urine, mucus, and saliva and preventing them from leaking out. Qi keeps the blood flowing within the vessels to avoid extravasation, controls the amount and time of the secretions and excretion of sweat, urine and saliva, and prevents body fluids from excessive loss. It also describes the maintenance of the structural integrity of the body, helping to keep organs in their proper places. Last but not least, qi consolidates sperm to prevent premature ejaculation.

When this function is disrupted it will lead to problems such as bleeding or excessive secretion of body fluids, i.e. spontaneous sweating, excessive sweating upon slight exertion, frequent urination, heavy bleeding during menstruation; or nocturnal emission, premature ejaculation, seminal emission; or a loss of structural integrity with prolapses of organs or body parts like is seen in cases of uterine prolapse or various hernias.

The securing and promoting functions work in a complementary manner. On the one hand, qi promotes the circulation of blood and body fluid, on the other hand, it also controls and adjusts the secretion of fluid substances to prevent their unnecessary loss. Only when these two functions are harmonized can the healthy blood and body fluid circulation be reached and maintained.

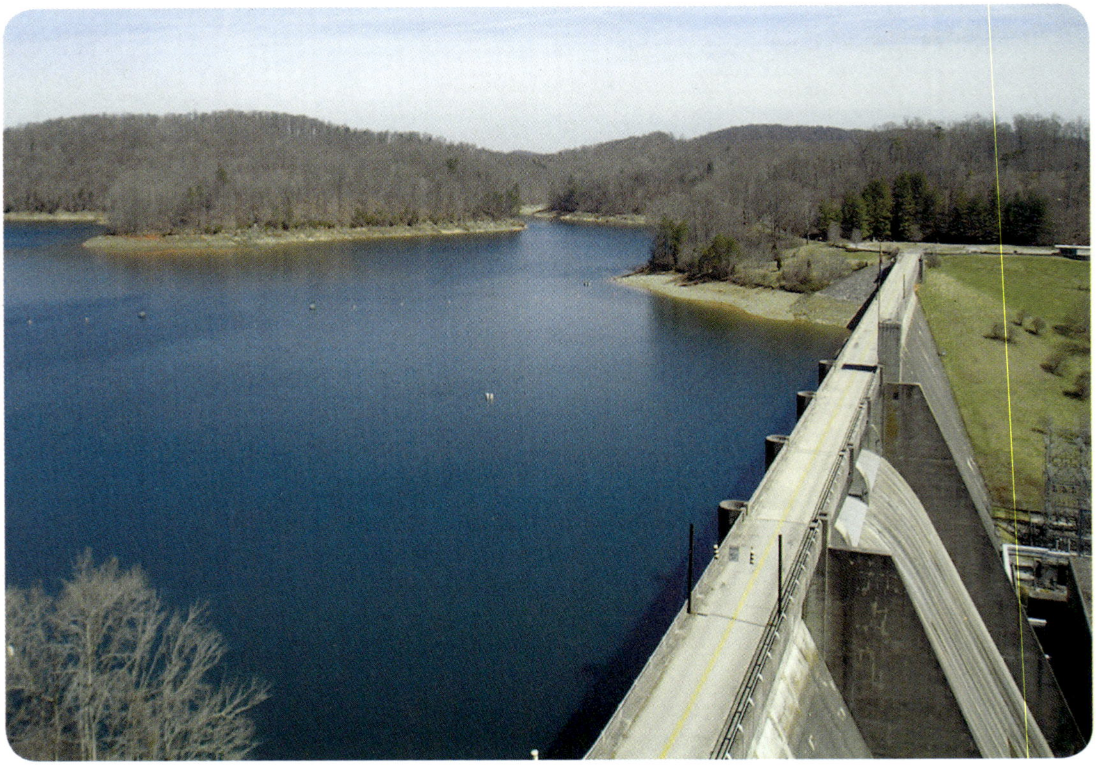

> Qi transforming

"Qi is the source of transformation."

Changes in the body and mind are ascribed to the transformative function of qi. This can be compared to metabolism in biomedical terminology. For example, food is ingested and transformed into bodily substances, and indigestible food and waste are also transformed into urine and stool for excretion. That is to say, any changes of substances can be considered the result of the transforming effect of qi. Emotional stress may influence the body and cause problems like headaches. For better or worse, these transformations are dependent on qi. Too much, too little, or improperly moving qi can cause different kinds of problems with the transformations that are managed by qi.

Although the above mentioned functions of qi differ from each other, they are all based on the basic property of qi. Qi flows throughout the whole body in four directions: ascending, descending, entering, and exiting. Generally, ascending refers to the upward movement of qi; descending means the downward flow of qi; entering indicates the inward movement of qi; and exiting means the outward movement of qi. Each organ has different specialized movements. For instance, spleen qi pertains to ascending while stomach qi, on the other hand, pertains to descending.

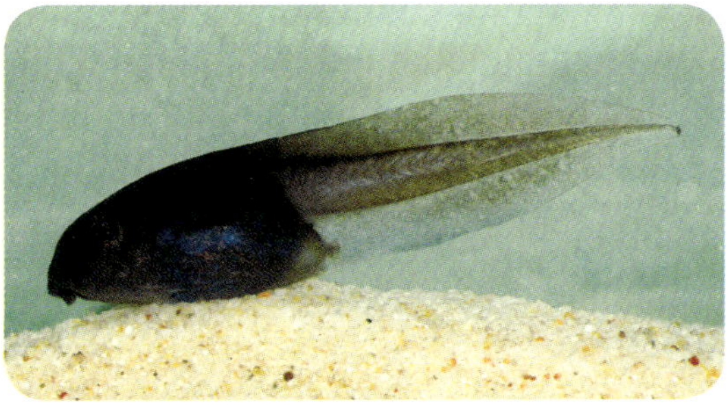

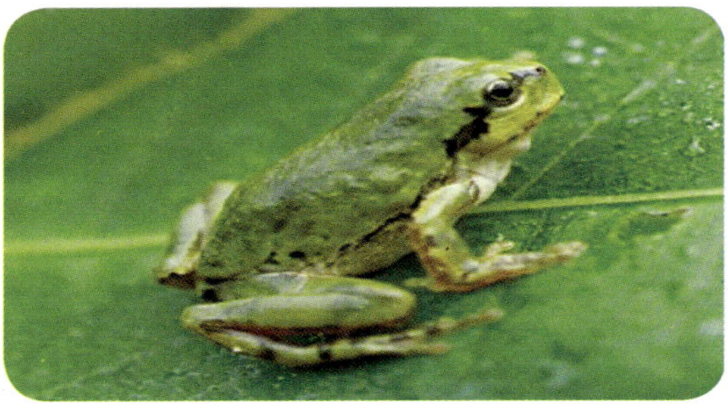

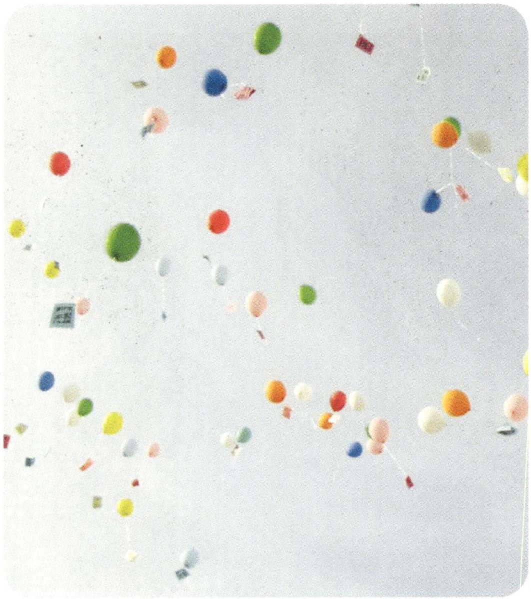

The different movements of qi must work in a coordinated manner to maintain a balance. Once this harmony is disrupted, it will lead to problems of the adverse upward flow of qi, collapse of qi, escape of qi, obstruction of qi, and stagnation of qi. For example, lung qi tends to go downward, so insufficient downward or adverse upward movement of lung qi can cause a cough. Collapse of qi often results from excessive descent or deficient ascent of qi. Escape of qi generally results from profuse sweating or severe bleeding and qi flows out with these substances. Obstruction of qi indicates that the pathways for qi to go outward are obstructed, marked by sudden occurrence of coma or syncope. And stagnation of qi refers to the stagnated flow of qi in the whole body or in a local area.

Qi, the most basic substance that constitutes the world, is often classified into four types according to what it acts on: primordial qi, pectoral qi, nutritive qi, and defensive qi.

> Primordial qi

Primordial qi, as its name indicates, is the most original and fundamental driving force for the growth and development of the human body and the function of *zang-fu* organs. The primordial qi is originated from the kidney where congenital essence from parents is stored and further nourished by acquired essence. Pathologically, the congenital defect and postnatal feeding problems will cause the deficiency of primordial qi, which, in turn, will impair the functional activities of the whole body. In

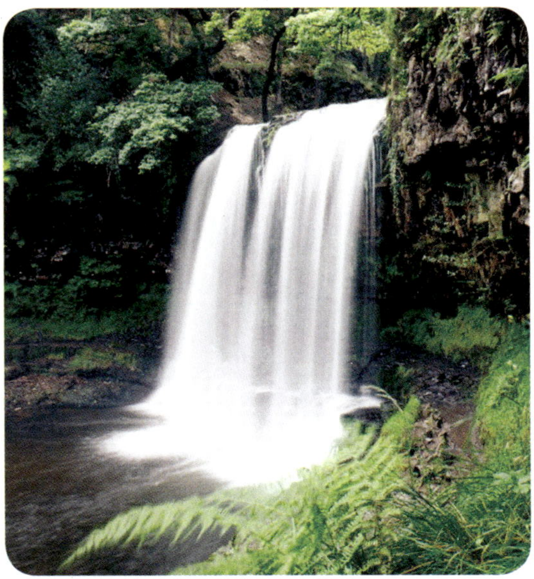

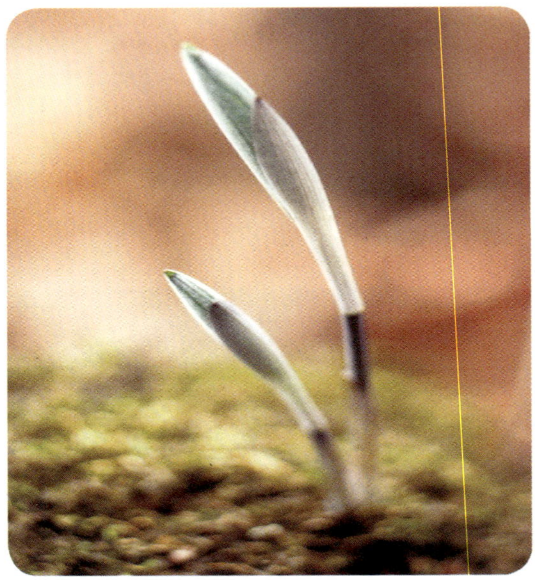

this case, supplementing spleen and stomach, known as the resources of postnatal essence, may be helpful to some extent.

> Pectoral qi

Pectoral qi, as its name indicates, is stored and concentrates in the chest. It is formed by combining fresh air inhaled by the lungs and food essence derived from spleen and stomach, and is distributed in the thorax, then to the blood vessels and the respiratory tract. By flowing through the respiratory tract, pectoral qi assists lungs in breathing and affects how strong the person's voice can be. Usually, unclear speech, a feeble voice, shallow breathing or shortness of breath are signs of deficiency of pectoral qi. While by flowing through the blood vessels and the heart, it plays an important role in regulating the heartbeat, the circulation of qi and blood, and the pulsation of vessels. Pectoral qi also works on keeping the body warm and the activities of the limbs nimble.

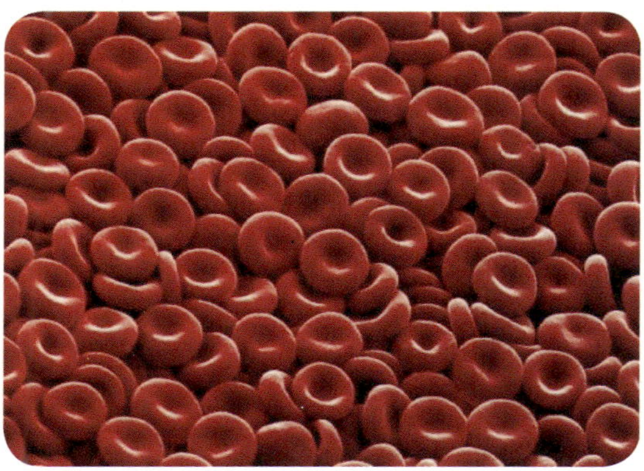

> Nutritive qi

Nutritive qi, as its name indicates, is rich in nutrients and supplies nourishment to the body. It flows inside the blood vessels with blood. Nutritive qi mainly comes from food essence produced by the transformation and transportation of spleen and stomach. Starting from the middle *jiao*, nutritive qi goes to the lungs where it enters the main circulation, with the primary functions of generating blood and providing the needed nutrients to nourishing the whole body.

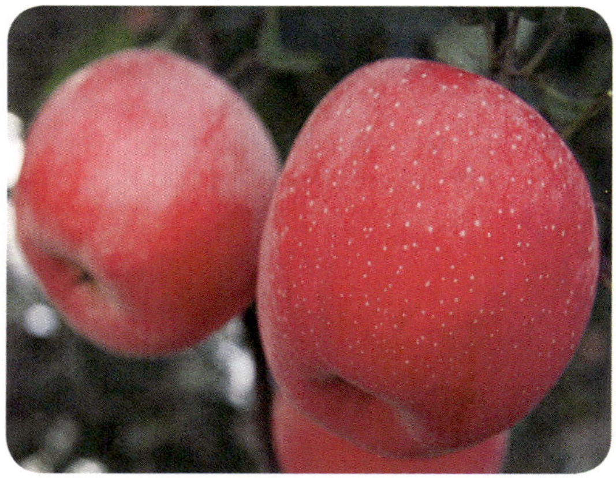

> Defensive qi

Defensive qi, as its name suggests, protects against pathogenic factors and helps prevent diseases from beginning or spreading. Defensive qi also comes from refined food essence but runs outside the blood vessels corresponding to the nutritive qi and circulates freely in different areas all over the body, including sweat glands, pores, skin, hair, muscles, etc. The major functions of defensive qi are to protect the body surface from the invasion of external pathogens, to warm and nourish *zang-fu*, skin and hair, muscles, etc., to keep the body temperature normal, ensure the normal functional activities of *zang-fu* and tissues, as well as to control the opening and closing of the sweat glands. It is worthwhile to note that although nutritive and protective qi are from the same origin of refined food essence transported and transformed by the spleen and stomach, their flows are opposite to each other. Only when balancing their nutritive (yin) and protective (yang) functions, can healthy sweat be discharged, normal body temperature be maintained and defense function and sound sleep be ensured.

In summary, qi is the general force that animates the body's functions. Qi is also the material basis on which different parts of the body can interact. When our qi is healthy and plentiful, we enjoy physical and emotional wellbeing. This healthy qi can be easily disrupted if we don't take constant care. These disruptions can be caused by sudden weather changes, stress, unhealthy food, or lack of proper physical activity. There are a variety of qi problems according to Chinese medicine. One is qi deficiency, which is often described in biomedical terms as chronic fatigue syndrome. Another common qi disturbance is qi stagnation, which may result in pain, headache, and stomachache. A well-trained Chinese medicine practitioner has the knowledge and capability to pinpoint which *zang-fu* organs have what kind of qi problems.

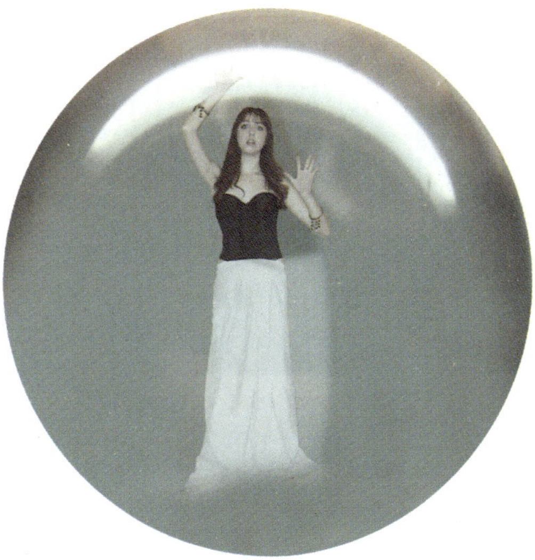

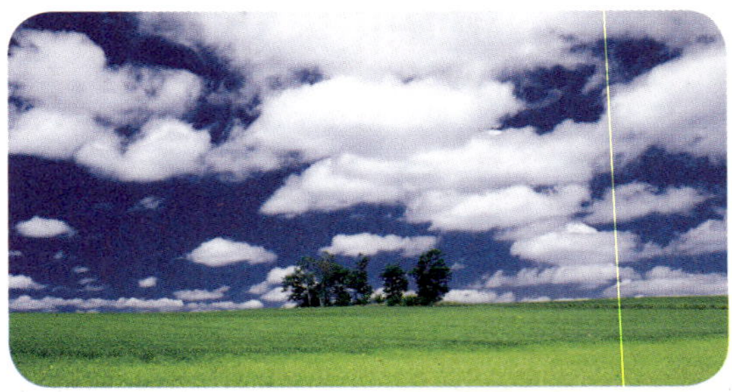

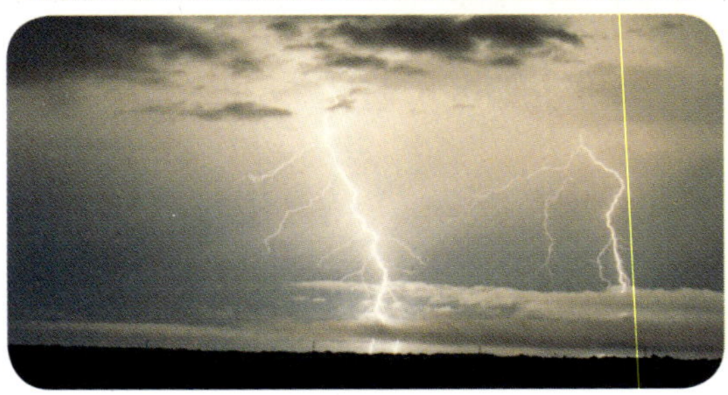

The qi of people with depression is often disturbed. The flow of qi and the mental condition are closely related to each other. Emotional instability may cause the stagnation of qi, like anger may lead to dizziness, headache, and distention and pain in the hypochondriac regions. The following graph outlines some qi disorders commonly found:

	Failure to promote	Failure to warm	Failure to defend	Failure to transform	Failure to secure
Pathological changes	-Hypofunction of *zang-fu* organs -Blood and body fluid obstruction	-Interior cold -Low temperature	-Poor immunity	-Disturbance of life activities	-Abnormal discharge of excretion and secretion
Signs and symptoms	-Fatigue -Abdominal distension -Indigestion	-Cold hands and limbs -Blood stasis on the tongue	-Susceptible to infection and colds or flu	-Fatigue -Hypodynamia	-Aconuresis -Encopresis -Metrorrhagia and metrostaxis

The basis of physiology, pathology, diagnosis, and treatment in Chinese medicine is the theory of essential qi. This theory's main principle is that essential qi is the basic substance that makes up the body. The physiological and pathological changes of the body are the results of normal and abnormal movements of qi. Analyzing the movements of qi is an important part of diagnosis in Chinese medicine, which is called pattern differentiation. Therefore, one purpose of therapeutic treatments is to adjust these abnormalities of qi.

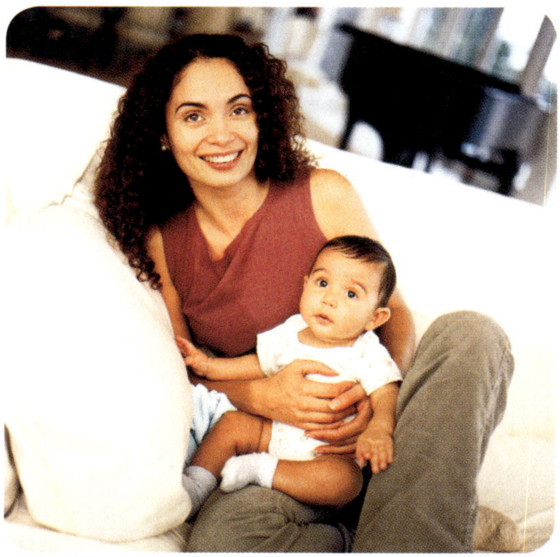

Besides this, metabolism of such essential materials as blood and fluids also depends on the action of qi. From the perspective of Chinese medicine, blood and qi are inseparable. As the "mother" of qi, blood carries qi and provides nutrition for its movement. In turn, qi is the "commander" of blood, which means qi is the power driving blood flow throughout the body and provides the force controlling it to the places where it should and needs to be.

The meaning of qi is many faceted. Qi is what links man and nature and is the material basis for all things. Chinese medicine has discovered that the qi of the internal organs can be reflected on the external parts of the body. The qi of the heart is evident on the tongue, the qi of the liver is manifested in the eyes, the qi of the spleen (pancreas) can be seen on the mouth, the qi of the lungs is visible on the nose, and the qi of the kidney can be observed on the ears. By observing the external manifestations, the functions of the internal organs can be inferred. Meanwhile, stimulus received externally can be conducted into the internal organs by qi. Acupuncture, moxibustion, and massage are all based on the concept that qi in the channels can act on the internal organs.

These internal organ and sense organ correspondences may sound strange to many readers. Please remember that the Chinese understanding of the functions organs perform is different from the understanding of modern biomedicine. The organs in Chinese medicine are more than the anatomical structures seen separately in biomedicine. The Chinese understanding is based not only on the actual physical object, but on functions that encompass a sphere of influence. These functions may seem unrelated, but all are linked by theory based on the natural world.

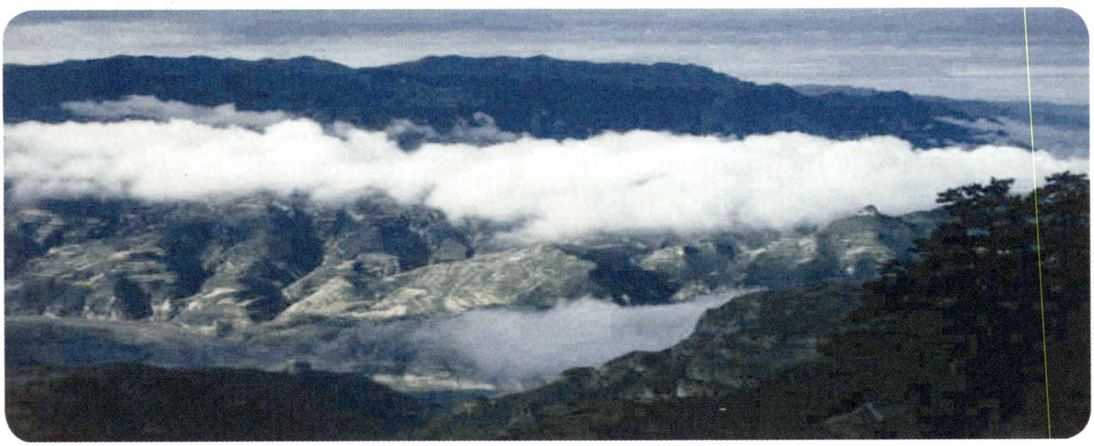

It is the fundamental, simple concepts that are most important and often neglected in learning. The idea of qi, along with yin-yang theory, is of utmost importance to Chinese medicine. Without qi there is death; with qi there is life. Try not to form a fixed idea about qi after this short explanation. Keep an open mind and deepen your understanding of qi as we explore more about Chinese medicine.

Case Two

A 31-year-old man suffered from depression for years. He took a lot of antibiotics as a child for his tonsilitis (most medications, including antibiotics, tend to weaken the liver). By the time he was in school he was hyperactive and was prescribed Ritalin. At age 25, he became very depressed and was on various anti-depressant medications for five years, to no avail. At age 31, he started with Chinese Bitters and Curcuma first. When he experienced significant relief in his symptoms in only a few weeks, he decided to do the complete program of liver and gallbladder cleansing. His depression never returned after he cleansed his liver and gallbladder. (Adopted from: http://www.sensible-health.com)

2. Yin–yang

Ancient Chinese people were extremely interested in and based much of their thinking on observations of nature, so it is no surprise to find that Chinese medicine draws extensively on natural metaphors. The theory of yin-yang fully articulates the metaphoric view. Originally, the words yin and yang were used to describe the sides of a mountain that predominately faced away or towards the sun respectively. The side facing the sun pertains to yang while the side facing away from the sun is yin. Due to the regular rotation of the earth, each individual mountain will have one side that mostly faces the sun, which is the yang side, and one side that usually faces away from the sun, which is the yin side.

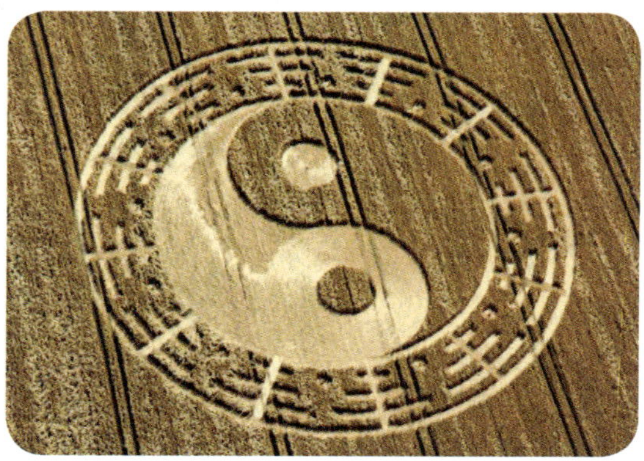

These two opposites in all objects and phenomena are not stationary but in constant motion and change. Indeed, because of the regular change from darkness to light due to the rotation of the earth, everything has an intrinsic yin aspect and yang aspect. The rotation of our planet has caused everything on it to evolve in such a way that it adapts to the cyclic coming of light and dark. For instance, winter (yin) transforms through the spring into summer (yang), which in turn transforms through autumn into winter. The gain, growth, and advance of the one means the loss, decline, and retreat of the other; and every natural phenomenon is balanced through the constant flux of alternating yin and yang. Yin and yang can change into and balance each other, for instance, day is yang and night is yin; as day fades away it turns into night, and as yin fades away it becomes yang. Yin and yang are inseparable characteristics of being part of planet Earth. The concept of unified duality is a central part of ancient Chinese culture, and the Chinese understanding of every natural and social phenomenon is based on this. There are always two (with a relationship), not an isolated one. Harmony is the balance between the two, and

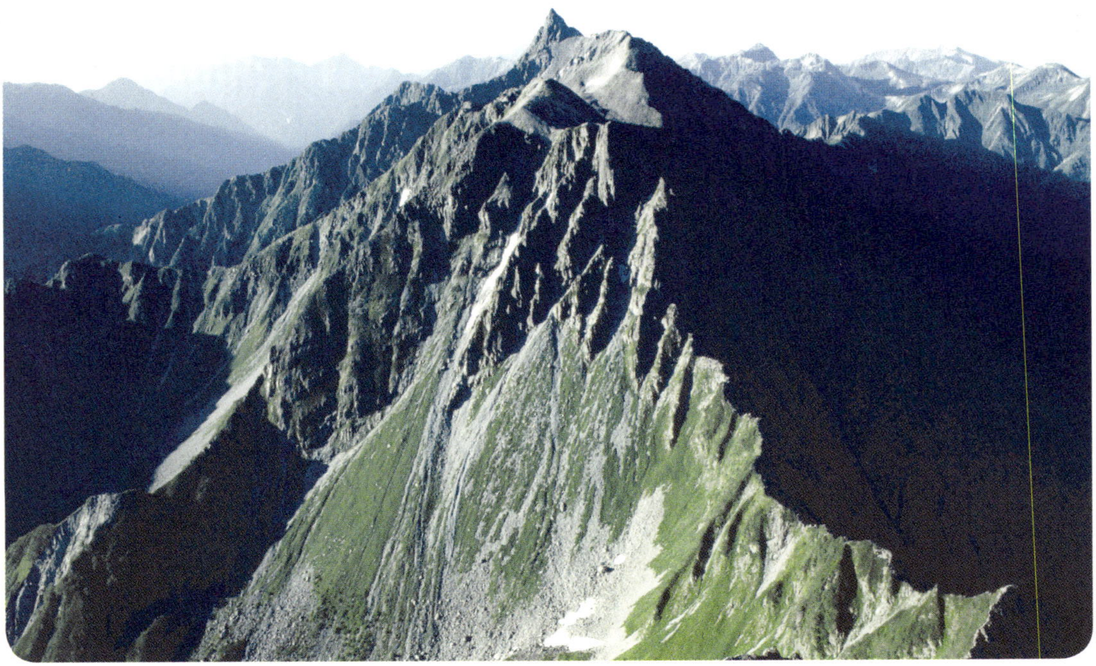

this is an ideal condition for yin and yang. Understanding harmony is an important part of understanding Chinese medicine. The words "balance" and "harmony" are sometimes interchangeable, but they are quite different in Chinese medicine, that is to say balance is merely the first step toward harmony. When two things are in harmony, they are not just of equal proportion but mixed together naturally into a whole.

The direct meanings of yin and yang in Chinese are bright and dark sides of a certain object. Chinese philosophers adopt yin and yang to represent a wider range of opposite properties in the universe. Yang is associated with qualities such as brightness and warmth while yin is associated with the opposing characteristics of darkness and cold. Some further examples are: daytime pertains to yang while night is yin; sunny weather is yang while cloudy weather is yin; spring and summer are yang and autumn and winter are yin; fire is yang while water is yin, and so on. Further expansion of this logic leads to the division of everything in the universe into yin or yang based on the quality, property, position, trend, function, or effect of the phenomena being classified. In general, anything that is moving, ascending, bright, progressing, hyperactive, including functional diseases, pertains to yang. While anything of stillness, descending, darkness, degeneration, hypoactivity, including organic diseases, pertains to yin.

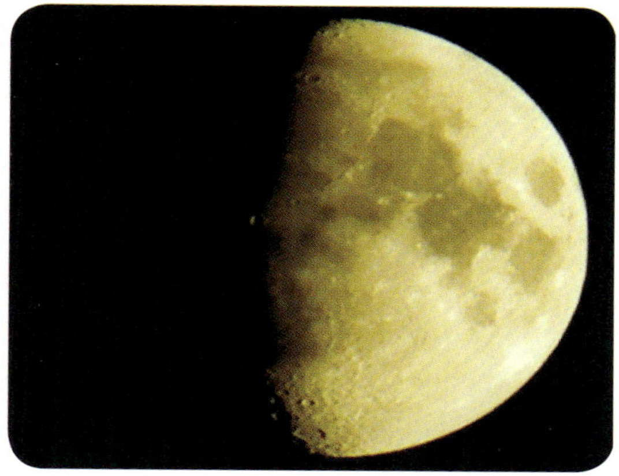

The concept of yin-yang is the general division of any given thing (including living things, inanimate objects, feelings, actions, etc.) into two polar attributes which are related to each other. Yin and yang can also be used to subdivide already classified categories. As stated in *The Yellow Emperor's Inner Classic* "Yin and yang can be counted in tens hundreds and thousands, and can be continued until infinity." For example, we already described summer as yang, but during summer there are days when it is extremely hot (more yang) and days when it is cloudy and cooler (more yin); day is yang and night is yin, but morning is defined as yang within yang, afternoon is yin within yang, evening before midnight is yin within yin, and the time after midnight is yang within yin. The complementary and opposing nature of yin and yang can be used as labels to describe two opposing things like sky and earth, or two opposing aspects contained within one thing. See the following table for a clearer picture of the division of yin and yang.

Examples of Yin-yang Categorization

Category	Yang	Yin
Time	Day	Night
Space	Heaven	Earth
Season	Spring, Summer	Autumn, Winter
Temperature	Hot	Cold
Weight	Light	Heavy
Speed	Fast	Slow
Motion	Up and out, vigorous	Down and in, subtle
Brightness	Light	Dark
Sex	Male	Female
Tissue and organs	Skin, hair	Bone, tendon
Disease	Acute	Chronic

In Chinese medicine the fundamental definition of health is when there is a good balance of yin and yang in the body. Diagnosis of disease and its treatment are all aimed at restoring this equilibrium. This may sound simplistic, but when you consider the fact that all organs, functions, emotions, fluids, and structures each have yin and yang aspects that must be balanced, you can see how the doctor's job of detecting every imbalance with using no more than the five senses is a very difficult task. But please try to keep what Zhang Jing-yue stated in his well-known *The Complete Works of Zhang Jing-yue* (*Jǐng Yuè Quán Shū*, 景岳全书) in mind, "Although medicine is complicated, it can be summed up in one word, namely: yin-yang."

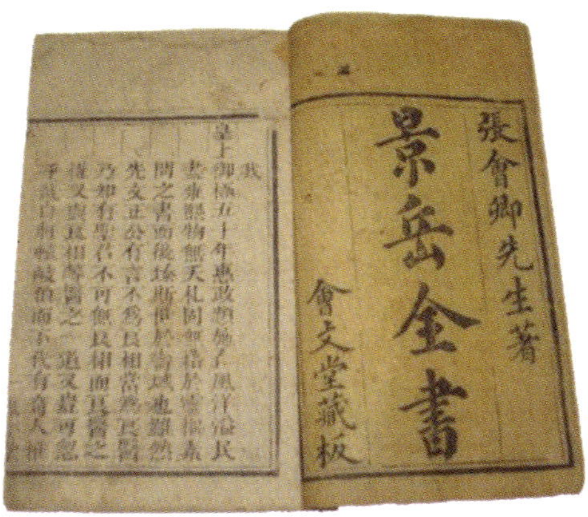

The Comple te Works of Zhang Jing-yue
(Jǐng Yuè Quán Shū)

Yin and yang are guided by the law of unity of the opposites. In other words, yin and yang are in conflict but meanwhile interdependent, since the nature of yin and yang is relative and neither of them can exist in isolation. The interrelationship between substance (yin) and function (yang) of the body is an example of yin-yang interdependence. Only with sufficient substance can the human body function in a healthy manner; and only when the functional processes are in good condition, can the essential substances be properly refreshed. The most illustrative example in Western medicine similar to the yin-yang interdependence is the interrelationship between anabolism and catabolism, without anabolism there would be no catabolism, and without catabolism there would be no anabolism. The interdependence of yin and yang also means that the condition of one will affect the other. If there is too little yin, then yang will appear to be in excess; and if there is too much yin, there will appear to be too little yang. The reverse is of course true for when there is too little or too much yang. A simple example can be seen when the body's temperature rises or falls too much. With fever there is a relative abundance of yang heat. This means the cool yin aspect of the body is not sufficient to counteract the heat. Therefore the practitioner must restore the balance of yin and yang by making the cool yin aspect of the body equal to the hot yang aspect. Likewise, when a person has hypothermia and a dangerously low body temperature, this means there is a relative abundance of yin cold in relation to yang heat.

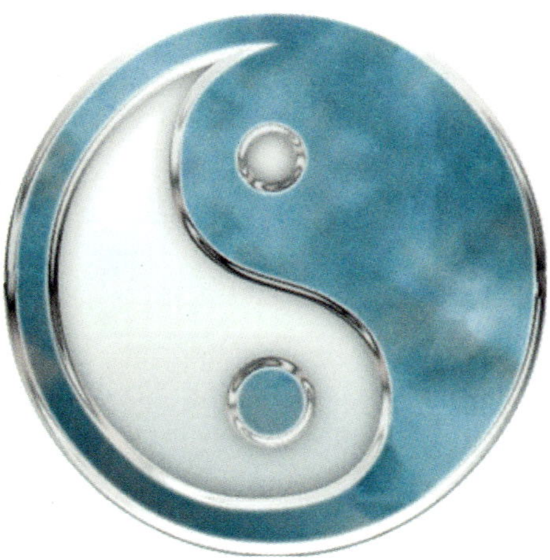

However, it is not enough to know merely which is the stronger of yin or yang and which is the weaker. If there is more yang than yin, for example, this could be due to either too much yang and thus yin is relatively weak, or it could be because there is not enough yin, therefore, yang appears to be in excess.

This is a difficult concept for any students of Chinese medicine at the beginning, so let us look at an example. A forest that has not had any rain for many months will be dry and probably hot. Dryness and heat are yang qualities as opposed to yin moisture and cold. A forest that is on fire is also in a condition of yang heat. In each case, the yang aspect is greater than the yin aspect. But to restore the yin-yang balance of both situations, one must choose different strategies. To restore the forest in drought it is necessary to add yin, meaning water. On the other hand, to balance a blazing fire, one has no other option but to remove the excess yang fire. In Chinese medicine, the dry forest would be said to be in a state of yin deficiency, where the heat is due to a relative abundance of yang. The forest fire is a state of yang excess, where yin may very well be normal. The other states are yang deficiency and yin excess. Chinese medicine holds that human life is not static but dynamic, so is the balance between yin and yang. In normal conditions, the waxing-waning of yin and yang changes at a gradual rate in a state of relative balance. When the balance is jeopardized, disease occurs. As stated in *The Yellow Emperor's Inner Classic*, "Yin in excess consumes yang, and yang in excess consumes yin." "Yin in excess causes cold syndromes, and yang in excess causes heat syndromes." Please see the diagrams to better understand the four different types of yin-yang imbalances: yang excess, yin excess, yang deficiency and yin deficiency.

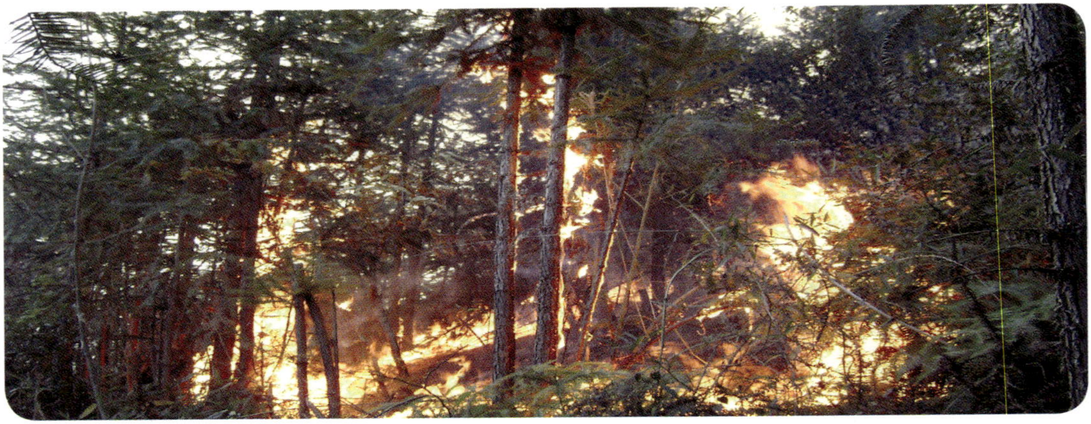

Typical Manifestations

Yang excess	Fever, aversion to heat, thirst, desire for cold drinks, reddish complexion, restlessness, yellowish-colored mucus, dark-colored urination, constipation, red tongue, yellowish tongue coating, rapid pulses
Yin excess	Aversion to cold, no thirst, desire for warm drinks, pale complexion, thin and watery mucus, loose stool, light-colored tongue, whitish tongue coating, slow or tense pulses
Yang deficiency	Preference for warmth, cold limbs, pale complexion, spontaneous sweating, fatigue, shortness of breath, loose stool, enlarged and light-colored tongue, whitish tongue coating, deep, slow, and weak pulses
Yin deficiency	Thirst, dry mouth and throat, hot feeling in the soles and palms, afternoon fever, night sweating, red tongue with little coating, rapid, and fine pulses

Yin and yang can transform into each other. This change does not take place at random, but only at a certain stage during the development process of certain things when both internal and external causes are ready. Pathologically, however, deficiency of either yin or yang may result in the depletion of the other, known as "impairment of yin influencing yang" and "impairment of yang influencing yin."

As one dialectic way of thinking, the theory of yin-yang can be applied to any field of medicine under the precondition of that the human body should be viewed as an organic whole. Diagnosis and treatment in Chinese medicine is usually more dynamic than with chronic diseases in biomedicine. Conditions may change daily, though with chronic disease it is usually safe to reevaluate once a week or more often. A patient diagnosed with an excess of yang will have yang-type symptoms such as high fever, restlessness, red complexion, rapid pulse, or yellowish tongue coating, since an excess of yang leads to heat. The heat of excess yang can damage the cool water of yin and can be seen when the patient has symptoms like dry mouth and throat, thirst, or a dry tongue.

In clinic, every patient may present a different pattern, or usually a combination of patterns, because every patient is different. Even for one patient, depending on the development of the disease, lifestyle modifications adopted, or environmental changes, the diagnosis will also have to be modified and refined at each specific stage.

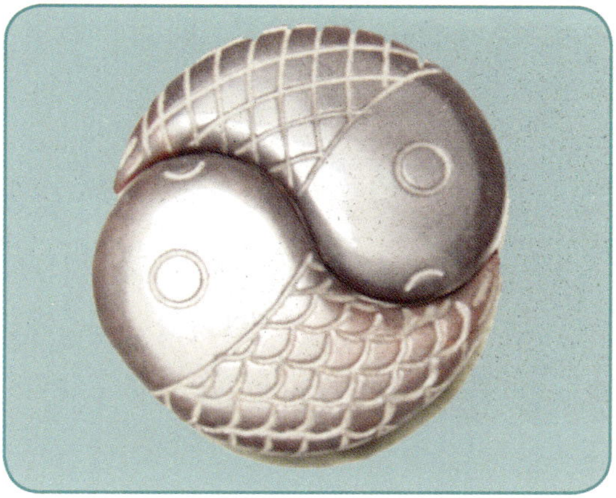

The diagnosis of yin or yang is based on an integrative and insightful analysis of all the signs and symptoms of each individual patient, and the point is to differentiate the yin and yang nature of the disease correctly and get a clear picture of the imbalance of yin and yang.

After all of the information about a patient is collected, the data will be vigorously analyzed and categorized by an experienced practitioner into different patterns of disharmony. The patterns can be numerous, and will vary with the individual, time, location, climate, and other factors involved. Corresponding treatment protocol will be made according to the specific patterns identified. Such therapeutic principles as "fortify what is in deficiency," "reduce what is in excess," "treat cold with warming measures," and

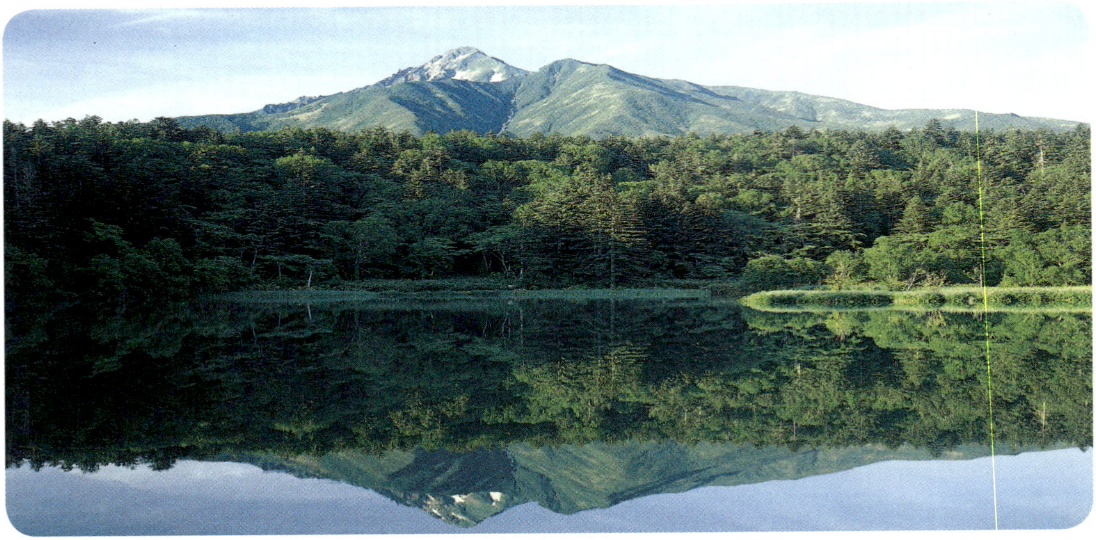

"treat heat with cooling measures" are the general rules with great therapeutic effects on restoring the balance of yin-yang. That is to say, for pathogenic factors with a yin nature, yang measures are appropriate, and for pathogenic factors with a yang nature, yin measures should be adopted; for deficiency syndromes, supplementing or reinforcing measures are necessary. In advanced cases, however, sometimes it is better to "treat the yang aspect for diseases of a yin nature," and "treat the yin aspect for diseases of a yang nature". Sometimes, acupuncturists needle the points of the yang channels for disorders of the yin channels, and the points of the yin channels for illnesses of the yang channels. Chinese medicine is aimed at highly individualized treatment -- the goal of all types of medicine. Chinese medicine's goal is the recovery of the innate function of the body -- a true medicine.

Case Three

A female patient, 35 years old, came to visit a practitioner of Chinese medicine. She complained about depression, difficulty in handling her job as an accountant, and difficulty communicating with people around her. She felt restless and pessimistic. Three months before she came here, her husband took her to a hospital for a psychological consultation, and her depression was evaluated at an integral value of Y-92. She said the antidepressants didn't work for her. She had a yellowish complexion, puffy swollen eyelids, chest pain, frequent sighs, insomnia, dreaminess, memory loss, poor appetite, pale tongue with thin coating and teeth marks, and thin and wiry pulses. According to all the information, she was diagnosed as having stagnation of liver qi and deficiency of heart and spleen. The corresponding therapeutic methods were to fortify the spleen, nourish the heart, and soothe the liver. A treatment combining acupuncture with medicinals was given; the selected acupoints were RN 12 (*zhōng wǎn*), ST 36 (*zú sān lǐ*), BL 20 (*pí shù*), BL 21 (*wèi shù*), BL 15 (*xīn shù*), HT 7 (*shén mén*), *yìn táng,* and LV 3 (*tài chōng*), and the formula was a modification of *Xiāo Yáo Sǎn* (Free Wanderer Powder). The patient felt relief from the depression two months after beginning treatment. Then, she continued with another five acupuncture treatments to consolidate the therapeutic effect.

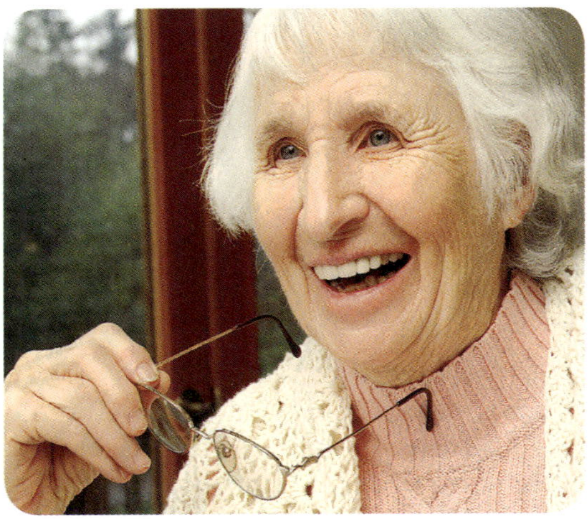

3. Five Phases

The original expression of five phases in Chinese medicine is "*wǔ xíng*" and the Chinese term "*xíng*" literally means movement and the process of one thing acting upon another. Hence, "*wǔ xíng*" refers to the constant movements of the five types of vital substances in the universe, representing the processes that are fundamental to the cycles of nature, and therefore correspond to the human body.

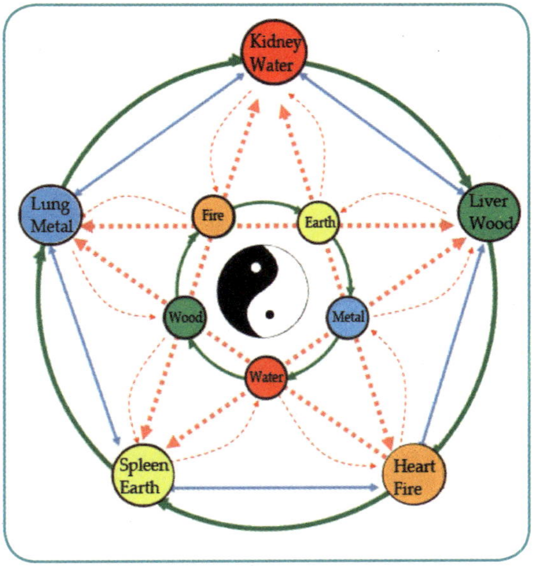

As one of pillar theories and one of the major diagnostic and treatment protocols of Chinese medicine, the five phases, also translated as five elements or five movements, are comprised of wood, fire, earth, metal, and water, revealing a series of constant movements, changes, and concordances. Through observing what happens in nature and adopting the methodology of "comparing similarity to expose phenomenon," ancient Chinese philosophers defined the dynamic characteristics of the five phases as follows:

Property of Five Phases

Category	Originally meaning	Transferred meaning	Personality
Wood	Flexing and extending	-Germination -Extension -Softness and harmony	-Creative -Strong and resilient
Fire	-Hot -Ascending - Light and energetic	-Scorching heat -Flaring -Things or phenomena that ascend -Change and activity	-Intelligent -Impulsive -Fervent and dynamic
Earth	-Productive -Fertile -Nourishing and growing	-Reproduction -Nourish -Solidity and grounding	-Firm and resolute -Down-to-earth -Practical -Hard-working and very conservative
Metal	-Restriction -Strike -Receivable and changeable	-Cleaning up -Killing -Strength and firmness	-Forceful -Strong and determined
Water	-Cold -Moisture -Descending and downward flowing	-Flowing downwards -Things or phenomena belonging to cold or with cold functions	-Fluent -Have deep feelings and strong intuitions or psychic powers as well

The observation of nature and the interrelationships in both the environment and within the human body laid a solid foundation for the five-phase theory, which were the correspondences of each phase to a variety of phenomena. And numerous correspondences were discovered. Things as different as human organs, tastes, emotions, sounds, directions, colors, seasons, climate factors, and stages of growth were found to have something in common. The commonest correspondences are listed in the table below:

Commonest Correspondences Between Nature and the Human Body

	Category	Wood	Fire	Earth	Metal	Water
Human	***Zang* Organs**	Liver	Heart	Spleen	Lungs	Kidneys
	***Fu* Organs**	Gall Bladder	Small Intestine	Stomach	Large Intestine	Bladder
	Sensory Organs	Eyes	Tongue	Mouth	Nose	Ears
	Tissues	Tendon	Vessel	Muscle	Skin	Bone
	Emotions	Anger	Joy	Worry/ Pensiveness	Grief/ Sadness	Fear
	Sounds	Shouting	Laughing	Singing	Crying	Groaning
	Fluids	Tear	Sweat	Saliva	Snivel	Urine
	Pulses	Taut	Bound	Moderate	Superficial	Deep
Nature	**Seasons**	Spring	Summer	Late Summer	Autumn	Winter
	Odors	Rancid	Scorched	Fragrant	Rotten	Putrid
	Colors	Green	Red	Yellow	White	Blue/ Black
	Tastes	Sour	Bitter	Sweet	Pungent	Salty
	Climate Factors	Wind	Heat	Damp	Arid	Cold
	Developmental stages	Germination	Growth	Transformation	Harvest	Storage
	Direction	East	South	Center	West	North

More than two thousand years ago, Basic Questions (*Sù Wèn*, 素问) stated that, "the east generates wind, wind generates wood, wood generates sour, sour generates liver, liver generates tendons...", that is to say the five-phase theory reveals the interrelation existing between and among those various things which are triggered by a particular phase and each phase has its whole set of relationships among the matters constituting the material world. It hence lays the theoretical basis for the unique bond between humanity and nature.

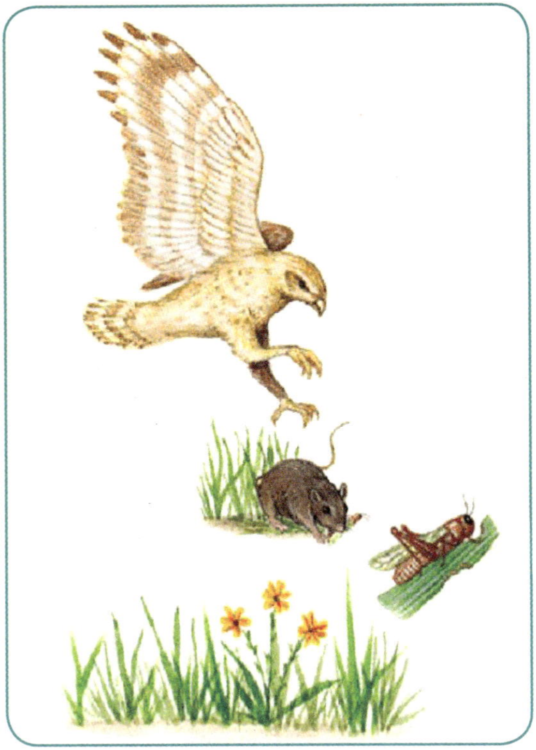

Chinese medicine holds that nothing in this universe exists alone, nor does it stand still, but instead remain in permanent and dynamic equilibriums. According to the five-phase theory, there are four main approaches through which the phases interact with each other, reflecting a dynamic process and cyclic movements.

> Generating cycle

The generating cycle, also translated as the *shēng* cycle, the nourishing cycle or the mother-son cycle, pictures the way in which each phase promotes the growth and development of the next phase. Each phase, serving as the mother to the next phase, offers the generative and driving force for the following child phase in a circular and endless way: water nourishes wood, wood feeds and fuels fire, fire produces ashes that make earth, earth yields metal, liquefied metal produces water. In

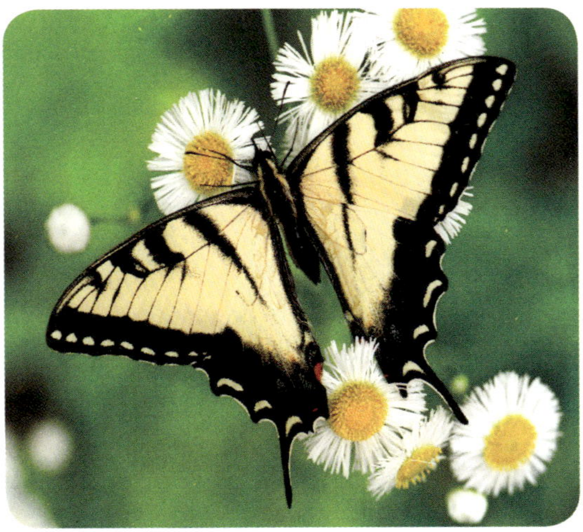

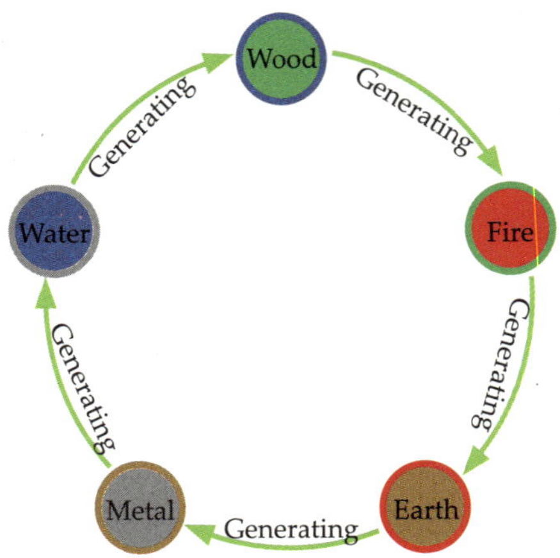

this way, each of the phases has the property of "generating" and "being generated." The one that generates is the "mother," the one being generated is the "son." Each of the five elements has a generating relationship with another. The clockwise sequence on the circle represents the generating cycle.

> Restricting cycle

The restricting cycle, also known as the *kè* cycle, regulating cycle, or restraint cycle, builds a system of checks and balances among all five phases. Namely, water puts out fire, fire melts metal, metal cuts wood, wood contains earth, and earth soaks up water. More specifically, water, for example, controls fire and is controlled by earth. This relationship has the properties of "being restricted" and "restricting." Each of the five elements also shares a restricting relationship with another. The clockwise sequence depicted by the pentagon stands for the restricting cycle.

Generating and restricting are two aspects that cannot be separated, As one of the Chinese medicine classics points out, "If there is no generation, then there is no growth and development. If there is no restriction, then endless growth and development will become harmful." This indicates both are fundamental for maintaining normal harmonious relations and constant circulation of natural elements. Thus the movement and change of all things exists through their mutual generating and restricting relationships. Whereas, over-restricting and counter-restricting are two approaches adverse to the normal restricting relationship and denote the mutual influence of the *zang-fu* organs and their pathological conditions.

> Over-restricting Cycle

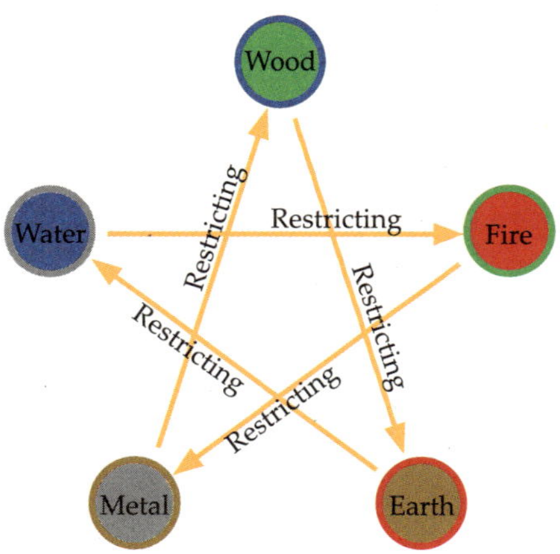

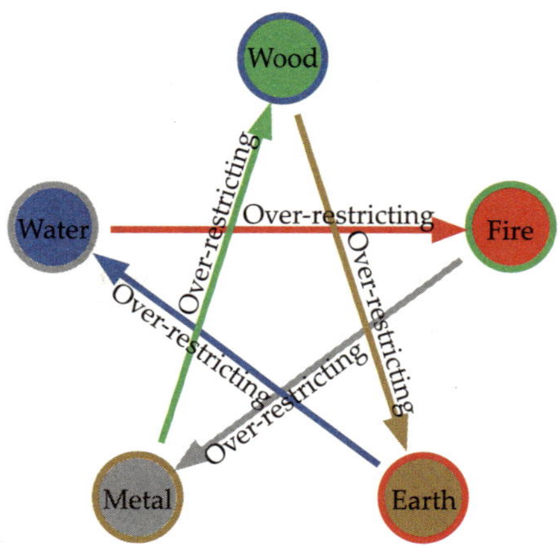

The over-restricting cycle, also translated as *chéng* cycle, over-restraint cycle, or over-acting cycle, represents an imbalance within the restricting cycle where certain phases provide too much restriction over and weaken the phase being controlled. It denotes that the restraint of one phase to another surpasses the normal level. For instance, the hyperactivity of wood phase may over-restrict the earth phase; the latter will be impaired in various manners. Clinically, you may encounter patients suffering from the disruptions in the digestive system due to the overactive liver-wood phase controlling the spleen-earth phase.

> Counter-restricting Cycle

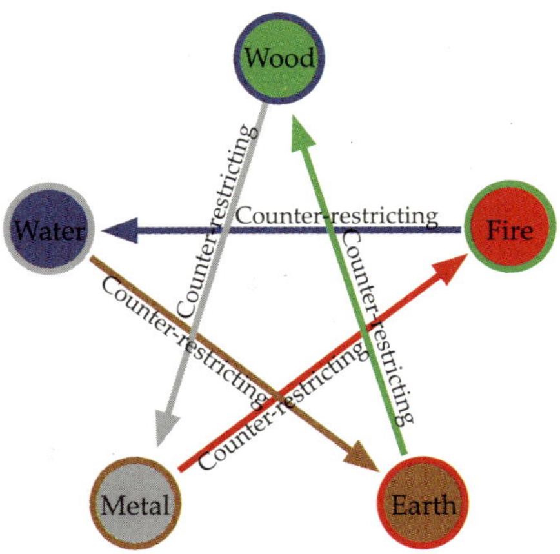

The counter-restricting cycle, also known as *wǔ* cycle, counter-controlling or insulting cycle, is also an imbalance within the restricting cycle when a certain phase offends or returns the restricting force generated by the phase that restricts. That is to say, one of the five phases restricts the other opposite to the normal order. For example, weak and insufficient metal may result in the hyperactivity of wood, and the latter will then counter-restrict the former. Clinically, you may see people with long-term fire syndromes that eventually affect the kidneys-water. In the Basic Questions, it states: "when one of the five phases is excessive, it will control its controlled phase and counter-control its controlling phase."

Practically speaking, the five-phase theory can be used in a variety of ways for addressing health problems. It can be applied to the classification of all phenomena. Wood, for example, symbolizes germination, extension, softness, and harmony, which infers that anything with those properties should be brought into the category of the wood phase. According to this theory, external appearances are mirror for the abnormal changes of the internal organ's functions and interrelationships. The signs, symptoms, complexion, voice, tastes, pulse, etc. are hints, since the organs inside have certain connections with colors, tones, five tastes, and changes in the pulse, etc. The five-phase theory is employed to analyze human body physiologically and pathologically by using generating and restricting relationships to guide clinical diagnosis and treatment. Specifically speaking, the five-phase theory not only explains the mutual relationships between and among different parts of human body, as well as between humanity and nature, giving expression to the holistic concept of Chinese medicine, but also demonstrates their mutual pathological influence. Let us take a look at how liver illness affects or can be affected by other organs from the perspective of Chinese medicine. Liver disease may impair spleen because wood may over-restrict earth, while spleen illness may affect the liver as earth can counter-restrict wood, liver disease may also impair heart as the mother-organ can affect the son-organ that derive from the mutual generation relationship. If the lung is also affected by liver disease, this is categorized as wood counter-restricting metal. If it is transmitted to the kidney, then it is considered as "son affecting mother" illness. In other words, the complicated interactions between the *zang-fu* organs, organs under pathological conditions are generally over-restriction, counter-restriction, mother affecting son, and son affecting mother illnesses. So clinically, the data collected by the four examination methods (inspection, auscultation and olfaction, inquiring, and palpation) can be analyzed in this way. From there, the basic property of illness can be analyzed and determined, and the theory may be conducive to help form a diagnosis when there are conflicting signs and symptoms, resulting in the formulation of a treatment principle and method. For patients with skin problems, for instance, the Chinese medicine practitioner understands that according to five-phase theory, the organ system of the lung and large intestine are involved because the skin is the tissue of the lung. Thus, one or both organs will be treated to heal the root cause, not just the symptom of the skin problem.

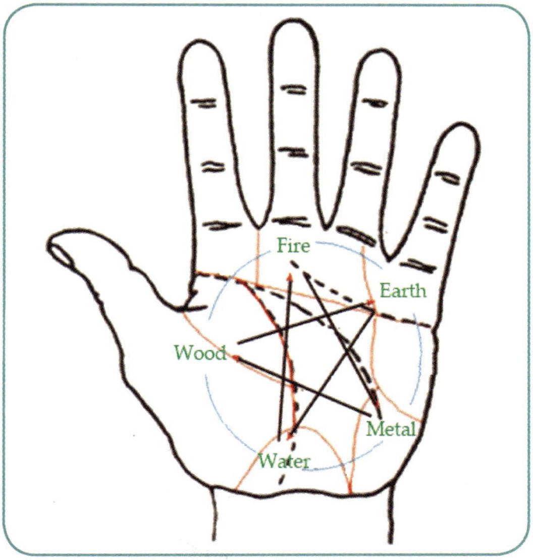

Moreover, clinical treatment should not only concentrate on the dysfunctional *zang* organ, but also be concerned about readjusting the relationships between the particular *zang* or *fu* organs in accordance with five-phase theory. The statement from *The Classic of Difficult Issues* (*Nàn Jīng*, 难经) that, "When the liver is diseased, the liver will transmit to the spleen, and so one should replenish the qi of the spleen," reflects the clinical application of five element's over-restricting theory. The four laws of five-phase theory have been used by generations of Chinese medicine practitioners creating more methods of treatment such as: "cultivating the earth in order to generate metal," "nourishing the water to conserve wood," "supporting the earth to restrict wood," etc.

Additionally, for acupuncturists, there are also mother and child points for each meridian and five *shù* (transporting) points reflecting the application of this theory to individual acupoints.

Last but not the least, the five-phase theory is useful for assisting patients with emotional problems, since the five-phase theory holds that the five human emotions: anger, joy, reflection, grief, and fear are still in the mutual generation and controlling relationships. And *zang-fu* organs are the material basis for mental, spiritual, and emotional expression, and unhealthy organs also manifest through unhealthy emotions such as depression.

In conclusion, the yin-yang and five-phase theories, reflecting the world view, philosophic thinking, and methodology of the ancient Chinese in terms of understanding and explaining nature and humanity, are used together as a guide to the diagnosis and treatment of disease in the clinic.

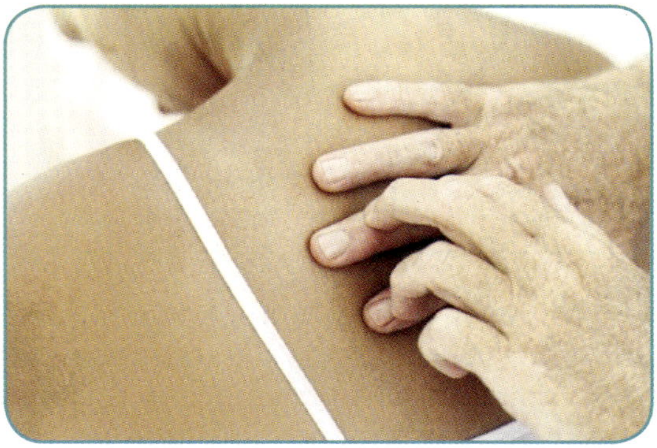

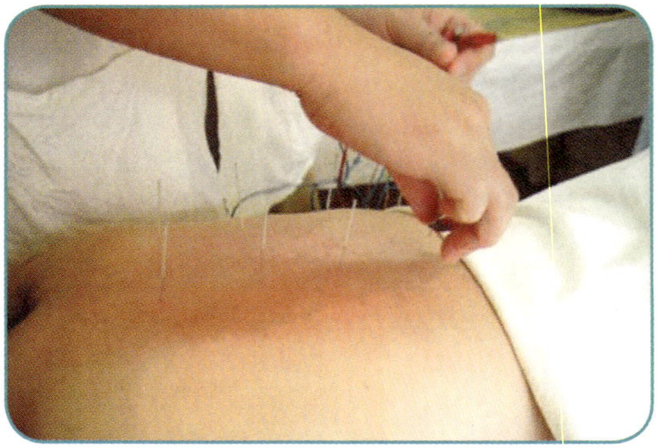

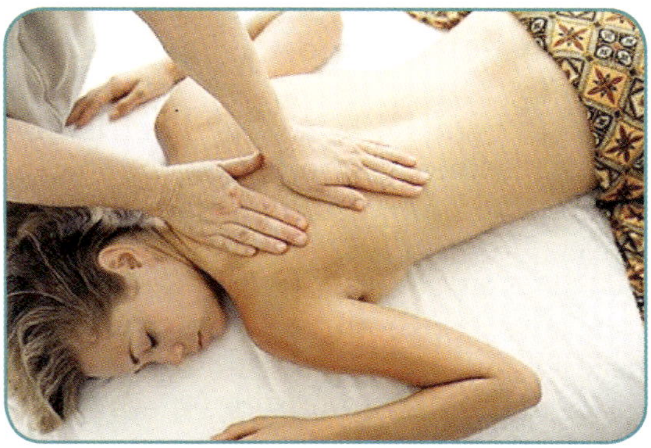

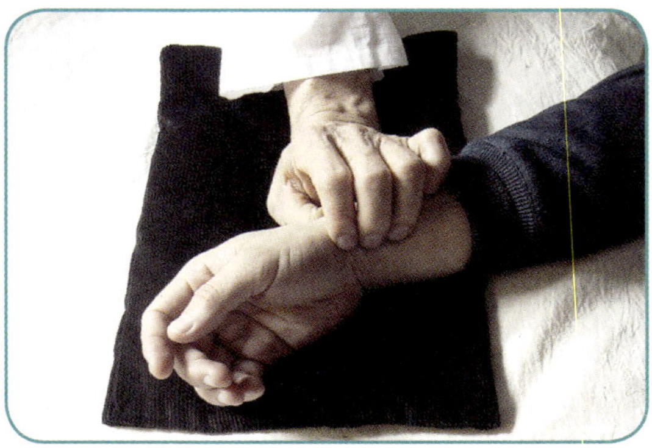

Depression in Chinese Medicine

Depressed moods, loss of interest in an activity that was once pleasurable, loss of emotional expression, feelings of guilt or low self-worth, disturbed sleep, loss of appetite with weight loss or overeating with weight gain, low energy, social withdrawal, and trouble concentrating are common mental disorders that appear linked to depression. It is not the same as a temporary blue mood, people with depression cannot simply cheer themselves up, pull themselves together and become better, hence immediate and appropriate treatment are necessary. At its worse, depression can recur or last for decades and can disable a person's capability to deal with his or her life on a daily basis. At its worst, it can lead to suicide. Three to five percent of the Chinese population has suffered from depression during their lifetime, while 10-15% of these people may attempt suicide.

From the perspective of biomedicine, the onset of depression may correlate with or predispose to such biological fac-

Figure 1. Percentage of persons 12 years of age and older with depression by demographic characteristics: United States, 2005-2006

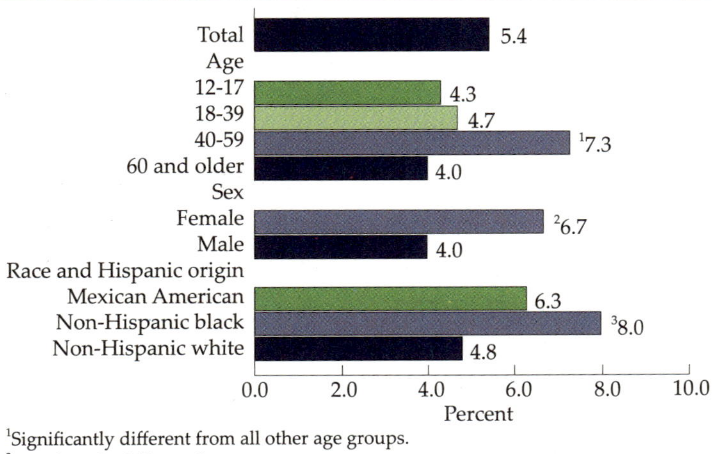

[1]Significantly different from all other age groups.
[2]Significantly different from men.
[3]Significantly different from non-hispanic while persons.
SOURCE: CDC/NCHS, National Health and Nutrition Examination Survey.

tors as biogenic amine, hypothalamus-pituitary-adrenal axis, and hypothalamus-pituitary-thyroid axis, genetic factors, and such psychosocial factors as cognition, personality, and gender. Although depression is the mental disorder that is most frequently studied, the truth is its etiology is still far from fully understood. While in Chinese medicine, depression is commonly defined as *yù zhèng* and the word "*yù*" literally in Chinese means accumulation, stagnation, and gestation. For thousands of years, Chinese medicine has held that "if qi and blood are in harmony, no disease will occur; however, once depression is present, various diseases will occur; hence most diseases in one's life are caused by depression." People's mental and emotional activities are closely related to *zang*-organ function, for instance, the heart is believed to store spirit and control happiness, and the liver is associated with anger. If there is an imbalance or blockage in any *zang* from any cause, a disturbed mental and emotional state will occur. Likewise, imbalanced emotional states such as excessive anger, anxiety, worry, or grief can cause *zang* disturbances. As *The Yellow Emperor's Inner Classic* written during the Warring States Period (457 B.C. - 221 B.C.) says, "Excessive contemplation leads to concentration of mind and spirit, which will result in sluggish flow of healthy qi and further qi stagnation." However, the spirit in Chinese medicine is different from that of the Western world; it is believed to reside in the heart instead of the brain and covers the dimensions of mind, spirit, consciousness, awareness, and vitality. It manifests in the pool of intelligence, mental status and activities such as perception, thinking, memory, and in the sphere of mind, emotions as well as the more spiritual and elusive aspects.

Etiology

Broadly speaking, depression in Chinese medicine is defined as a disorder resulting from both exogenous evils and emotional problems, which was the popular view before the period of Jin and Yuan Dynasty (1,115 - 1,368 A.D.). While narrowly speaking, it refers to an illness using emotional disturbances as an etiology and the stagnation of qi movements as basic pathology, which was recognized after the Ming Dynasty (1,368 - 1,644 A.D.).

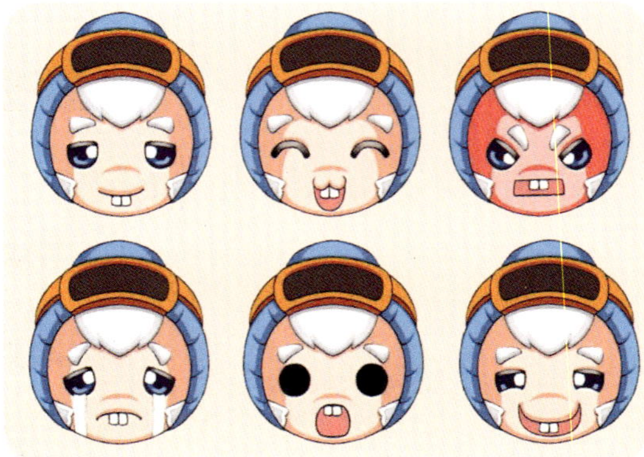

Generally, depression is induced by emotional and mental disturbance, and the basic pathological change is the stagnated flow of qi. Its onset and development also closely relates to the disharmony of qi and blood, and dysfunction of *zang* organs. Alongside or as a result of qi stagnation, blood stasis, internal fire, phlegm coagulation, and food retention may occur. The specific pathomechanisms are liver failing to regulate the free flow of qi, spleen failing to transport and transform, and heart failing to get nourishment as well as a disordered flow of fundamental substances in the body. The *zang* most frequently affected are liver, heart, and spleen; other organs may also be involved. Initially, the pathological change tends to be excessive, if it goes untreated, it will change into either a combination of excess and deficiency patterns or a deficiency pattern. Usually, people start by experiencing an imbalance in one organ, untreated or improperly treated, the disorder will spread, involving other organs. And that is the reason why Chinese medicine emphasizes early diagnosis and early preventive treatment of imbalances.

To be more specific, the primary etiologies for depression are as follows:

➡ Liver qi stagnation due to excessive anger

Emotional disturbances such as hate, resentment, and anger make the liver lose its ability to maintain the free flow of qi, leading to liver qi stagnation. The stagnant qi can inhibit the circulation of blood since qi is the commander of blood, which in turn leads to depression named *xuè yù* (blood depression). If liver qi stagnation is left untreated for a long period, it will turn into fire and cause depression named *huǒ yù* (fire depression). The stagnant qi can inhibit the free flow of body fluid, letting them accumulate in any part of the body and causing depression named *tán yù* (phlegm depression). The fire produced by liver qi stagnation consumes the yin of liver. All these can lead to functional disturbance and pathological changes in the mind and body.

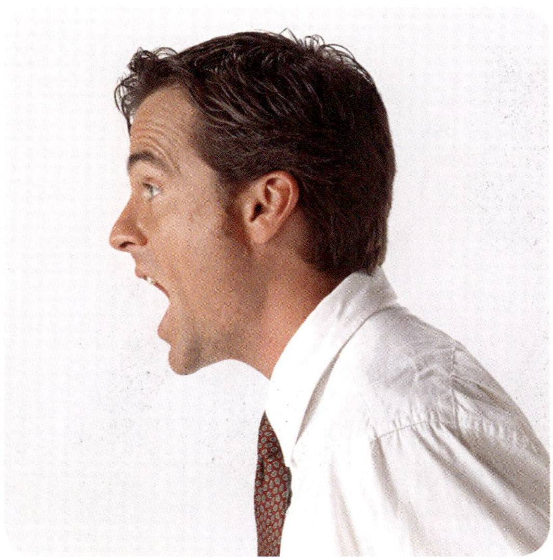

➡ Dysfunction of spleen to transport and transform due to excessive contemplation

Emotional disturbances like overthinking, anxiety, and nervousness cause the stagnation of spleen qi, so does long-term stagnation of liver qi, both can make the spleen fail to transport and transform, thus affecting food digestion and body fluid circulation. It will lead to food accumulation and the retention of body fluid. The accumulative dampness inside the body will congeal into phlegm that will bring about depression named *tán yù* (phlegm depression). The dysfunctional spleen provides poor resource for the production of qi and blood, making the heart, the house of the spirit, lack nutrients and resulting in deficiency of both heart and spleen.

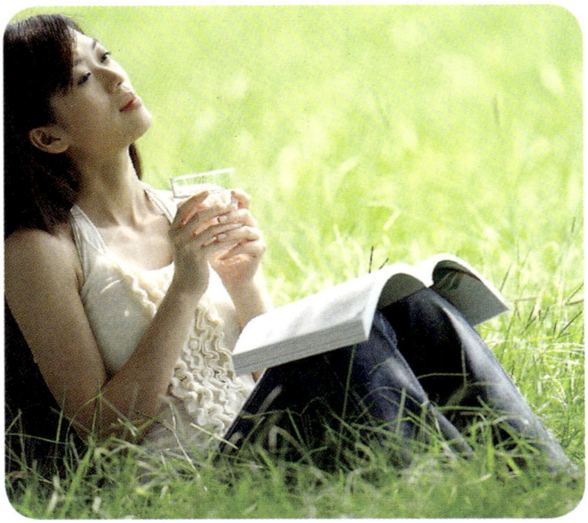

➡ Impairment of heart due to excessive emotional stimulation

Such strong emotional stimulation as stress caused by the the failure to realize one's dream, unhappy family life, or unfortunate events either sudden or long-term can impair the function of the heart to get nourishment, which in turn damages the spirit and leads to a series of pathological changes affecting other *zang* organs, since the heart is the monarch organ.

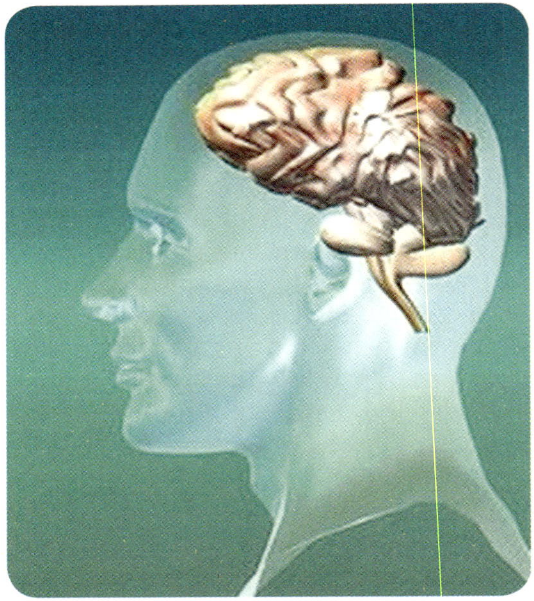

Yet, in spite of what is described above, there are some interesting new insights into the etiology and pathology of depression proposed by contemporary Chinese medicine doctors. Some researchers point out that yang and qi deficiency of the heart, gall bladder, and liver is the constitutional basis determining an individual's susceptibility to depression, since the heart is the house of spirit, the liver is the commander of strategy and planning, and the gallbladder is the governor of decision-making. When people with such a constitution experience unexpected emotional issues, he or she will develop malnourishment of the brain spirit, qi stagnation, and phlegm retention, and a dim state of mind; so the pathologies of depression are yang deficiency of the heart and gall bladder, malnourishment of the brain spirit, liver deficiency with qi stagnation, and phlegm retention binding spirit.[10] In light of the clinical manifestation of depression, some researchers state that it is caused by the seven emotional problems and mainly involved the liver, the emotional problems are the main reasons for liver stagnation.[11] Some researchers say that the information feedback axis of the brain-spirit, heart-spirit, five-*zang*-spirit, and emotion-activity is the mechanism for the occurrence of depression.[12] Other researchers hold that senile depression results from *zang-fu* degeneration, disharmony of qi and blood, as well as emotional stimulus, such organs as the heart, liver, and spleen are most frequently affected, and the primary pathology is the inordinate flow of qi and blood.[13]

There is no doubt that emotional factors are a major pathogenesis for depression, but the occurrence of depression not only depends on the intensity and time spent on emotional stimulation, but also relies on the health condition of the human body. As *Wondrous Lantern for Peering into the Origin and Development of Miscellaneous Diseases* (*Zá Bìng Yuán Liú Xī Zhú*, 杂病源流犀烛) states that, "all kinds of depression are attributed to weak and dysfunctional *zang* organs, excessive contemplation combining with weak *zang* organs lead to six kinds of depression, namely: qi, blood, dampness, heat, food, and phlegm depression," indicating the weak *zang* organs are endopathic causes for the onset of depression. Therefore, the healthy state of the body, adequate nutrition and harmony in all respects are prerequisites for the spirit to stay at peace. When inappropriate diet and physical exercise, extreme emotions, psychological trauma, and diseases pose negative influences on the body, the spirit does not have a comfortable and peaceful place to rest. Consequently, we should address the underlying causes of the depression and meanwhile calm the disturbed spirit so as to make the patient happier and more at peace.

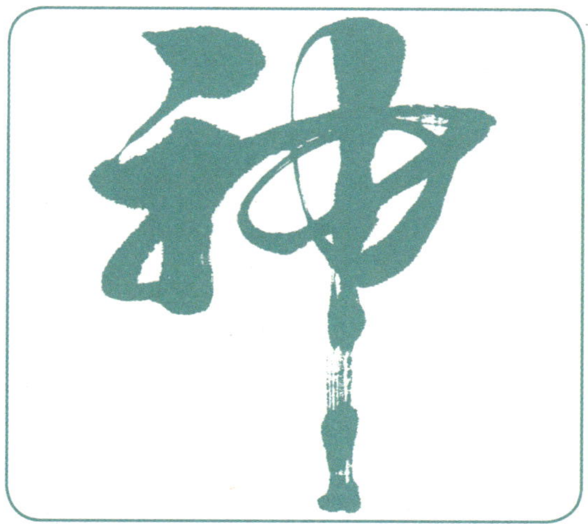

Pattern Differentiation

Chinese medical treatment gives priority to treatment based on pattern differentiation (*Biàn Zhèng Lùn Zhì*, 辨证论

治), which is an essential principle, a specific diagnosis and treatment method, and one of the basic features of time-honored Chinese medicine. Pattern differentiation is the prerequisite and basis for choosing treatment, while the treatment, as the process to fight disease, is to test whether the previous differentiation is right or not, they are interrelated, indispensable and inseparable during the process of diagnosing and treating disease and reflect the integration of theory and practice. Pattern differentiation means to analyze, induce, synthesize, differentiate, and summarize the clinical data of symptoms, signs, the tongue appearance, and the types of pulses collected through the four diagnostic methods and categorized into certain patterns. Then accordingly, appropriate therapeutic principles and approaches are decided. This is the way that Chinese medicine categorizes, understands, and treats all types of illnesses. It is a highly individualized principle and is always integrated with the disease diagnosis.

So what is a pattern (*zhèng*, 证)?

A pattern, similar to the concept of syndrome, is a group of interrelated signs and symptoms that together reveal the fundamental characteristics of a patient's condition. It should be noted that pattern is a summary of the pathological changes of a disease at a certain stage in its course of development, including the cause, location, and nature of a disease, as well as the mutual conflict between pathogenic factors and healthy qi. Chinese medicine believes that manifestations (signs and symptoms) mirror the performance of internal organs. So a pattern is the reflection of an underlying pathomechanism, often called the root of the disease. Over thousands of years, Chinese medicine has accumulated a large amount of experience in summarizing and categorizing these patterns in the most innovative ways. It now uses them as the guidelines in prescribing treatment. Disease diagnosis and pattern diagnosis go together and guide the practitioner to the proper treatment. There is a saying in Chinese medicine, "Different diseases, same treatment; same disease, different treatment." This saying underscores the importance of individualized pattern diagnosis in Chinese medicine.

During the process of diagnosing a patient's condition, four basic diagnostic techniques: inspection, auscultation and olfaction, inquiry, and pulse taking and palpation will provide useful and sufficient information. In addition to the patient's complaints, the practitioner will ask detailed questions that will offer clues to the nature of their imbalances. Such issues as occupation, quality of sleep, dreams, appetite, preferred foods, possible stress, even the temperature of the air conditioner will be asked. Concerning pulse taking, the Chinese medicine physician feels superficially, moderately, and deeply along the radial artery at specific points which correspond to the specific internal organs. For instance, pulses on the left wrist correspond from top to bottom (distal to proximal) to the heart, liver, and kidney. Generally, the quality of the pulse is evaluated in terms of frequency, rhythm, speed, and volume. With a time-honored history, Chinese medicine has developed an elaborate vocabulary to define a pulse, such as floating, wiry, hollow, thready, and slippery. Additionally, the tongue is also a mirror of human health and Chinese medicine has an elaborate system to note the condition of the tongue with respect to the color, texture, shape, size, and coating. For instance, a red tongue indicates excessive internal heat in many cases, and a white tongue reflects qi and blood deficiency. More specifically, each part of the tongue corresponds to a certain *zang-fu* organ. The middle of the tongue, for example, represents the spleen and stomach organs.

The patterns described below are some of the most typically encountered for patients with depression.[14]

Common Patterns in Depression

Patterns	Signs and Symptoms	Tongue	Pulse
Liver Qi Stagnation	-Depression -Restlessness -Chest stuffiness -Distention and unfixed pain in hypochondria -Epigastrium stuffiness and belching -Frequently sighing -Poor appetite -Irregular menstruation	Thin and greasy tongue coating	Wiry pulses
Fire due to Prolonged Liver Qi Stagnation	-Rashness -Bad temper -Distension and fullness in chest and hypochondria -Gastric upset and acid regurgitation -Bitter and dry mouth -Constipation -Headache with hot sensation -Tinnitus -Red and painful eyes	Red tongue with yellow coating	Wiry and fast pulses
Qi and Phlegm Stagnation	-Depression -Chest stuffiness -The sensation of a foreign body in the throat which can be neither swallowed nor expectorated	White and greasy tongue coating	Wiry and slippery pulses

Patterns	Signs and Symptoms	Tongue	Pulse
Long-term Stagnation Impairing Spirit	-Absent-minded -Vexation -Frequent sighing -Palpitation -Insomnia	Thin and white tongue coating	Wiry and thin pulses
Deficiency of Spleen and Heart	-Over-thinking -Over-suspicious -Vertigo and dizziness -Palpitation -Timidity -Lusterless complexion -Fatigue -Poor appetite -Insomnia -Forgetfulness	-Pale tongue -Thin and white tongue coating	Thin and weak pulses
Fire Caused by Yin Deficiency	-Restlessness -Hypochondriac pain -Dry mouth and throat -Vertigo -Palpitation -Vexation -Insomnia -Forgetfulness -Waist soreness -Spermatorrhea -Irregular menstruation	Red tongue with little coating	-Wiry, thin and fast pulses
Heart yin deficiency	-Restlessness -Palpitation -Forgetfulness -Insomnia -Dreaminess -Burning sensation in the chest, palms, and soles -Night sweats -Dry mouth and throat	Red tongue with little fluid	Thin and fast pulses

These are only some of the most frequently seen patterns. Usually, any pattern will not be as simple and straightforward as those listed above, and will usually have multiple facets. Furthermore, the patterns related to depression may be mixed with other underlying conditions and diseases. In the clinic, patients will often present other patterns or a combination of the above patterns. The point of this division is to highlight the major symptoms and the reason for them. The treatment will be different for each pattern and each patient. Practitioners will decide how to vary treatment according to the diversity and severity of the symptoms.

General Treatment Principles

Basically, the primary therapeutic principle for depression is to soothe the liver, regulate qi, and relieve depression. The *Treatise on Medical Formulas (Yī Fāng Lùn,* 医方论) states, "The disordered qi is the root cause for depression. If qi and circulation are back to normal, there is no cradle for the depression." Usually from the perspective of Chinese medicine, at first your practitioner will determine whether the nature of the pattern is deficient or excessive, then they will decide which specific therapeutic methods should be involved under the guidance of the primary therapeutic principle. For excessive pattern, which lead to vicious cycles, specific treatment methods may include, for example, promoting blood circulation, eliminating fire, removing phlegm, relieving dampness, and promoting digestion since problems such as formation of blood stagnation, fire, dampness, phlegm, and food retention may result from or exist along with the qi stagnation. It is worthy to note that there should be no consumption of qi when regulating qi, no exhaustion of blood when promoting qi circulation, no impairment of stomach qi when eliminating heat, and no wasting of healthy qi when removing phlegm. For deficient patterns, treatment may focus on nourishing the heart and calming the spirit, or tonifying the spleen and heart, or strengthening the liver and kidney based on the specific organs being involved and the condition of qi, blood, yin, and yang. Please remember, do not use too many medicinals that are dry in nature when nourishing the heart and spleen and do not use too many medicinals greasy in nature when tonifying the liver and kidney. Concerning the complex pattern of deficiency and excess, equal attention should be paid to the two aspects and top priority should be given to the predominant aspect. Some patients notice some improvement almost immediately after receiving Chinese medicine treatment. In addition to medical treatment, psychotherapy is of great importance. Removing the emotional stimulus helps patients understand and deal with their disease properly, and increasing their confidence in fighting depression is conducive to their recovery from the disease.

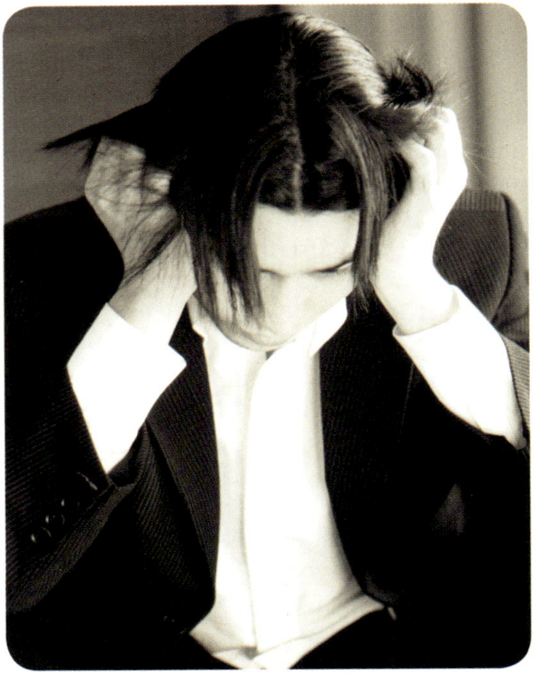

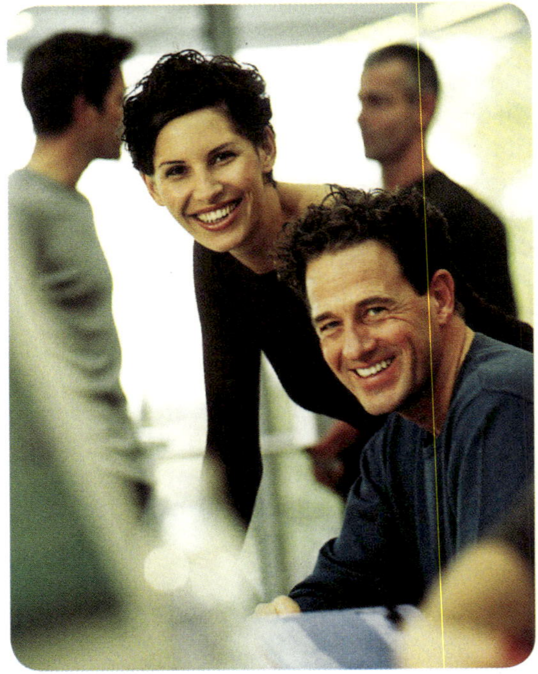

With treatment based on correct pattern differentiation, emotional regulation, psychological counseling, and attention to lifestyle habits, depression can be reduced and the progression of other diseases can be slowed or even stopped. Pattern identification and evaluation of treatments become more precise with the use of lab tests and the ability to track levels of various bodily substances. Whether you are depressed or are under overwhelming life changes, Chinese medicine as one of the oldest medical systems that acknowledge the holism of mind-body-spirit, employs a variety of approaches to help you return to balance both physically and psychologically. The names of acupoints embody mind-body connections, such as spirit's door (H 7), soul's door (UB 42) and will's residence (UB 44),[15] as they are approaches to mental and emotional illness. It is reported that acupuncture can markedly ease depression and that stimulation of specific acupoints can positively influence neurotransmitter production in the brain. It has also been shown that acupuncture enhances the positive effects of anti-depressant medications.[16] Treatment of depression with Chinese medicine has been developing over thousands of years. Its methods and theories are not fixed or stagnant and will continue to develop over time.

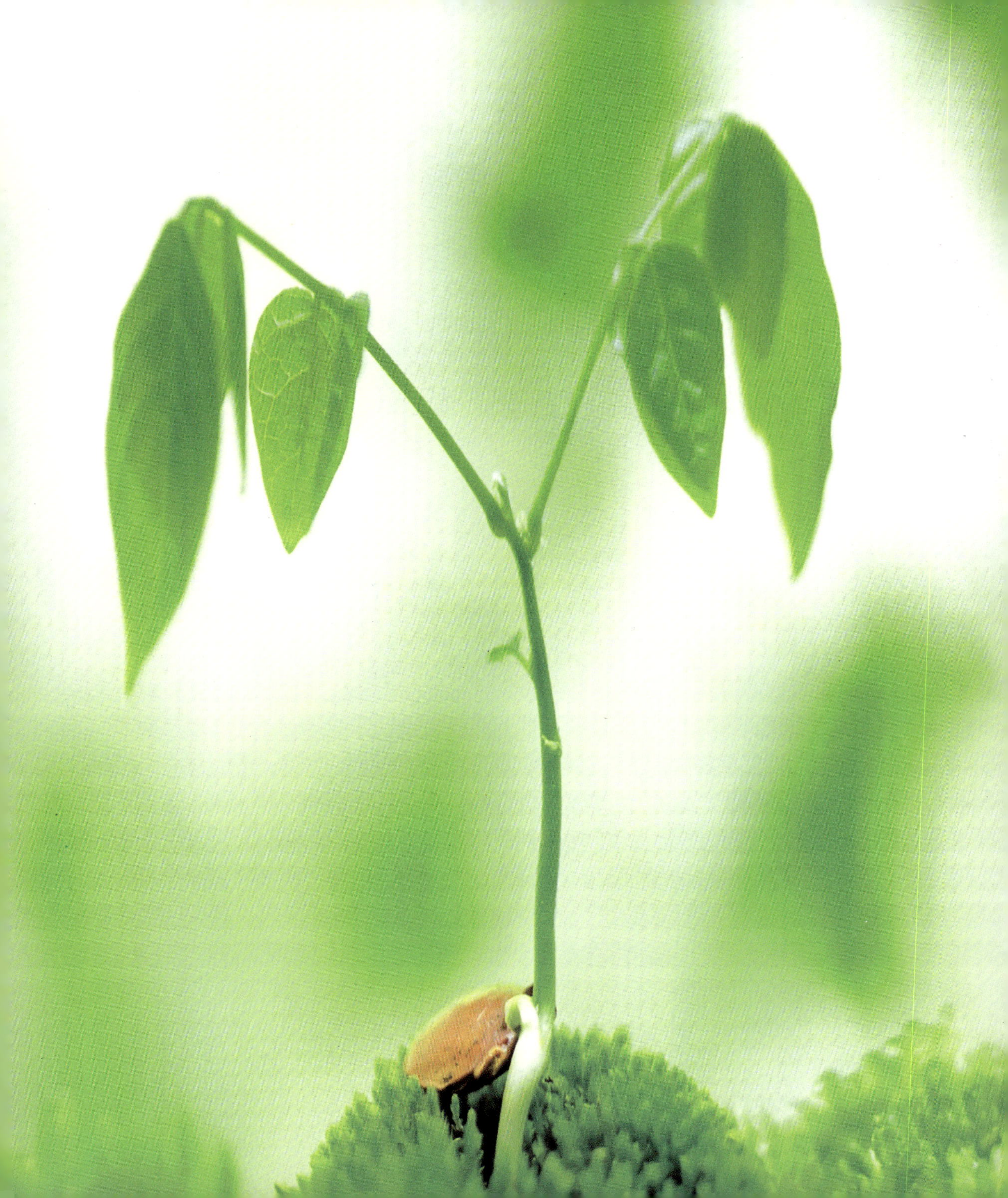

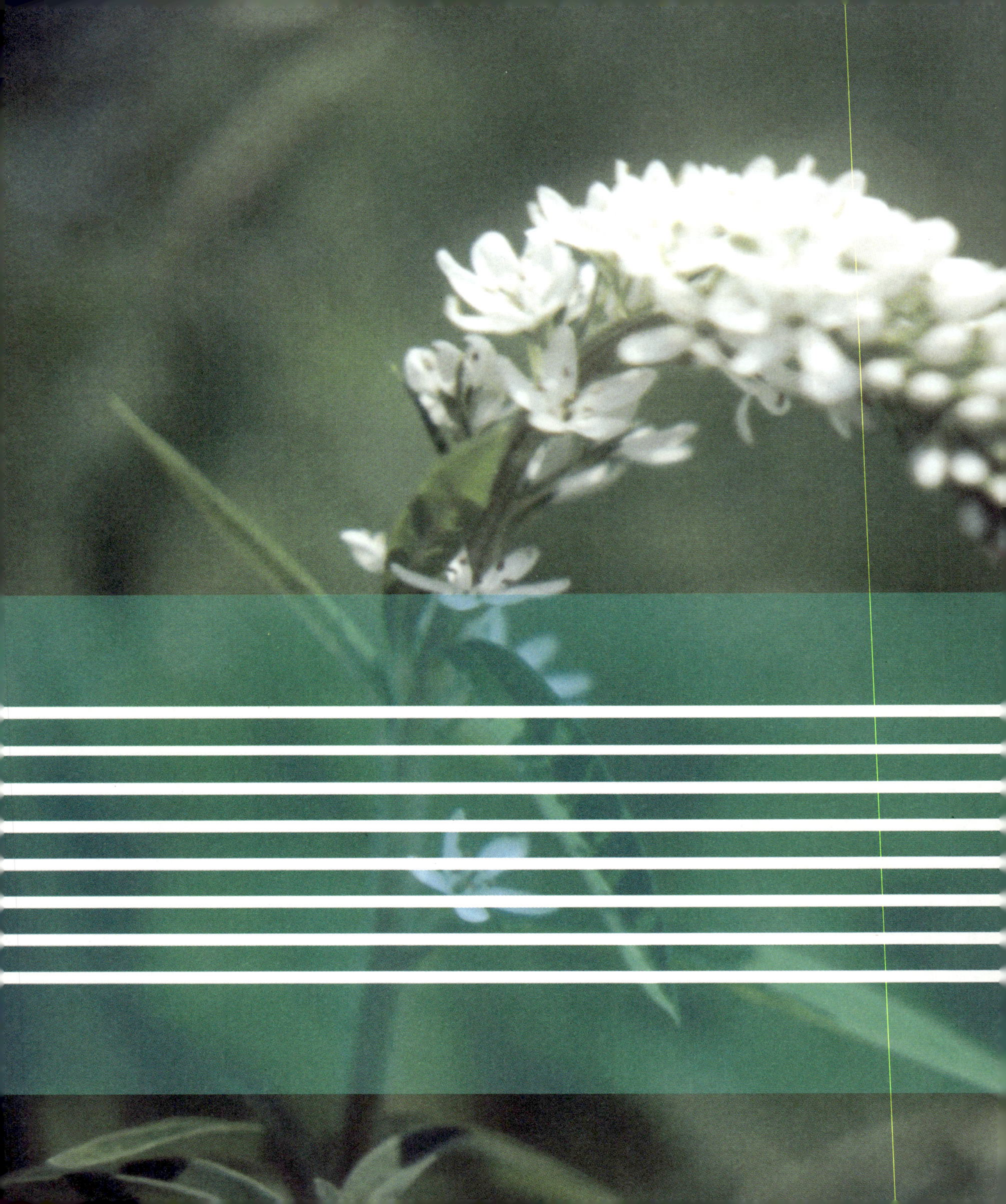

Chapter 3

How Can Depression Be Prevented?

Depression is the "quiet epidemic," people with depression are liable to be uncertain, less productive, excessively pessimistic and without hope, unable to concentrate on work, less interested in family affairs, unable to express love, or enjoy social gatherings. Being depressed increases the possibility of becoming disabled or killed as a result of suicide. The more severe the depression is, the greater the disability or the desirability of killing oneself is. Furthermore, depression not only hurts the depressed person, but also his family, friends, and communities. Another alarming truth is that currently more and more people are suffering and dying from the effects of depression than ever before. Therefore the problem of treating and more importantly preventing depression has become a social problem, not just an individual concern.

As previously explained, all natural phenomena have yin and yang aspects, and there is constant interaction between the human body and the natural environment. Health is believed to rely on the balance of these forces. That balance is easily affected by the food you eat, your lifestyle choices, the amount of exercise and rest you get, and how you manage your emotions. Your genetic predisposition also plays a role. If you tend towards spleen deficiency, you can strengthen your spleen by eating foods that support digestion and boost qi or by doing exercises that boost qi and preserve essence.

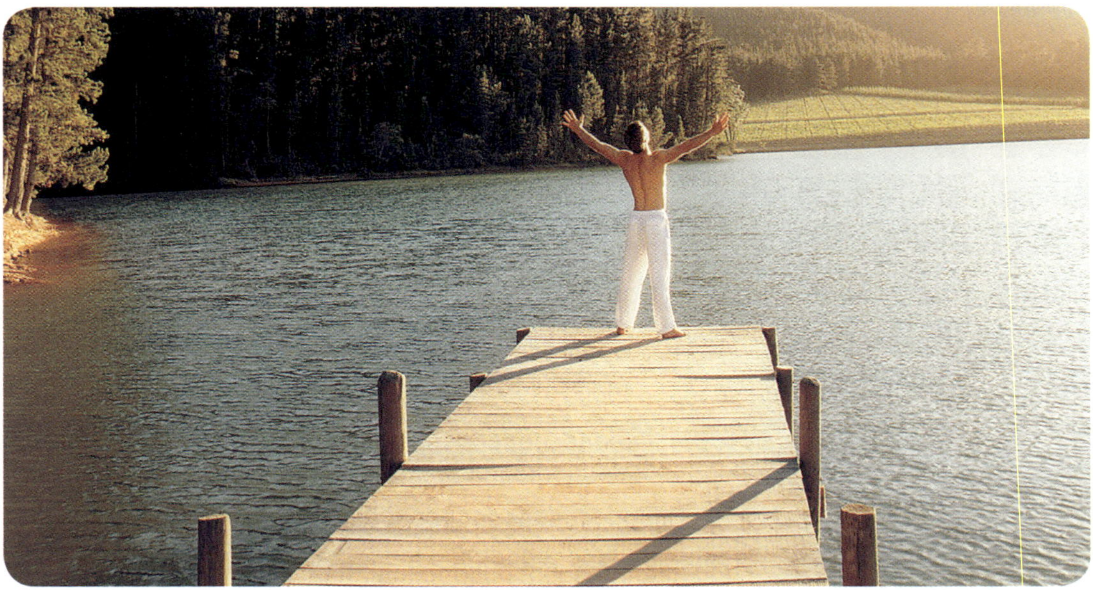

The maintenance of psychological health is important but beyond the scope of this book. Chinese medicine stresses the importance of a peaceful mind for the prevention of disease, since the body and mind are inseparable, and physical health and mental health mutually affect each other. Emotional extremes tax the *zang-fu* organs and lead to the formation of heat or fire which damage yin or exhaust qi. We all have our own experience on what we eat and how much exercise affects our moods, so sticking to a balanced diet and getting regular exercise will go a long way to maintaining a calm mind. Chinese medicine directly acts on the *zang-fu* organs to erase hypo or hyper states, and thereby restore equilibrium to the mind.

Just like any other disease, depression is due to an imbalance of yin and yang. So how can one maintain a balance of yin and yang in daily life?

The answer is through health preservation. It is a concept in Chinese medicine regarding how to enhance human physical fitness, how to prevent diseases, how to postpone aging and how to prolong human life by a variety of methods. *The Yellow Emperor's Inner Classic* says, "The sages in ancient times who knew the *dào* (the tenet for preserving health, 道) followed the rules of yin-yang and adjusted *shù shǔ* (the ways to preserve health, 术数). They were moderate in eating and drinking, regular in working and resting,

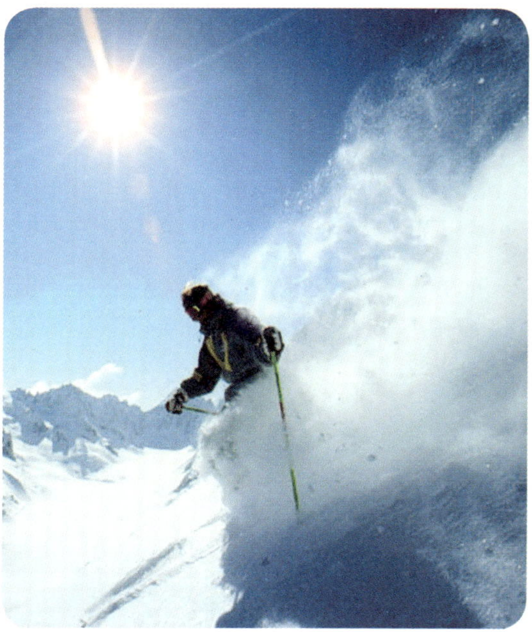

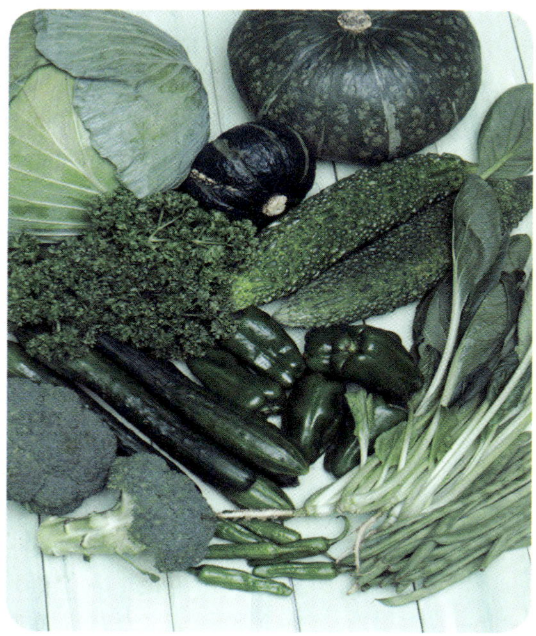

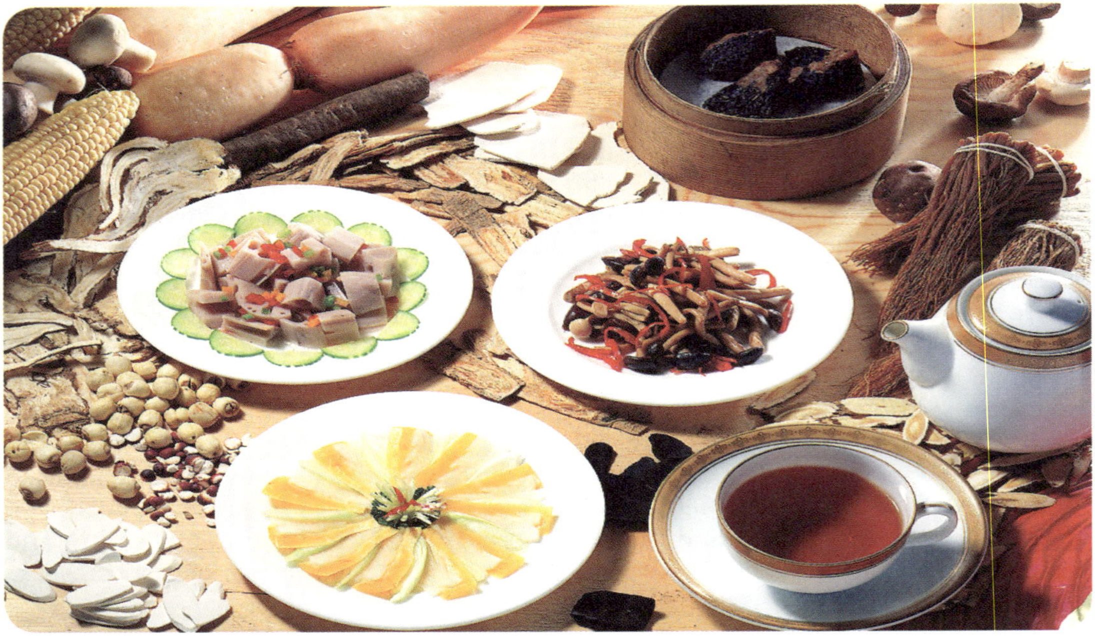

and avoided any overstrain. That is why they could maintain a desirable harmony between the spirit and the body, enjoying good health and a longer life." That is to say if we can take care of ourselves better, it is possible for us to enjoy 100 years of health and happiness.

Health preservation in Chinese medicine holds that people should understand the basic law of nature - live with nature and abide by yin-yang in the four seasons – namely: germination in spring, growth in summer, harvest in autumn, and storage in winter. It is advisable for different individuals from different regions in different seasons to choose different ways to maintain their health. Chinese medicine has specific principles guiding the practice of preserving health, such as co-improvement of body and spirit, coordination of yin and yang, abidance by nature, regulation of diet, formation of good daily life habits, harmony of *zang-fu* organs, free circulation of channels and collaterals, restoration of essence through controlling sexual activity, regulation of qi and breath, and a moderate range of exercise, and rest. For depression, a variety of methods are available and popular with people in need, such as health preservation of *zang-fu* organs, dietary and exercise approach to health preservation, health preservation through changing daily life habits, as well as health preservation with Chinese medicinals.[15]

Nourishing the Heart - An Organ of Monarch

The heart is located in the chest between the two lobes of the lungs, occupying the highest place among the five *zang* organs and governing the life activities of the whole body. This is why the heart is called "an organ of monarch" in *The Yellow Emperor's Inner Classic*.

The "heart governing blood" means that the heart propels blood to circulate in the vessels and that the heart is related to the production of blood. Only when heart qi is sufficient can a normal heartbeat be maintained and can blood circulate within the vessels normally and constantly to nourish every single part of the body thus maintaining the normal physiological function of all *zang-fu* organ systems with the manifestation of full vitality, lustrous and bright complexion, as well as moderate and forceful pulses, etc. Moreover, the normal circulation of blood fully depends upon the sufficient heart qi and blood and unobstructed vessels.

Heart controlling spirit is also known as heart storing spirit. The normal function of the heart to control the spirit relies on the nourishment and moistening functions of heart blood and heart yin, which are essentially the substantial basis for the spirit. Heart qi and heart yang work together to cheer heart spirit up, which also plays an important role. If the heart's function of controlling the spirit is normal, people will be full of vigor, clear in mind, mentally agile, and quick in response. If not, it will inevitably result in symptoms such as insomnia, dreaminess, listlessness, even coma, delirium, and unconsciousness. It is worth pointing out that Chinese medicine, centered on five *zang* organs, attributes the motivation of the spirit to the heart, and the concept of the heart in Chinese medicine actually includes certain functions of the brain.

Specifically, for people with depression, it is essential to nourish the heart in terms of yin, yang, qi, and blood. By doing so, the material basis of the heart spirit can be restored, then the place for the spirit to stay can regain its peace and eventually the patient can recover from the disease.

Calm Spirit and Regulate Breath; Aerobic Exercise and Tonify Heart

One method to calm spirit and regulate breath: sit up straight, square your shoulders and pull your belly in, adduct your lower jaw, put your right hand on the heart area, close your eyes, and quiet your spirit. Regulate your breathing gradually, make your breath slow and deep, then use your right hand to rub the heart area moderately and clockwise in line with the rate of respiration. One single breath comprises one inhalation and one exhalation, rub one circle with a single breath, do it 36 times. This plays a role in activating the circulation of qi and blood and providing nutrition to the heart.[17]

Do aerobic exercises to tonify heart methods: People, no matter with or without depression, should do some aerobic exercises according to their own physical condition on a daily basis. Sports such as walking, jogging, tai ji, and swimming are beneficial for maintaining a healthy cardiovascular system and enhancing cardiac function when done moderately. Nothing should be overdone.

Another method to tranquilizing the mind: close the eyes, breathe calmly and naturally, and relax the whole body. When inhaling, the tongue touches the upper palate; when exhaling, make a sound like "ke" (pronounced like the word "cup" without the final "p" ending) and the tongue leaves the upper palate with the air flow. Keep your breath deep, long, and moderate. Practice ten breath cycles (ten inhales and exhales). This is for tranquilizing the mind and relieving mental disturbance.[18]

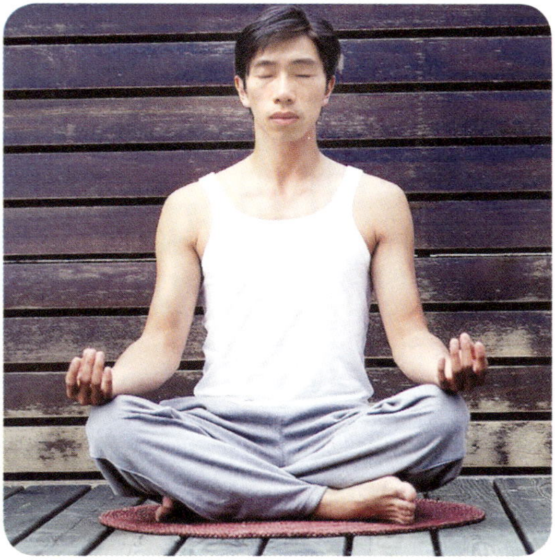

Acupoints Protecting the Heart

➡ Press PC 6 (*nèi guān*, 内关): PC 6 is located on the inside of your forearm, at two *cun* above the transverse crease of the wrist and between the tendons of palmaris longus muscle and flexor radialis muscle. This translates to about two finger-widths (widest point) proximal to the wrist crease on the palm surface of your forearm. Sit up straight, press and knead PC 6 on your left arm hard 30 times, then do the same thing for your right PC 6.

➡ Press PC 4 (*xì mén*, 郄门): PC 4 is located on the inside of your forearm, at five *cun* above the transverse crease of the wrist and between the tendons of palmaris longus muscle and flexor radialis muscle. This translates to about five finger-widths (widest point) proximal to the wrist crease on the palm surface of your forearm. Press and knead PC 4 on your left arm hard 30 times, then do the same thing to your right PC 4.

➡ Knead heart area: Place your left hand over your heart area, use your right hand to press the left hand, massage the heart area in a clockwise manner 30 times, then do it in a counterclockwise manner 30 times. It can free the circulation of qi and blood, nourish the heart and strengthen the cardiac function.

Heart-healthy Diet

The basic principle is taking more light and bland food, minimizing the intake of less nutritious foods such as sweets and fatty foods. Smoking and alcohol are prohibited, so are fatty and greasy foods or overeating. these medicinals should be available in any Chinatown at a Chinese pharmacy.

➡ *Bǎi zǐ rén* tea (柏子仁, Semen Platycladi oriental arborvitael, arborvitae seed): Fry and mash 10 g arborvitae seeds, then soak it in boiled water for five minutes and add a proper amount of sugar. It has tonifying heart, calming spirit, and moistening large intestine to relieve constipation functions; it is applicable for middle-aged and elderly patients with heart qi deficiency pattern, palpitation, insomnia, and constipation.

➡ *Lóng yǎn ròu* (龙眼肉, Arillus Longan, longan, flesh of the longan fruit) porridge: Cook 15 g flesh of the longan fruit, seven pieces of jujube, and 100 g rice into porridge. It has nourishing the heart, tranquilizing spirit, strengthening spleen, and enriching blood functions, it is the right one for palpitation, panic, insomnia, poor memory, anemia, etc. caused by deficiency pattern of heart blood.

➡ *Fú xiǎo mài* (浮小麦, Fructus Tritici Levis, blighted wheat) porridge: Cook 30 g blighted wheat, 100 g of rice, and ten pieces of jujube into a porridge. It can nourish heart spirit, tonify the spleen and stomach, relieve spontaneous sweating, and its indications include palpitation, insomnia, etc. due to heart qi deficiency.

➡ *Suān zǎo rén* (酸枣仁, Semen Ziziphi Spinosae, spiney date seed) porridge: Grind 10 g spiney date seed into tiny pieces and cook it with 100 g rice into porridge. It has nourishing yin, tranquilizing heart spirit, tonifying liver, and soothing spirit functions, so it is applicable for restlessness, insomnia, palpitation, and spontaneous sweating resulting from the blood deficiency pattern of heart and liver.

➡ Royal jelly: Mix 200 mg royal jelly in cooled boiled water for drinking. It has nourishing the heart, improving spleen, and strengthening the body functions, and it can be used for a deficiency pattern of heart and spleen with manifestations of panic, shortness of breath, insufficiency of spirit, fatigue, insomnia, poor memory, weakness, etc.

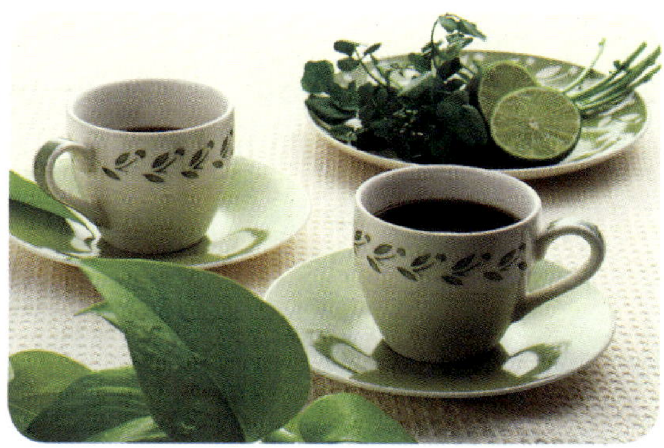

Diet

Let food be your medicine and medicine be your food.
-Hippocrates

The concept that food is medicine is also deeply rooted in the Chinese culture, which, as stated in *The Yellow Emperor's Inner Classic*: "The five grains are essential, the five fruits are beneficial, the five meats are helpful, and the five vegetables are supplemental", encourages people to eat a balanced diet. The reasons for depression are as numerous as there are differences in personality, but there is one thing we know for sure: nutrient deficiencies can alter brain function which lead to and tend to exacerbate depression. Besides this, certain vitamin or mineral deficiencies play a very important part in depression, such as deficiencies in zinc, vitamin C, folic acid, vitamin B-12, and vitamin B-6.

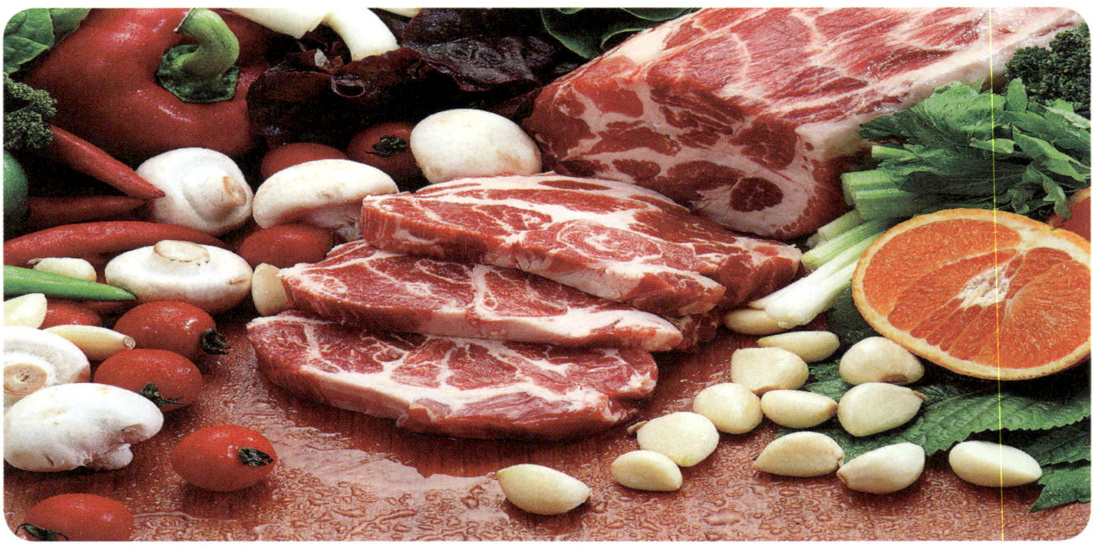

The *Records of Health Cultivation* (*Yǎng Shēng Lù*, 养生录) proposes six favorable means for keeping healthy through dietary changes: eat dinner earlier, eat food warm, do not overeat, eat bland food, eat slowly, and take soft food. Lu You (1,125 - 1,210), the famous poet of the Southern Song Dynasty (1,127-1,279), was enthused about taking bland, warm, and soft porridge. And you can tell from his poem: "Each of us yearns for longevity with good health and vitality, but just a few of us are aware of the method for obtaining longevity in our daily life; thanks to the *Porridge Book* of Zhang Lei (张耒), I take porridge on a daily basis, which in turn makes me happy and healthy like a fairy."

1. Chinese Dietary Theory Essentials

Maintaining health, strengthening the body, preventing disease, and treating the patient through dietary therapy is central to the philosophy and practice of Chinese medicine. A Chinese medicated diet is not a simple combination of food and Chinese medicine, but a specially designed dish that is prepared under the guidance of Chinese diet theory based on syndrome differentiation. It assesses foods in terms of not only nutritional components, but also its color, taste, texture, and shape. Foods with different tastes have different func-

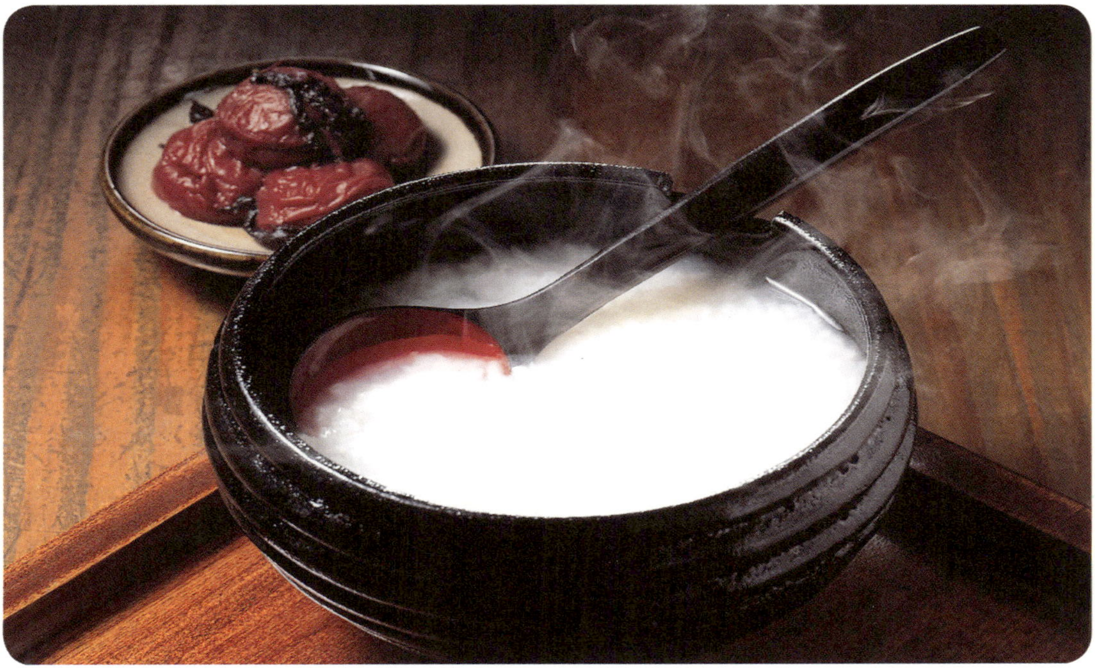

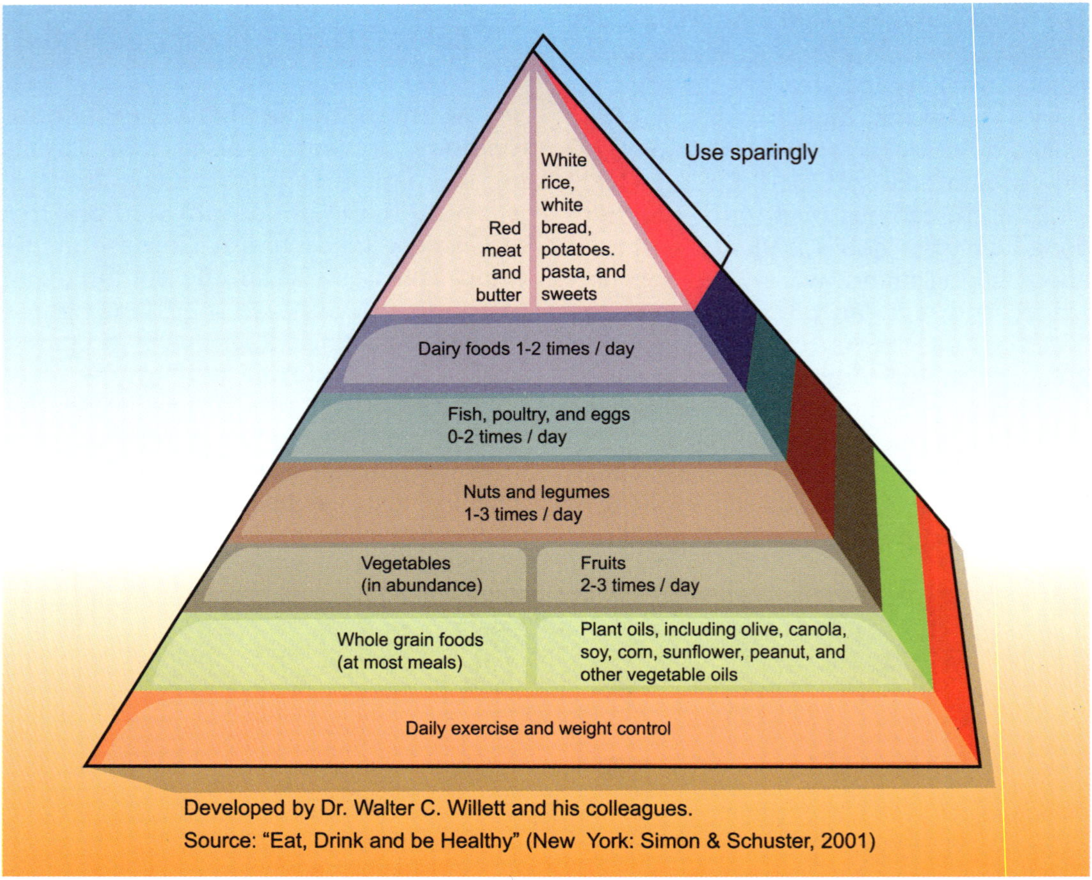

Alternative Food Pyramid

tions. For instance, spicy food is applied to disperse, sour to restrain, sweet to strengthen and moderate, bitter to purge and dry, and salty to soften and relax. According to the theory of five-phase, foods with specific colors, tastes, and shapes can fortify specific parts of the body and correct specific imbalances.

Dietary therapy is essential to the treatment of depression according to both Chinese medicine and biomedicine. Because of the vital part that nutrition plays in our overall health, Chinese medicine holds that food is the best medicine. The things we eat are natural substances that have their own unique qi (properties) just like Chinese medicinals. The properties of Chinese medicinals are used to correct any imbalance of qi, blood, yin, or yang. The properties of food can be used in a similar way. As much as possible, it is better to use food as medicine rather than taking any kind of medication, be it Chinese medicinals or pharmaceuticals. Eating is the most convenient, economic, and delicious prescription a doctor can give. Generally speaking, the Chinese percept to diet is to optimize digestion, increase qi and blood, and improve the *zang-fu* organ function. In this sense, it can be regarded as an extension of Chinese medicinals.

Each food item has its own properties and is selected based on the patient's pattern to treat disease or preserve health. Biomedical nutritional therapy separates food by content: carbohydrates, protein, fat, vitamins, etc. Chinese medicine concentrates on the qualities of each food item by dividing foods into the categories of taste and temperature. As an example, biomedicine would put most grains in the same category due to their high carbohydrate content. Chinese medicine, while also recognizing familiar food categories like grains, meat, vegetables, etc., also divides grains into different categories based on their temperature and taste.

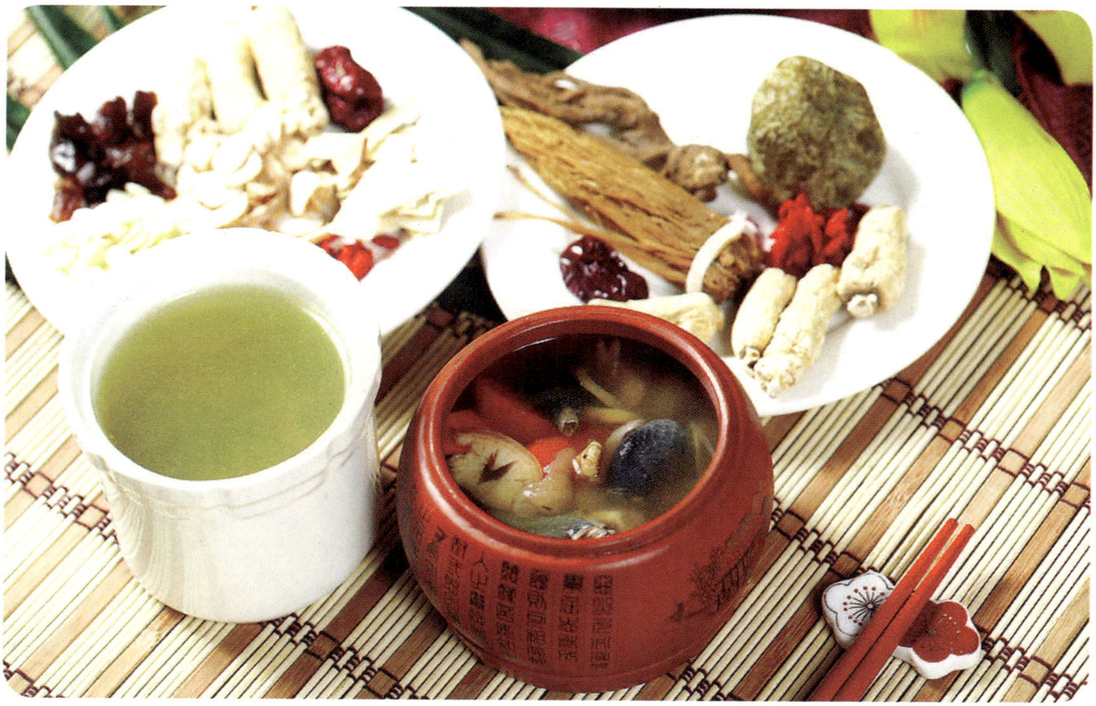

Foods are defined as yin and yang, warming and cooling, drying and moistening. Certain foods are better for some people than others. Looking at food from the Chinese perspective, beef, onions, and walnuts are all considered warm. Biomedicine on the other hand, would find little in common with these three foods. With the combination of modern nutrition and Chinese dietary theory, food therapy can be very effective.

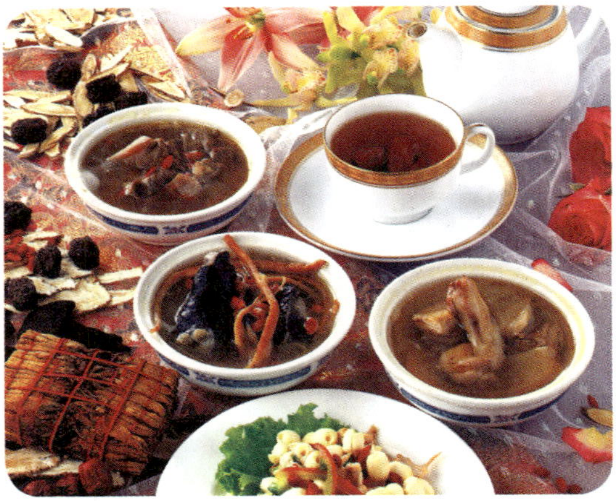

This classification of foods follows the same criteria used for medicinals and the application of food therapy follows the same diagnostic principles and procedures as well. Foods act on the internal organs and influence the qi of the body, which can be used to preserve health and treat disease. The main difference between food and medicinal substances is that food is generally milder. That's why food is taken daily and medicinals only when necessary.

Eating a balanced diet, in terms of Chinese medicine, is to balance the qi of the food. A diet too lopsided in one direction or the other for too long will eventually cause an imbalance of qi, blood, yin, and/or yang. Properly chosen, food can be used as medicine. Some Chinese medicinals can be used as food and added into your diet. Indeed, many common spices (cinnamon, cardamom, ginger, garlic) are commonly used in medicinal treatment. In Chinese medicine, the line between food and medicine is a blurry one. For those already suffering from disease, special foods are chosen based on the patient's individual condition. Dietary prescriptions in Chinese medicine are made according to individual pattern identification. Biomedicine calculates the calories, vitamins, fat content, etc. precisely. When combined, a very well-designed dietary regimen is possible.

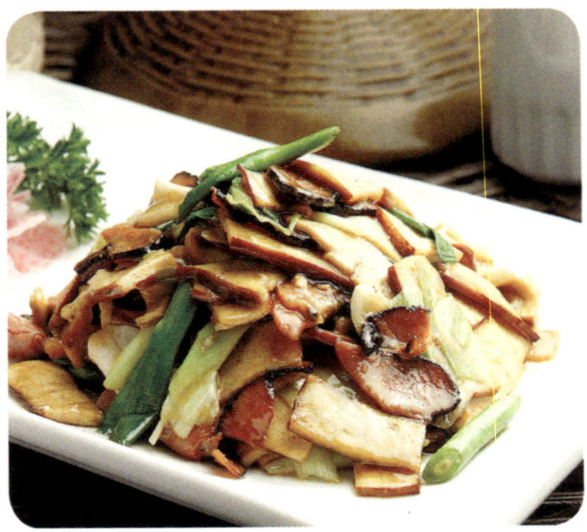

Two major dietary principles related to balancing yin and yang are the four properties of food and the five flavors of food. The former refers to the property of cold, cool, warm, and hot, and there is also a category neutral in property. Practically speaking, Chinese medicine categorizes food into three groups: cold / cool, neutral, and warm / hot. Hot foods like peppers and chicken have a warming effect on the body, strengthen yang, invigorate blood circulation, open stagnated meridians, and relieve cold; while cold foods like bittermelon and watermelon have a cooling effect on the body, clear heat and fire, cool blood, and eliminate toxins. Neutral foods don't have much influence on the body, and are an important part of maintaining a healthy balance. For example, rice is neutral and thus can be consumed daily, providing nourishment while not having a drastic effect on the body's function.

Different processing, cooking, and eating methods can change the properties of food. For example, Beijing roast duck, which is now considered one of China's national dishes, is cold in property in Chinese medicine, but its property is changed

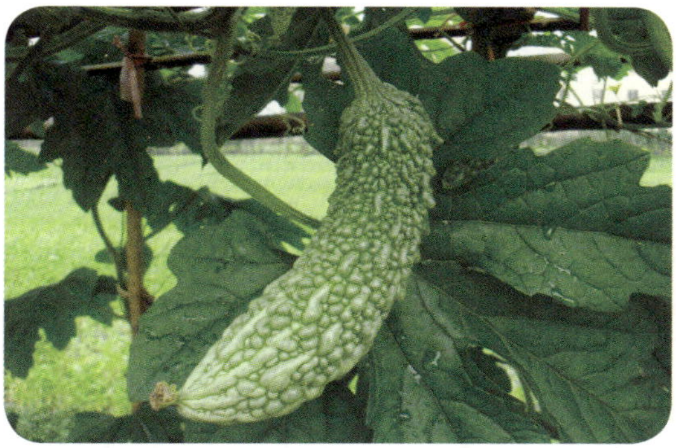

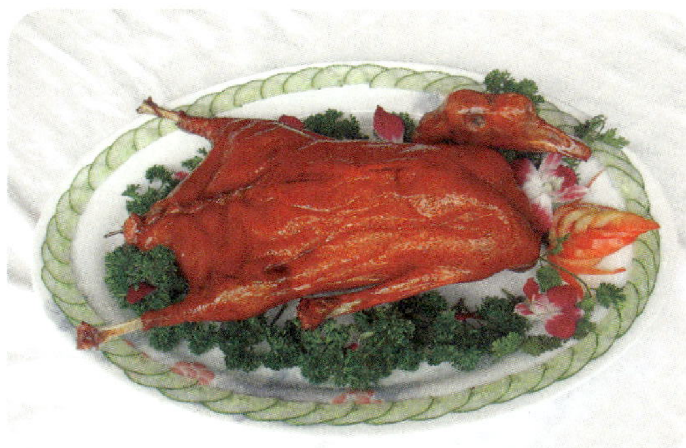

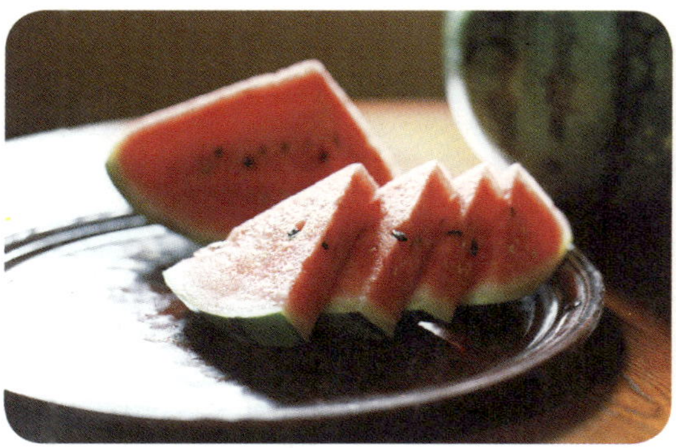

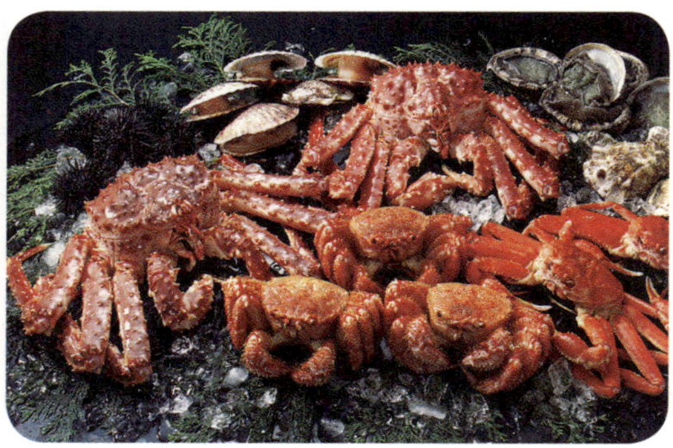

to neutral after being roasted in the oven, so that is why people can eat it anytime -- even in the coldest winter. Another case is eating crab with yellow wine, crab is cold in property, and yellow wine is hot in property, therefore eating them together changes their property to be healthy.

The following are some examples of common food items and their properties. A complete list of food properties is beyond the scope of this book. We hope that the list below will provide a good general outline, and help you make educated guesses about unlisted foods by comparing them to related items on the list.

Common Foods and Their Properties

Category	Hot	Warm	Neutral	Cool	Cold
Beverages	Alcohol	-Cocoa -Coffee -Wine -Black tea	Water	-Green tea -Fruit juices -Peppermint tea -Soy milk	Ice
Dairy		-Butter -Goat cheese	Cheese	Yogurt	Cow's milk
Fruit and vegetables		-Cherry -Fennel -Leek -Peach -Onion	-Carrot -Cauliflower -Grape -Fig -Plum -Potato	-Celery -Cucumber -Soy bean -Sprouts -Spinach -Zucchini	-Asparagus -Banana -Orange -Rhubarb -Seaweed -Tomato -Watermelon
Medicinals and spices	-Cinnamon -Chili -Curry -Garlic -Ginger -Paprika -Pepper	-Anise -Basil -Rosemary		Tarragon	-Dandelion -Yellow gentian

Adapted from p23, Joerg Kastner, *Chinese Nutrition Therapy*, Thieme, Stuttgart, New York, 2004

For depression patients, Chinese medicine physicians often ask the patients to keep a three-to-five-day dietary record, to evaluate the factors in the diet which can contribute to depression. If a person suffers from the cold-induced pattern, he/she will be strongly advised to take warming food instead of cold and raw food. Spleen yang deficiency, for instance, may present such symptoms as fatigue, poor appetite, abdominal distension, cold hands and feet, as well as watery diarrhea, indicating the function of spleen to transform and transport are obstructed by cold and dampness. In this case, warming the spleen and draining dampness are required, and the appropriate food should be warm in property and soft in texture, since the cold and raw foods will compel the spleen to deplete its diminishing reserves of energy during the process to warm and "cook" the food.

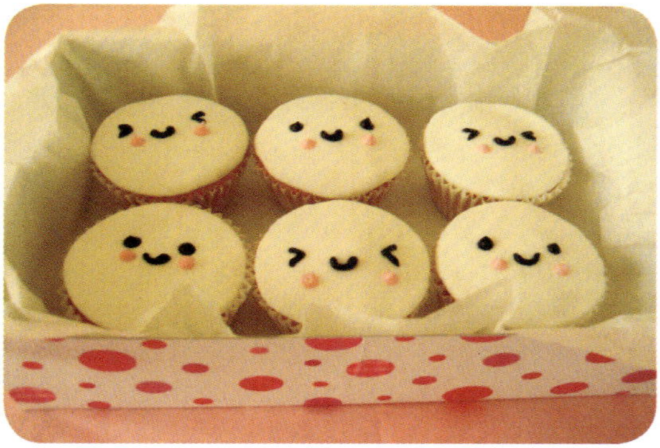

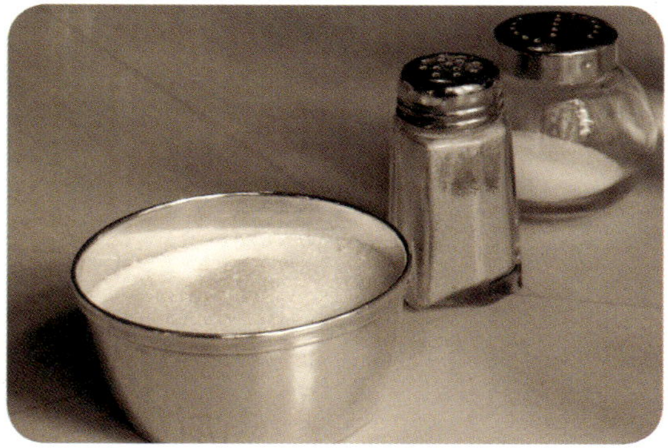

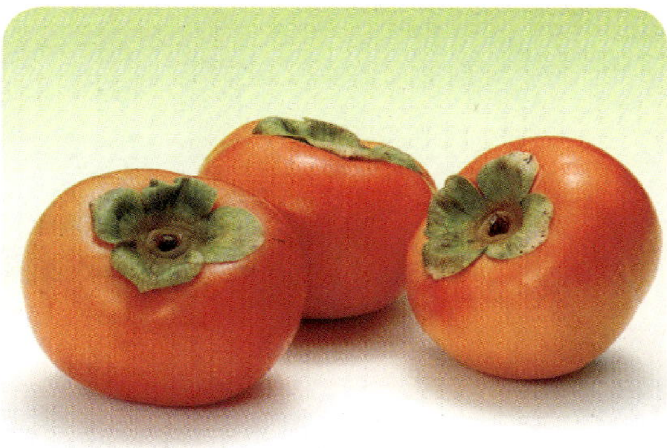

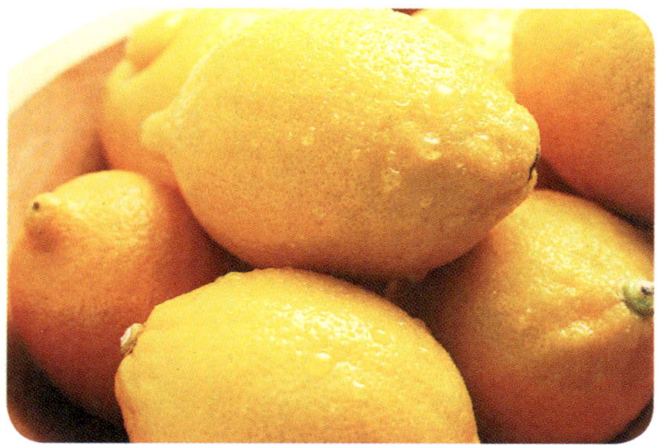

The five flavor theory refers to the flavors of sour, bitter, sweet, pungent, and salty. They are applied to foods in the same way as medicinals and they do not exist alone due to their specific corresponding relationship with certain organs and meridians according to the five-phase theory. More specifically, each taste has a different therapeutic effect. Sour-tasting foods constrain sweat, stop cough, and relieve diarrhea; bitter foods impel qi to flow downwards, dry dampness, expel toxicity, purge fire, and clear heat; sweet foods harmonize, tonify, and relieve pain and spasms; pungent foods disperse, move qi, and invigorate blood; salty foods soften masses, and nourish blood and yin. Additionally, there are two categories of "aromatic" foods and "plain tasting" foods.

Generally, flavor that we prefer reflects our physical needs. If you really crave a flavor badly, you can have some, since Chinese medicine holds that different food types can benefit different body organs. Nature gives people five climate factors, the earth provides people with five flavors, and humankind is raised by nature and earth. In addition, the five flavors have their corresponding internal organs, namely: sweet to spleen, sour to liver, acrid to lung, salty to kidney, and bitter to heart. Nevertheless, do not overeat one. Sometimes, a craving for a flavor helps you understand what is happening inside your body. Some pregnant women, for instance, crave sour food; that is because her blood surges to nourish the fetus that results in both liver yin and blood deficiency, and the sour flavor enters the liver, which is the depository of blood. So, food flavors are associated with the internal organs, and influence them just like medicinals do. The essence of Chinese dietary therapy is to choose proper food items and add certain medicinals to the diet that will help to restore the body's harmony. In many cases, foods and medicinals are mixed and cooked together for hours, thereby the nutritional value has been processed and the mixture is highly effective on various diseases.

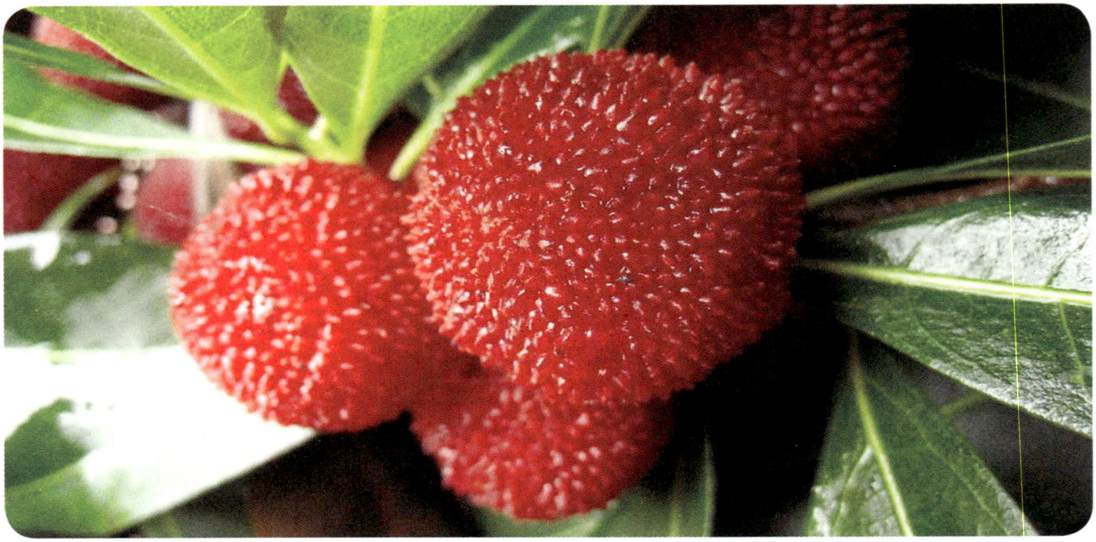

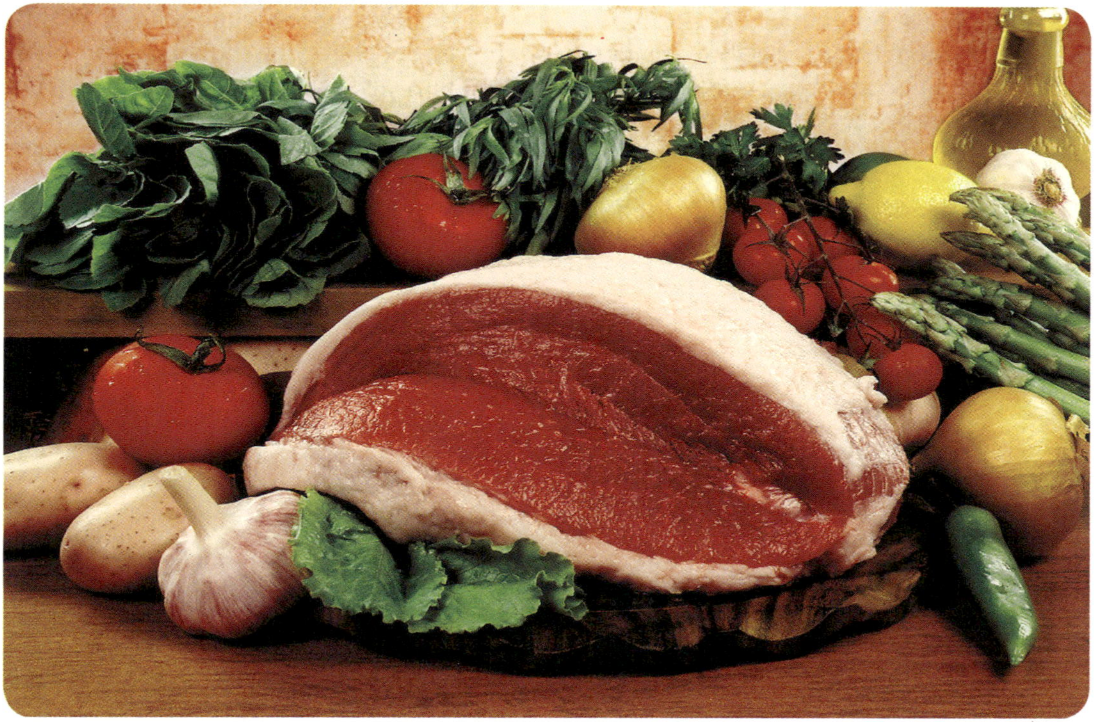

Besides this, Chinese medicine holds that seasonal food is better. China is a large agricultural nation that experiences pronounced seasonal changes. Taoism, one of the oldest Chinese cultural traditions, holds that the closer we stay to the rhythms and cycles of nature, the healthier we can be, so we should eat seasonal food. For instance, summer is hot in property, which consumes energy and body fluids, thus fruits and vegetables with cool property are most helpful. In addition, we should "cultivating yang in spring and summer and nourishing yin in autumn and winter." In Chinese medicine, spring is the period when yang qi ascends, which is marked by lengthening days. It is also known as *shaoyang*, indicating the yang qi at that time is less strong. Everything in nature is germinating, and yang qi in the body is also rising. According to the five-phase theory, spring corresponds to sour in the five flavors, blue in the five colors, and tendons and liver in the human body. In spring, yang qi should rise, the liver qi should regulate, vegetables and fruits blue in color and sour in taste should be consumed, and some moderate exercise should be done.

In Chinese medicine, regulating the diet means matching foods to a person's internal condition and the external environment. The following describes the different properties, flavors, and functions of some common foods that are highly recommended by Chinese medicine practitioners. They are common to the Western diet and because they are so helpful in helping manage depression, patients are strongly advised to find these wonderful foods and integrate them into their diets. Many of them can be found in Asian supermarkets or natural food stores. Some of them are available in concentrated form as pills or powders. In order to help you find them, we have tried to include various common names.

> Deep sea fish

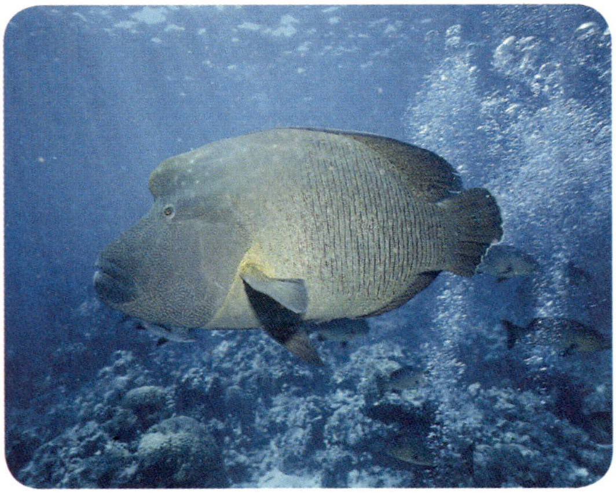

Property: cool
Flavor: salty
Function: strengthen the kidney and heart

Studies suggest that omega-3 fatty acids in deep sea fish functions the same as lithium carbonate, one of the most commonly-used antidepressants for helping calm nerves and promoting the secretion of serotonin.

> Chicken

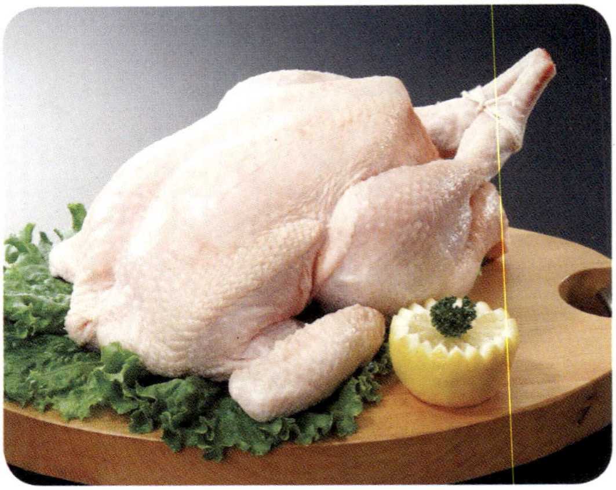

Property: warm
Flavor: sweet
Function: warm the digestive system, replenish qi and nourish blood, invigorate the kidney, and replenish essence and marrow

Chicken is rich in and is a major source of selenium. There is no evidence to support selenium as a treatment for depression, but a study in the United Kingdom found that when normal people were given selenium supplements, their mood improved.

> Banana

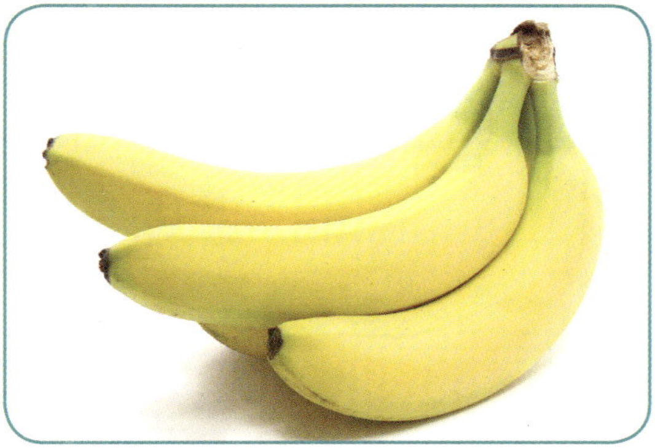

Property: cold
Flavor: sweet
Function: clear heat, moisten large intestine, and remove toxic material

Banana contains a natural chemical compound called alkaloid, which cheers people up and boosts their confidence. Moreover, banana is the best source of tryptophan and vitamin B6, which can help the brain manufacture serotonin thereby reducing depression.

> Grapefruit

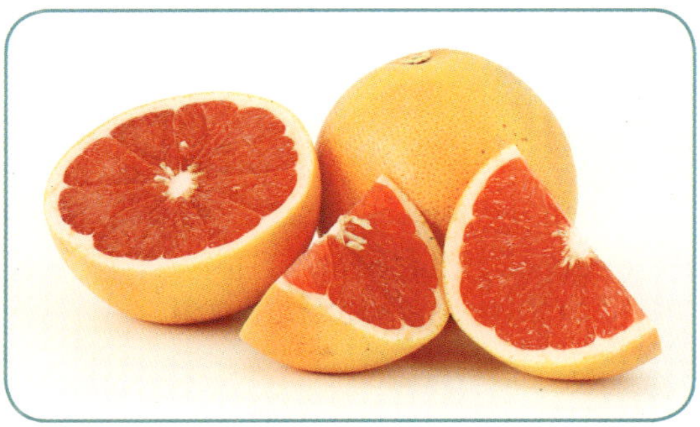

Property: slightly cold
Flavor: sweet
Function: strengthen qi and blood, fortify muscles and tendons, and induce urination

Grapefruit purifies complex thoughts and refreshes the mind. It is also rich in vitamin C, which helps maintain the density of red blood cells to improve physical resistance and is an excellent guard against stress. Moreover, vitamin C is one of the indispensable elements in making dopamine and adrenalin, both of which can stimulate excitement.

> Cherry

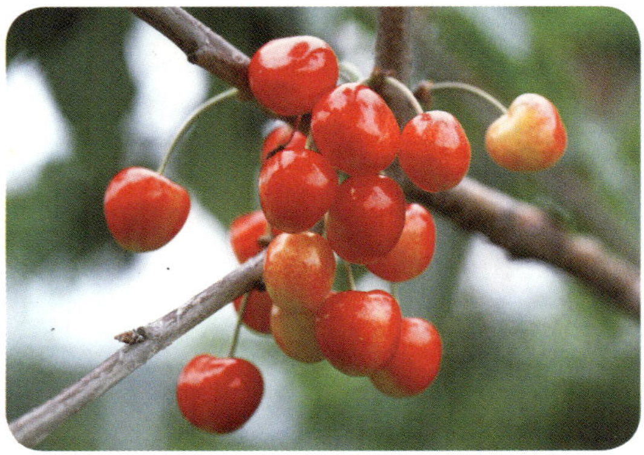

Property: warm
Flavor: sweet
Function: promote the production of body fluid, moisten the lungs, relieve restlessness, and improve appetite

A study found that cherries contain a material called anthocyanin, which can reduce inflammation, relieve pain, and make people happier. Experts say that eating 20 cherries is more effective than taking aspirin to relieve pain, and researchers at the University of Michigan point out that eating 20 cherries is more effective than taking medicines to relieve depression.

> Spinach

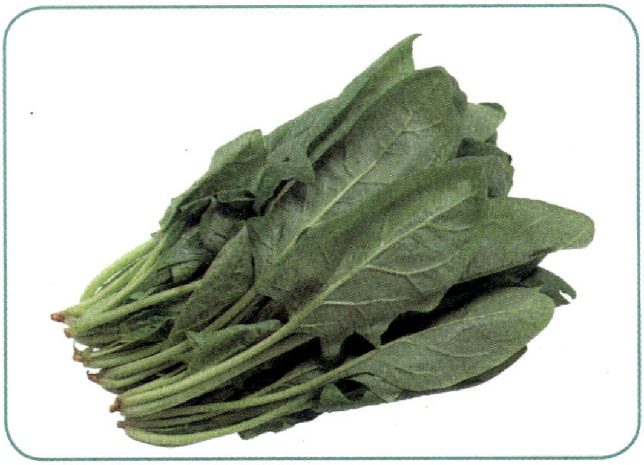

Property: cool
Flavor: sweet
Function: nourish the blood and stop bleeding, open the bowel, moisten dryness and quench thirst, and treat blood in the stool

In addition to large quantities of iron, spinach contains abundant folic acid. The lack of folic acid will lead to mental illness, including depression, Alzheimer's, etc. Researchers found that those who fail to get enough folic acid have difficulty falling asleep or staying asleep even 5 months later with symptoms such as forgetfulness and anxiety. And lack of folic acid directly leads to a fall in serotonin, which may lead to depression.

> Garlic

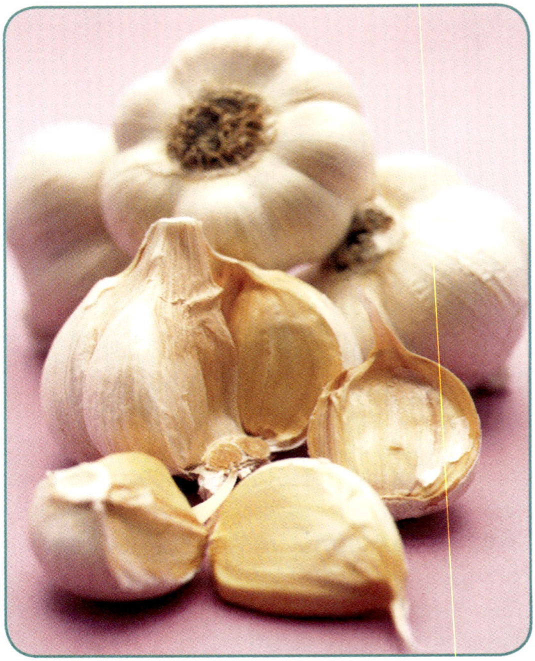

Property: warm
Flavor: spicy
Function: warm the digestive system and invigorate the stomach, promote digestion and the movement of qi, expel parasites, and detoxify

Research in Germany investigating the effect of garlic on lowering cholesterol found that when people eat garlic, they are less likely to be fatigued, anxious, or angry.

> Pumpkin

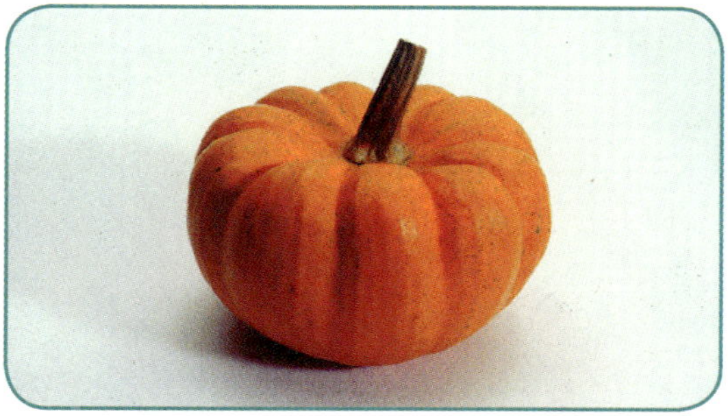

Property: warm
Flavor: sweet
Function: strengthen the digestive system and boost qi, detoxify, expel parasites, open the bowel, and prevent diabetes

Eating pumpkin can create good moods because it is rich in vitamin B6 and iron; both materials can help transform the blood sugar stored in the body into glucose, which is the only fuel for the brain and beneficial for the maintenance of strong energy.

> Skimmed or low fat milk

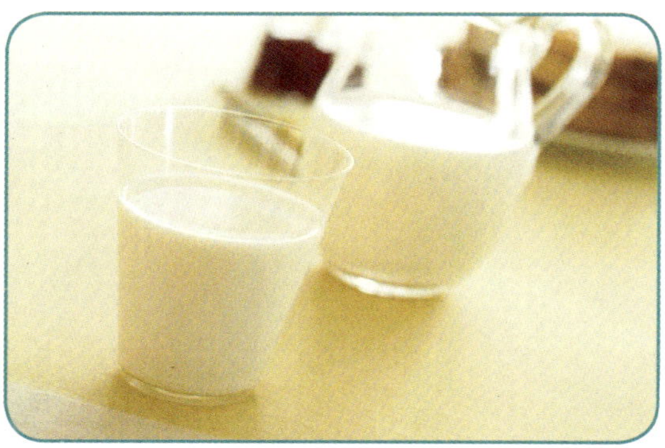

Property: neutral
Flavor: sweet
Function: invigorate qi and supplement blood, strengthen the lung and nourish the stomach, and promote body fluids to moisten the intestines

Low fat or skimmed milk is the major source of calcium. A study in the United States found that after taking 1,000 mg calcium pills for three months, three out of four women with pre-menstrual syndrome are less likely to be nervous, irritable, and anxious.

> Edible mushroom

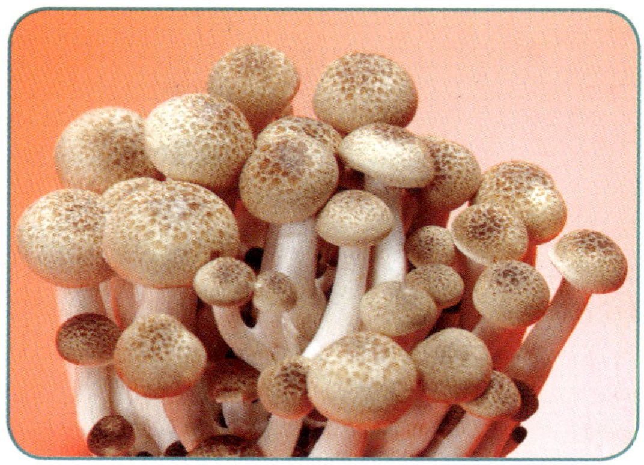

Property: neutral
Flavor: sweet
Function: reinforce the spleen, replenish qi, and thrust out skin eruptions

Edible mushrooms are used extensively in many Chinese cuisines. Many species of edible mushrooms are high in fiber and provide vitamins such as thiamine, riboflavin, niacin, biotin, cobalamins, and ascorbic acid. It is also a source of some minerals, including iron, selenium, potassium, and phosphorus.

> Wheat bread

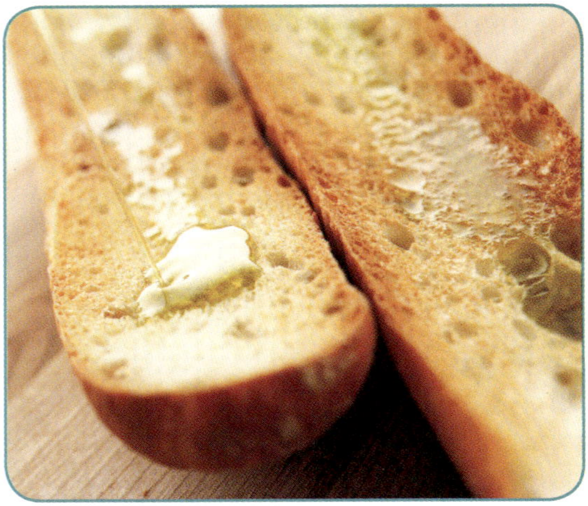

Property: slightly cold
Flavor: sweet
Function: nourish the heart and kidney, relieve mental strain, strengthen the kidney, invigorate the spleen, eliminate heat, and quench thirst

A carbohydrate-rich diet can enhance the secretion of serotonin. Many researchers believe an imbalance in serotonin levels may lead to depression, and Massachusetts Institute of Technology researchers state it makes good sense that some people eat desserts and food made with flour as anti-depression drugs.

> Walnut

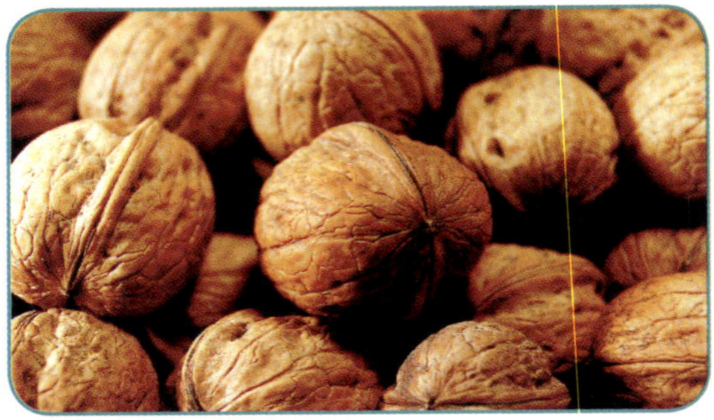

Property: warm
Flavor: sweet
Function: tonify the kidney to secure the essence, warm the lung to relieve arthma, and moisturize the large interstine to relieve constipation

Walnut is one of the best vegetarian sources of Omega 3 fatty acids, and an increased intake of Omega 3 has been shown to be very helpful in fighting depression. Just one quarter cup of walnuts can provide you with 91% of the daily recommended intake of Omega-3 fatty acids.

> Brown rice

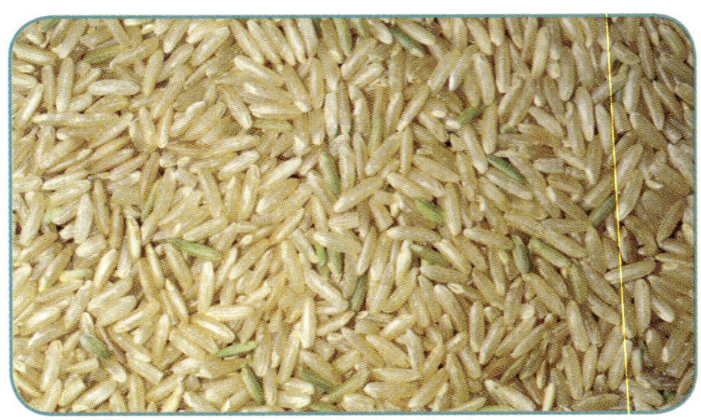

Property: neutral
Flavor: sweet
Function: invigorate middle *jiao*, replenish qi, tonify the spleen and stomach, strengthen qi, relieve thirst and restlessness, and arrest dysentery and diarrhea

Brown rice contains vitamins B1, B3, iror, magnesium, folic acid, etc. It has gradual releases of glucose into the bloodstream to prevent sugar lows and mood swings, and also provides many of the minerals we need to function properly. This high-fiber food can also keep the digestive system healthy and lower cholesterol.

Chinese medicine believes that everyone is born with a particular constitution that is inherited from one's parents. Moreover, the population can be classified into eight constitutions, namely constitutions with superabundant yang, superabundant yin, deficiency of yang, deficiency of yin, deficiency of qi, deficiency of blood, exuberant dampness, or blood stasis. Those constitutions pertain to determining what sort of disorders you are prone to have and how you react to them. Specifically, superiority of yang refers to heat constitution or heat diseases, while superiority of yin refers to cold constitution or cold diseases. Interestingly, foods can also be classified into cold, cool, warm, and hot. The food cold or cool in property is right for yang superiority, while the food warm or hot in property is applicable for yin superiority. Typically, Chinese medicine practitioners will consider your constitution to prevent disease and imbalance. The victims of depression often suffer from constrained liver qi due to mood swings. Their conditions may get aggravated and complicated when taking food either warm-acrid in property, such as leek, Chinese green onion, garlic, pepper, Chinese toon, fennel, and ginger, or food sweet-warm in property with the function of assisting fire, such as mutton and beef, which plays a negative role of "adding fuel to the fire." Therefore, patients should take more digestible and nutritious food cold-neutral in property while exposing themselves to drug therapy and psychotherapy. The foods of this kind include oatmeal, polished round-grained rice, corn, sweet potato, soybean, mustard, carrot, lotus root, boiled peanut, lettuce, head lettuce, Jew's ear, rape, Chinese cabbage, bean curd, pea, orange, day lily, pear, potato, black sesame, rice bean, etc. A proper diet can sometimes play a complementary role in a medical treatment.

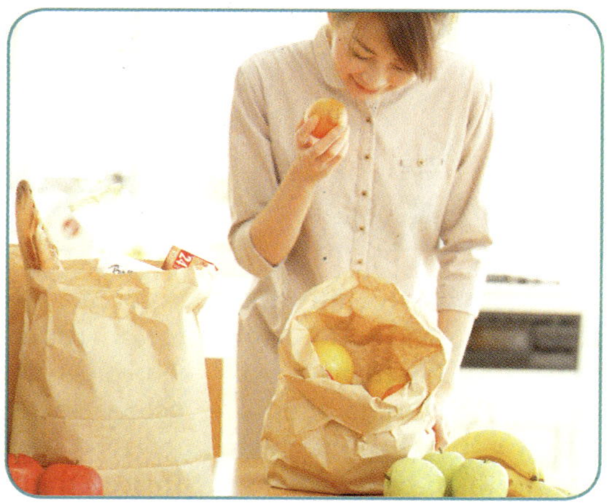

2. Specifics and Recipes

For people with depression, exposing yourself to a Chinese medical diet on a daily basis shows the great magnitude by which food plays in strengthening the house of the spirit. Eating a Chinese medicinal diet should abide by such laws as tonifying the spleen and kidney because the former is the postnatal foundation of life while the latter is the prenatal foundation of life, combining tonification and regulation in small amounts each time.

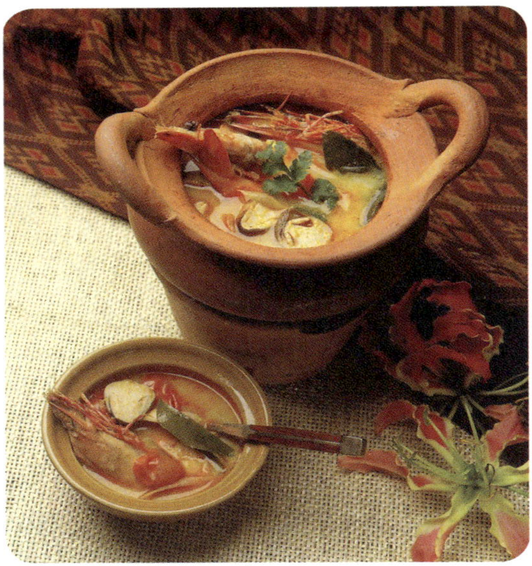

Below are some suggestions on medicinal ingredients and common foods that can be used in simple recipes. Many of the medicinals cited are mildly sweet or fairly bland so they won't impart a very strong taste to the dishes. Most of them are best used in soups and stews, though more specific cooking information is listed below. We hope that with the advice of your practitioner, you can learn which recipes and ingredients are right for you and incorporate them into your daily routine. You should be able to buy the medicinals in small amounts to be used in cooking from your practitioner or at an Asian supermarket.The amounts given are in grams and liters. To convert to ounces and cups, 30 grams is roughly equal to one ounce, and one liter is about four cups.

3. Porridge

Rice porridge is a simple dish usually made by boiling rice in water. As one of the easiest ways to digest grains, it is often served as a breakfast dish. Traditionally, rice porridge is used as a food to nurse the sick back to health. Porridge is a part of daily life, and there is a Laba Festival, which falls on the eighth day of the 12th lunar month on the traditional Chinese lunar calendar, that marks the official start of the Spring Festival. Usually, Chinese celebrate the day by eating Laba porridge, which is made with rice, nuts, cereals, and dried fruit. There is a legend about the porridge, the founder of Buddhism, Sakyamuni, fainted from hunger and exhaustion during his journey to find virtue. He was saved by a passing shepherdess who fed him porridge. Sakyamuni then went on to become Buddha on the eighth day of the 12 lunar month.

> Chinese date (jujube) porridge

Cook ten pieces jujube and 15 g Indian bread with hostwood first, then remove dregs from the decoction; cook 100 g millet with the remnant liquid into porridge. It is capable of tonifying qi, strengthening the stomach, and tranquilizing the mind. Warm porridge is recommended when breakfast and dinner is served.

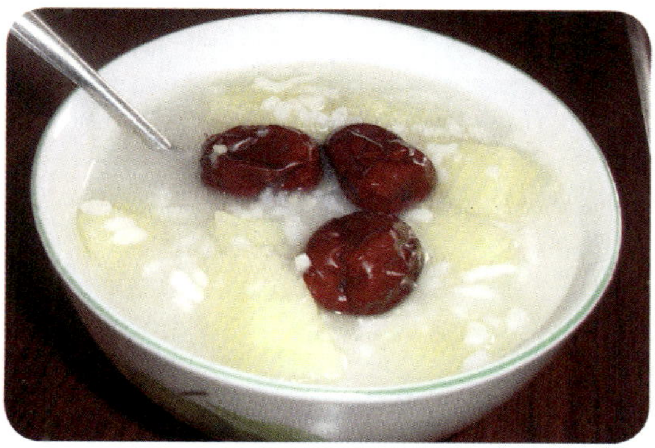

> *Gān mài dà zǎo* porridge

Cook 15 g licorice root first, remove its dregs from the decoction, and cook 15 g wheat and ten pieces jujube with remnant liquid into a porridge. It is capable of tonifying qi, nourishing the heart, and tranquilizing the mind. Warm porridge is recommended when you are hungry.

> Walnut porridge

Cook 150 g rice, 30 g walnut kernel, 10 g lily bulb, 20 g black sesame, and water into porridge. It is capable of strengthening deficiency, nourishing yin, and tonifying intelligence.

> Sesame porridge

Fry and mince 50 g sesame seeds, cook 100 g rice into porridge, then add the ground sesame seeds into the porridge. It is applicable for dizziness, poor memory, and premature senility.

> Lotus seed and jujube porridge

Peel and de-seed 30 g lotus seed, cook with water until the lotus seeds are soft, add 60 g rice and 10 pieces of jujube, cook them together into porridge. It can tonify the spleen to stop diarrhea, strengthen the kidney to control essence, and nourish the heart to tranquilize the spirit.

> Lily bulb porridge

Grind 30 g lily bulb, then cook lily bulb and 50 g of sticky rice into a porridge, and add rock sugar before serving. It can nourish yin to moisten lung and tranquilize the heart to calm the spirit.

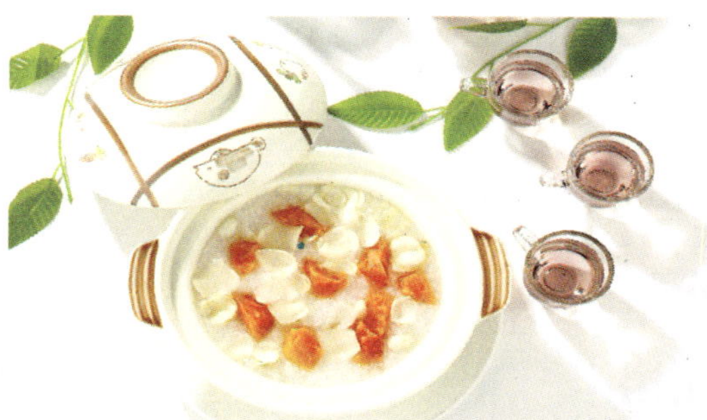

4. Recipes for Different Patterns

The patterns listed below are simple ones and you may have two or more of the patterns mentioned below.[19] If that is the case, please choose freely from any recipe that pertains to your pattern.

> Qi deficiency pattern

Signs and symptoms: lassitude, shortness of breath, no desire to talk, asthma at slight exertion, spontaneous sweating, pale complexion, poor appetite, loose stool, pale or reddish tongue with white moist coating, and feeble pulses
Therapeutic principle: fortify qi

Medicinals That Can Be Used in Cooking

Chinese Name	Common Name	Pinyin	Latin Name
黄芪	Astragalus	*huáng qí*	Radix Astragali
人参	Ginseng	*rén shēn*	Radix Ginseng
党参	Codonopsis root	*dǎng shēn*	Radix Codonopsis
西洋参	American ginseng	*xī yáng shēn*	Radix Panacis Quinquefolii
白术	(White) Atractylodes rhizome / ovate atractylodes	*bái zhú*	Rhizoma Atractylodis Macrocephalae
红景天	Gold theragran / integripetal rhodiola medicinal	*hóng jǐng tiān*	Radix et Rhizoma Rhodiolae Crenulatae
甘草	Glycyrrhizae licorice root	*gān cǎo*	Radix et Rhizoma Glycyrrhizae

Recommended recipes:

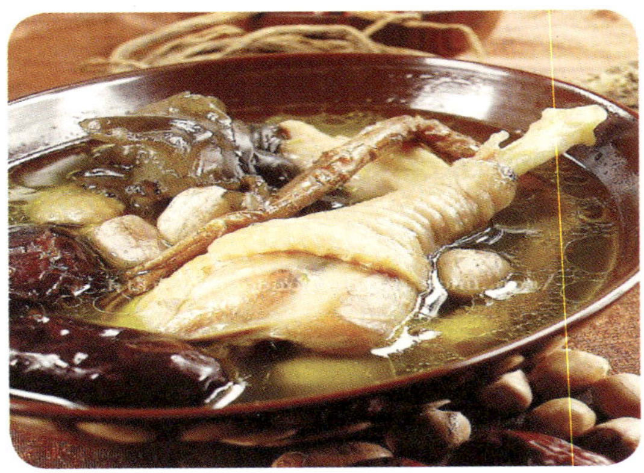

Ginseng porridge

Cut 10 g ginseng into pieces, soak it in one litre of water for 40 minutes, and then put it in an earthenware pot. Heat it over a strong fire until the water boils, then change to a gentle fire and keep heating for about two hours; put 100-150 g rice into the ginseng decoction and then boil until very soft. It is capable of reinforcing the middle jiao, replenishing qi, and invigorating the spleen.

Chicken soup stewed with Astragalus

Scald the prepared 750 g black-bone chicken in boiling water until the the folds on the skin smooth, wash it in cold water and drain. Cut 30 g Astragalus into sections 6-7 cm long, put them tidily into the abdominal cavity of the chicken. Cut the 10 g clean scallion and 10 g ginger into section and slices respectively; put the chicken and 1.5 litres of water into an earthenware pot and heat it over a strong fire for 50 minutes. Then remove the scallion, ginger, and astragalus out before eating. This soup can fortify qi, elevate yang, nourish the blood, and strengthen deficiency.

> Yang deficiency pattern

Signs and symptoms: cold limbs and hands; tinnitus; vertigo; lassitude or cold-pain in the loins and knees; impotence; premature ejaculation; sterility; clear urine; loose stool; pale complexion; fatigue; pale tongue; deep, thready, and feeble pulses
Therapeutic principle: strengthen yang

Medicinals That Can Be Used in Cooking

Chinese Name	Common Name	Pinyin	Latin Name
肉苁蓉	Desert cistanche	*ròu cōng róng*	Medicinala Cistanches
人参	Ginseng	*rén shēn*	Radix Ginseng
白附片	White aconite accessory root slices	*bái fù piàn*	Radix Aconiti Lateralis Praeparata
肉桂	Cassia bark	*ròu guì*	Cortex Cinnamomi
鹿茸	Deer velvet	*lù róng*	Cornu Cervi Pantotrichum
杜仲	Eucommia bark	*dù zhòng*	Cortex Eucommiae
干姜	Dried ginger rhizome	*gān jiāng*	Rhizoma Zingiberis

Recommended recipes:

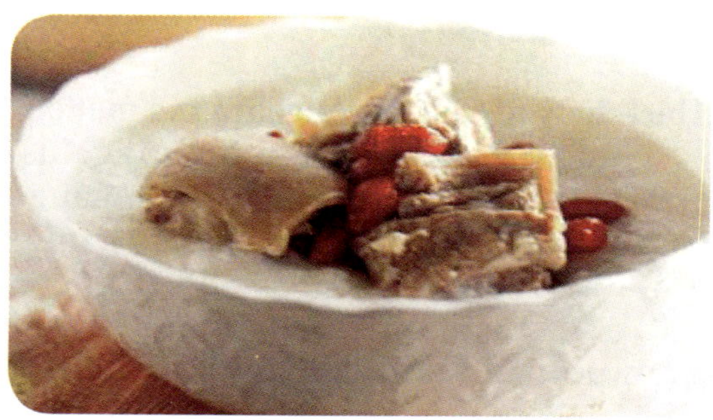

Desert cistanche and mutton porridge

Cut 10 g desert cistanche and 60 g prepared mutton into slices. Decoct desert cistanche in an earthenware pot to obtain the extract and remove the dregs. Then put the mutton, 60 g rice, water, salt, scallion stalks, and fresh ginger into the pot to make porridge. It can replenish the kidney, invigorate yang, improve the function of spleen and stomach, and loosen bowel movements to relieve constipation.

Extract of Cherokee rose fruit

Add an appropriate amount of water to decoct 100 g Cherokee rose fruit, pour off the extract two hours later, and add water to decoct it again. Repeat the process four times, then squeeze out and separate the extract from the dregs. Cook all the extract together to make it more condensed, then add 200 g honey and mix it thoroughly. Cool it and remove the froth on the surface. This can strengthen the kidney and tonify the essence of life.

> Blood deficiency pattern

Signs and symptoms: vertigo, dizziness, fatigue, limb numbness, palpitation, insominia, bad memory, sallow complexion, pale lips and nails, thready and rapid or unsmooth pulses

Therapeutic principle: nourish blood

Medicinals That Can Be Used in Cooking

Chinese Name	Common Name	Pinyin	Latin Name
当归	Chinese Angelica	*dāng guī*	Radix Angelicae Sinensis
制何首乌	Prepared fleeceflower root	*zhì hé shǒu wū*	Radix Polygoni Multiflori Praeparata cum Succo Glycines Sotae
阿胶	Donkey-hide gelatin	*ē jiāo*	Colla Corii Asini
白芍药	White peony root; peony	*bái sháo yào*	Radix Paeoniae Alba
熟地黄	Prepared rehmannia root	*shú dì huáng*	Radix Rehmanniae Praeparata
龙眼肉	Longan / flesh of the longan fruit	*lóng yǎn ròu*	Arillus Longan

Recommended recipes:

Thick soup of Chinese Angelica and mutton

Put 15 g Angelica, 25 g Astragalus, and 25 g Codonopsis Root into a gauze bag and tie up its opening; put 500 g mutton, the medicinal bag, scallion, ginger, salt, and cooking wine into an earthenware pot, and add the right amount of water. Heat it over a strong fire until it reaches the boiling point, and then let it simmer gently until the mutton is completely soft. It can nourish the blood and fortify the deficiency.

Drink of longyan and spine date seed

Pound 10 g spine date seeds into pieces and put them into a gauze bag. Put

12 g euryale seeds into 500 ml water to boil for about half an hour, then add longan and spine date seeds, and boil them together for another 30 minutes. Take out the bag of spine date seeds and add the right amount of white sugar. Filter to get the extract. It can nourish the blood, tranquilize the mind, tonify the kidney, and control the vital essence.

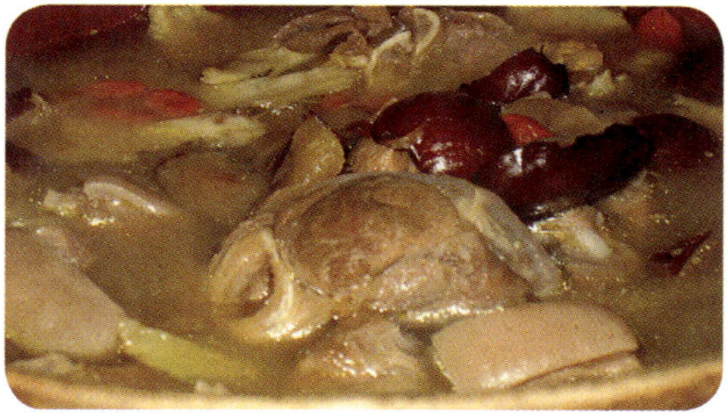

> Yin deficiency pattern

Signs and symptoms: emaciation; dizziness; vertigo; dry mouth and throat; insomnia due to vexation; burning sensation of the chest, palms, and soles; night sweats; redness in the zygomatic region; red lips; lassitude in the loins and knees; emission; forgetfulness; red tongue with little coating; thready and fast pulses

Therapeutic principle: nourish yin

Medicinals That Can Be Used in Cooking

Chinese Name	Common Name	Pinyin	Latin Name
北沙参	Root of straight ladybell / glehnia root	*běi shā shēn*	Radix Glehniae
枸杞子	Chinese wolfberry fruit / lycium fruit / matrimony wine fruit	*gǒu qǐ zǐ*	Fructus Lycii
鳖甲	Turtle carapace	*biē jiǎ*	Carapax Trionycis
玉竹	Fragrant solomonseal rhizome	*yù zhú*	Rhizoma Polygonati Odorati
山茱萸	Asiatic cornelian cherry fruit / cornus	*shān zhū yú*	Fructus Corni

Recommended recipes:

Cornus porridge

Wash 15-20 g cornus and get rid of the kernel. Boil it with 60 g rice and 1 litre of water until very soft. Add white sugar when the porridge is about to be done and keep cooking for a while. This porridge is able to replenish the yin of liver and kidney, restore essence, and treat excessive sweating.

Asparagus tuber porridge

Decoct 15 g asparagus in water to get concentrated extract and remove the dregs. Put 60 g rice and the right amount of water into the extract and boil it into the porridge. Add crystal sugar after it has boiled and keep cooking for a while. It can nourish yin, moisten the lungs, and promote production of body fluid to relieve cough.

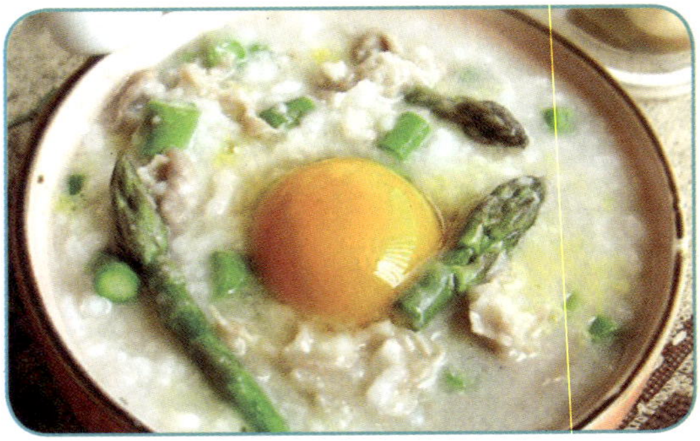

> Heat pattern

Signs and symptoms: aversion to heat, agitation and insomnia with nightmares, fever, red face, constipation, desire for cold drinks, red and dry tongue with yellow coating, rapid and full pulses

Therapeutic principle: clear heat

Medicinals That Can Be Used in Cooking

Chinese Name	Common Name	Pinyin	Latin Name
金银花	Honeysuckle flower	*jīn yín huā*	Flos Lonicerae Japonicae
板蓝根	Isatis root	*bǎn lán gēn*	Radix Isatidis
绿豆	Mung bean / phaseolus	*lǜ dòu*	Semen Phaseoli Radiati
野菊花	Wild chrysanthemum flower	*yě jú huā*	Flos Chrysanthemi Indici
紫花地丁	Tokyo violet medicinal	*zǐ huā dì dīng*	Medicinala Violae
竹叶	Lophatherum stem and leaves / henon bamboo leaf	*zhú yè*	Folium Phyllostachydis Henonis

Recommended recipes:

Mung beans soup

Soak 50 g beans overnight or at least for four hours, in plenty of water. Place the beans in a large pot and add 2 liters of water. Bring to a boil, stir, and simmer for one hour. Let cool, refrigerate for 30 minutes, serve, and season with rock sugar. Mung beans, according to Chinese medi-

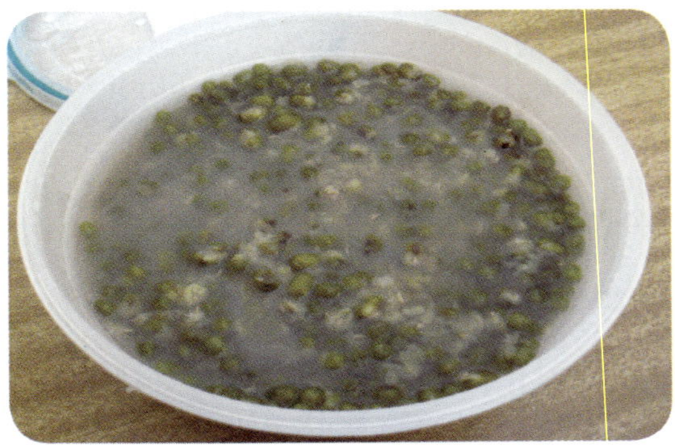

cine, have a cooling effect on the body, so this is a very popular dish to clear heat, especially in summer.

Fried bittermelon

Wash the bittermelons, peel and cut in half lengthwise, deseed and thinly slice them. Heat the oil in a deep saucepan, when the oil becomes very hot, lower the heat and add sliced bitter melons and salt to the oil. Deep fry until they become pale gold. This dish can clear heat, relieve toxin, as well as lower blood sugar.

> Dampness pattern

Signs and symptoms: heaviness of the head and body, dizziness, poor appetite, stuffy chest, excessive mucus, and poor health

Therapeutic principle: remove dampness

Medicinals That Can Be Used in Cooking

Chinese Name	Common Name	Pinyin	Latin Name
茯苓	Indian bread	*fú líng*	Poria
冬瓜皮	Chinese waxgourd peel	*dōng guā pí*	Exocarpium Benincasae
玉米须	Cornsilk	*yù mǐ xū*	Stigma Maydis
薏苡仁	Coix seed	*yì yǐ rén*	Semen Coicis
金钱草	Lysimachia; christina loosestrife	*jīn qián cǎo*	Medicinala Lysimachiae
藿香	Agastache	*huò xiāng*	Medicinala Agastachis

Recommended recipes

Coix seed porridge

Rinse 50 g coix seed and 30 g red beans. Soak in water for about two or three hours. Rinse 50 g unpolished rice and soak in water. Cook coix seed, red beans, and rice in half a pot of water. Turn down the heat and cook for two hours, season with rock sugar or salt. It invigorates the spleen, improves water circulation, reduces swelling, and promotes urination.

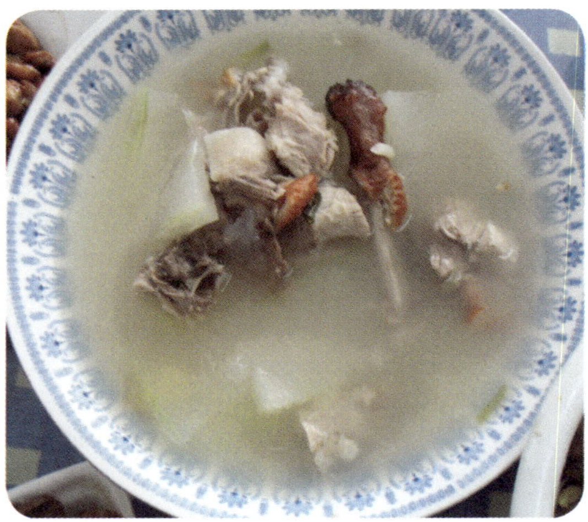

Chinese waxgourd and chicken soup

Put 50 g chicken breast into water and boil it for five minutes. Remove the chicken and rinse it. Bring 2.5 liters of water to boil, and then add 300 g Chinese wintermelon and 50 g Coix seed, and some salt. Continue to boil the soup over low heat till 1 liter of water remains and the other ingredients are soft.

> Blood stagnation pattern

Signs and symptoms: fixed stabbing pain, dark complexion, fixed masses, bleeding clots, purple lips and nails, purple tongue with petechia, wiry, and choppy pulses

Therapeutic principle: activate blood circulation to relieve stagnation

Medicinals That Can Be Used in Cooking

Chinese Name	Common Name	Pinyin	Latin Name
丹参	Danshen root	*dān shēn*	Radix et Rhizoma Salviae Miltiorrhizae
川芎	Sichuan lovage root	*chuān xiōng*	Rhizoma Chuanxiong
桃仁	Peach seed	*táo rén*	Semen Persicae
三七	Pseudoginseng root	*sān qī*	Radix et Rhizoma Notoginseng
益母草	Motherwort Medicinal	*yì mŭ căo*	Medicinala Leonuri
郁金	Turmeric root tuber	*yù jīn*	Radix Curcumae

Recommended recipes:

Pseudoginseng root chicken soup

Bring 2.5 liters of water to a boil in a stockpot. Rinse, skin, and halve 750 g fresh chicken, then scald with boiling water. Add the chicken, 30 g rinsed pseudoginseng root and 3 slices fresh ginger root, cook over high heat for 15-20 minutes. Turn down the heat and simmer uncovered for two hours, then season with salt. Serve hot. It is an effective mover of blood stagnation, improves blood circulation, eliminates pain and eases bruises, improves the skin texture, refreshes the mind, and energizes the body.

Peach seed and hawthorn tea

Grind the ingredients of 60 g peach seed and 120 g hawthorn and put the mixture in ten tea bags. Drink one bag every day and season with rock sugar to taste. It is applicable for patients with coronary heart disease marked by obvious symptoms of blood stasis.

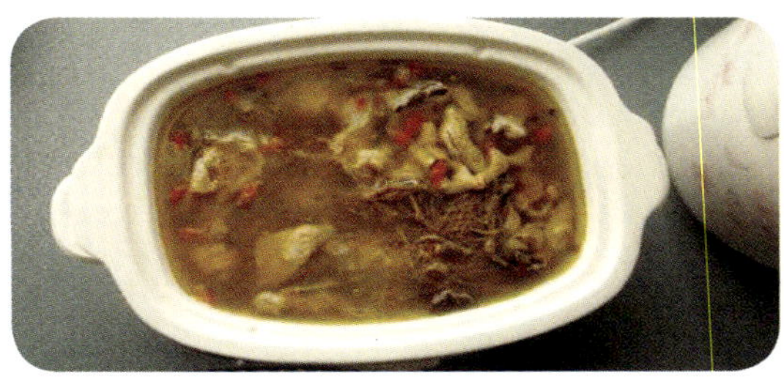

> Qi stagnation pattern

Signs and symptoms: distending pain that moves around, depression, irritability, purple tongue, and wiry pulses
Therapeutic principle: promote qi circulation to eliminate stagnation

Medicinals That Can Be Used in Cooking

Chinese Name	Common Name	Pinyin	Latin Name
陈皮	Aged tangerine peel / citrus	*chén pí*	Pericarpium Citri Reticulatae
荔枝核	Lychee seed	*lì zhī hé*	Semen Litchi
玫瑰花	Rose flower	*méi guì huā*	Flos Rosae Rugosae
青皮	Green tangerine peel	*qīng pí*	Pericarpium Citri Reticulatae Viride
刀豆	Sword bean / canavalia gladiata / jack bean	*dāo dòu*	Semen Canavaliae
柿蒂	Persimmon calyx / kaki	*shì dì*	Calyx Kaki

Recommended recipes:

Rose flower tea

Boil a mixture of 6 g rose flowers and 3 g aged tangerine peel in a pot for 10 minutes; add rock sugar to taste, and drink the filtrate. This tea may help relieve qi stagnation and improve spirit.

Aged tangerine peel duck

Boil 10 g tangerine peel and simmer it for 20 minutes. Rinse and wipe 100 g duck breast, cut into slices, add 4 slices of ginger into hot oil, and fry until it turns pale gold; add two tablespoons of Shao Xing wine, dark soya sauce, rock sugar, and the decoction of tangerine peel; cover and simmer it for approximately 30 minutes or until tender. This dish can strengthen the spleen and stomach, relieve dampness, and disperse qi stagnation.

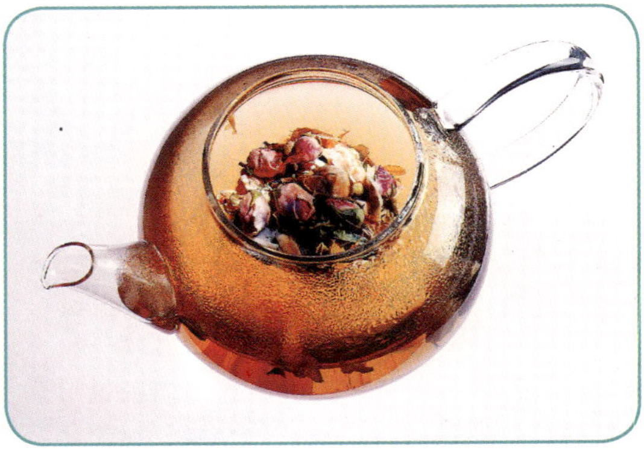

> Food retention pattern

Signs and symptoms: stomach and abdominal stuffiness and pain, belching and regurgitation, poor appetite and vomiting, diarrhea, thick greasy tongue coating, and slippery pulses
Therapeutic principle: promote digestion to alleviate retention

Medicinals That Can Be Used in Cooking

Chinese Name	Common Name	Pinyin	Latin Name
山楂	Chinese hawthorn fruit	*shān zhā*	Fructus Crataegi
神曲	Medicated leaven	*shén qū*	Massa Medicata Fermentata
麦芽	Germinated barley	*mài yá*	Fructus Hordei Germinatus
鸡内金	Chicken gizzard lining	*jī nèi jīn*	Endothelium Corneum Gigeriae Galli
谷芽	Grain sprout	*gŭ yá*	Fructus Setariae Germinatus

Recommended recipes:

Lotus leaf and hawthorn fruit tea

Soak 5 g lotus leaf, 5 g hawthorn fruit, and 3 g coix in boiling water. This medicinal tea promotes digestion, improves bowel movements, as well as reduces fat and weight.

Food retention relieving cake

Grind 100 g crataegus, 100 g barley sprout, and 100 g medicated leaven into fine powders. Boil 7 g radish seed, 7 g prunella spike, and 7 g cassia seed with 500 ml water for 15 minutes. Mix the powder and the strained decoction together to make small cakes, steam 10-15 minutes or until the cake is done. The cake can invigorate the spleen, promote digestion and relieve food retention,

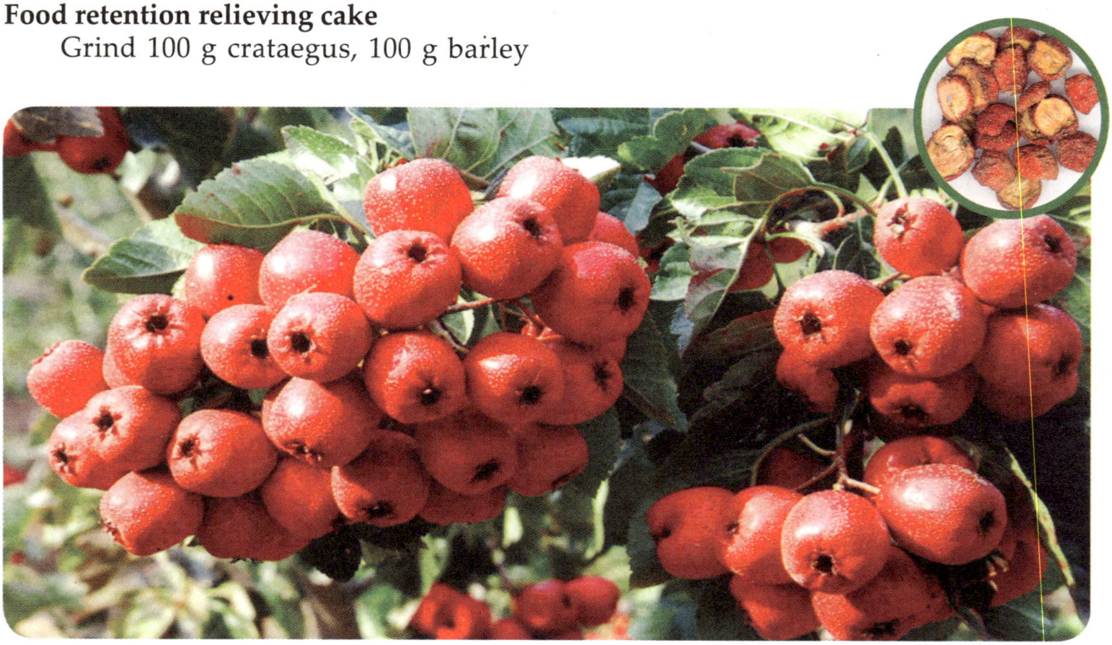

Exercise

1. What Kinds of Exercises Are Helpful and What Should Be Avoided?

In Chinese, there is a saying that, "running water never gets stale, a door-hinge is never worm-eaten." This means keeping things moving will prevent damage. Movement and change are fundamental to all objects in the universe; motion is absolute, but stasis is relative. Wherever one looks, from galaxies to the inside of cells, motion exists everywhere. The above idiom emphasizes the importance of motion in even simple objects. The *Book of Changes* (*Yì Jīng*, 易经, a.k.a I Ching) is a "reflection of the universe in miniature." The word "*Yì*" stands for ease and simplicity, change and transformation, and invariability. Thus the three principles underlying the *Yì Jīng* are: simplicity, variability, and persistency. Concerning the traditional exercises of Chinese medicine, the basic principles and requirements include the combination of motion and stillness, persistent and moderate exercises, learning to walk before you run, and doing the right exercise at the right time -- an individual-oriented exercise.

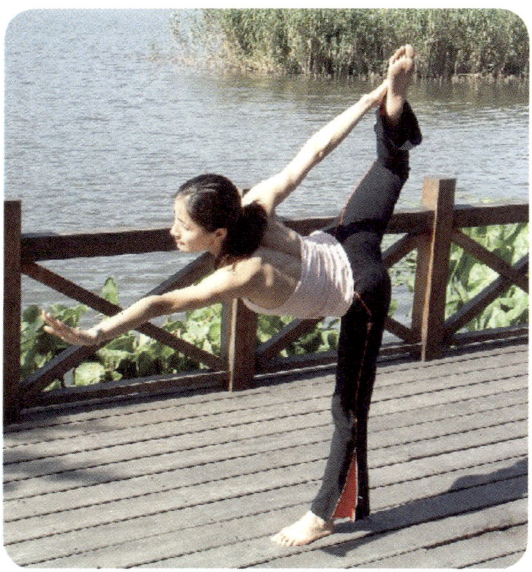

Physical activity is extremely beneficial for those trying to get rid of depression. Together with dietary therapy it is an essential part of long-term successful anti-depression treatment. A.L. Brosse, et al.[20] critically reviewed the evidence that exercise is effective in treating depression in adults, and found out that available evidence provides considerable support for the value of exercise in reducing depressive symptoms in both healthy and clinical populations. Regular exercise can change the brain chemistry and lead to feelings of wellbeing. Psychologically, doing exercises can restore your sense of mastery and accomplishment; it will increase the feeling of social support when doing exercise with friends or with an enjoyable group. What's more, any form of exercise is a potential distraction from worries and negative thoughts that make depression worse. Exercise can improve sleep, which helps alleviate depression in some people; exercise may influence the metabolism and availability of central neurotransmitters, as well as hormones associated with mood—affecting brain chemistry beneficially; exercise increases the body's metabolic rate and decreases blood pressure, thus increasing energy—a great way to fight fatigue.

Experts strongly stress the importance of outdoor activity in the process of treating depression. Enough exposure to sunshine will help the brain secrete 5-hydroxytryptamine (5-HT), known as the hormone of alleviating, delighting, and stabilizing mood, which will in turn influence the secretion of endorphin.

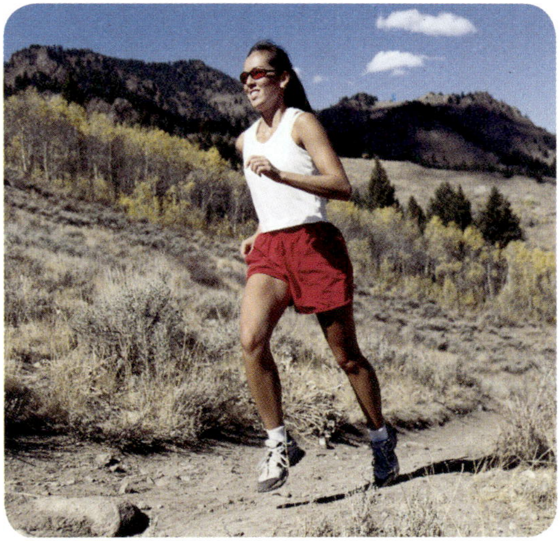

2. Tai Ji and Qi Gong

Tai Ji Quan

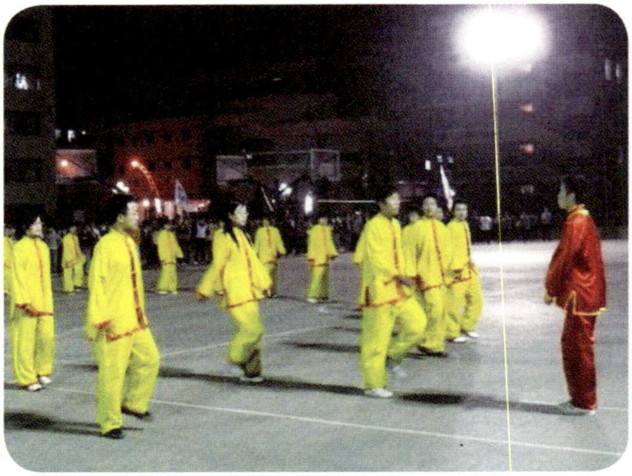

On August 8, 2008, in the opening ceremonies of the 2008 Beijing Olympic Games, 2008, tai ji performers practiced their form in perfect synchronicity.

"The 2,008 performers doing tai chi in a circle that surrounds a rectangle is an epitome of the notion of 'heaven is round and the earth is square.' And the boxing itself perfectly illustrates Lao Tzu's teaching – 'The soft and pliable will defeat the hard and strong.'" *(China Daily)*

"Amid forests of sheer fabric on which shifting images of water and light skittered, tai ji dancers offered a glimpse of a peculiarly Chinese environmentalism – the unity of mankind and nature." *(The Wall Street Journal)*

Tai ji quan, a unique body-mind exercise, is based on martial arts, Daoist philosophy, and yin-yang theory. The principle of tai ji quan is using softness to overcome force. It is a special kind of *kung fu* practiced to maintain health and for self-defense. Because it doesn't demand a lot of bodily energy or strength to learn, it is suitable for both young and old, and makes a great aerobic exercise. The more you practice, the better you will understand your own body, helping to coordinate and clear your body and mind. You will feel peace and grace physically, psychologically, and emotionally after practicing tai ji quan. Modern research has shown it to boost immunity, reduce weight, relieve complications, and create an improvement in the overall sense of wellbeing. Studies also suggest that tai ji quan is effective in improving the elasticity of blood vessels, enhancing the function of the nervous system to help you feel better and re-balance energy and vitality, promoting the respiratory function to expand vital capacity, reopening the channels and collaterals, as well as strengthening the vital qi.

There have been many schools of practice during its development over the past centuries. Presently the five major schools are Yang (杨), Chen (陈), Wu (吴), Sun (孙), and Wu / Hao (武/郝). A possibly new, sixth school of tai qi quan that has a following is Zhao Bao (赵堡) style. Whichever school you study, you will be taught similar slow, graceful, smooth movements. The essence of tai ji quan is its harmonious and natural movements representing the constant, harmonious transformation and interaction of yin and yang. Its movements are simple but subtle. It takes time, discipline, and persistence to master the forms.

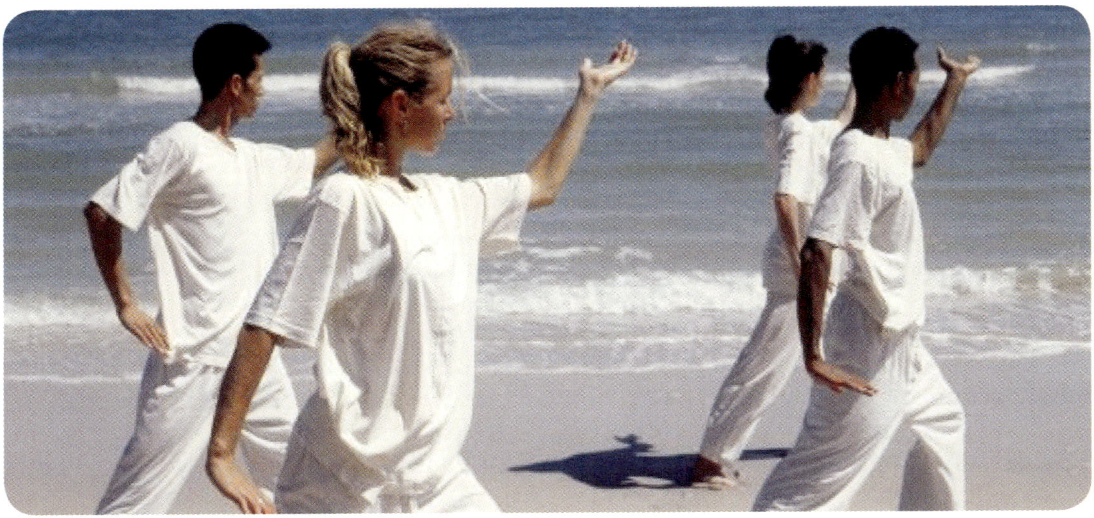

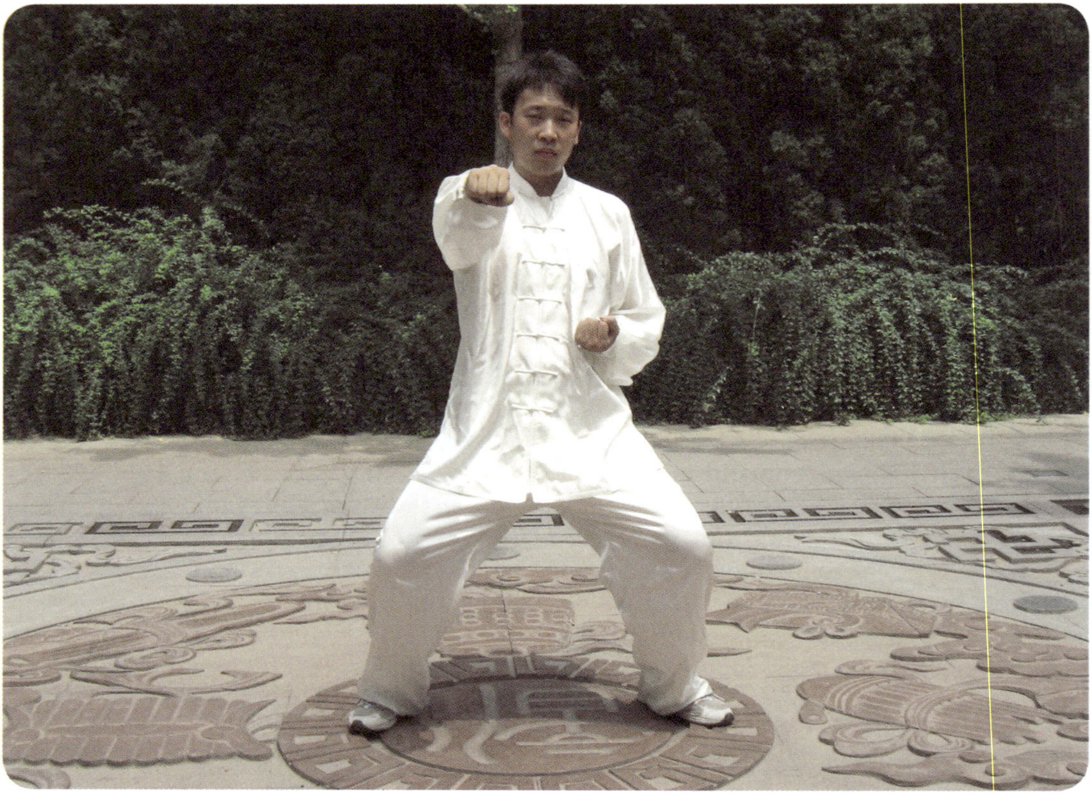

It is highly recommended that you learn tai ji from a qualified instructor. A recording can help you get a rough idea about the basic movements and the sequence. But tai ji is not dancing or modeling, where the external form is most important; nor is it aerobics where the point is simply to get the heart rate going. You need an experienced instructor to guide you through the internal process as well as the external movements. You need to practice on a regular basis. Find a quiet place with fresh air. After you become familiar with the movements you will start to feel the subtle difference it makes on your body.

With a calm mind, guide your movements consciously, breathing slowly, deeply, and naturally. Your movements should be stable, constant, gentle, and fluent. By learning to move slowly but consistently, your body can be trained to follow the subtle instructions of the brain. Gradually, coordination between your body and mind will be improved. A practitioner who had been learning tai ji for five years once fell down from a moving bicycle and to her surprise, she was not hurt at all. As she hit the ground, her body naturally folded into the best position to avoid a head injury. The ability to adjust to the environment like this indicates a higher level of vitality and leads to a greater state of health.

Tai ji quan is both yin and yang: moving and still, hard and gentle, backward and forward, and flexible and firm. Practicing tai ji can boost your qi and harmonize the yin and yang of your body. Practicing tai ji can make you feel refreshed, relaxed, and increase your awareness and enthusiasm for life. Tai ji is a door into the world of rediscovering your own body and how it relates to the world outside. It is for everyone.

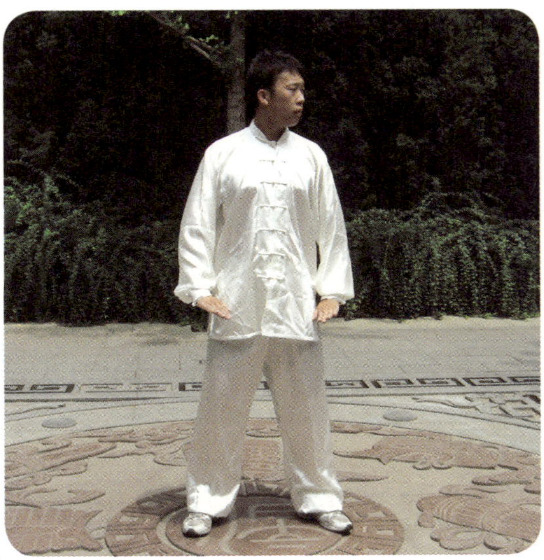

There are no specially designed tai ji routines for the prevention of depression, but tai ji is a kind of aerobic exercise. As was explained above, aerobic exercise can help reduce depression, because the movements of tai ji are slow and gentle, so they can regulate the flow of qi and blood leading to better organ function, and a stronger metabolism. Practicing tai ji in nature is an ideal form of exercise for a stressful life.

Pushing hands is known as an important part of tai ji quan and refers to the pair exercise routine in internal Chinese martial arts. Pushing hands can untie people's nature of fighting against force with force, and make the body yield to the force and redirect it. It allows people to develop the sensitivity of feeling the direction and strength of the outsider (partner), and to learn how to generate, coordinate and deliver strength to others and how to neutralize the offensive power in an effective and safe manner. This may partially explain how the softness of tai ji overcome hardness. The practicing of pushing hands includes eight gates (*bā mén,* 八门) that are said to be associated with the eight trigrams (*bā guà,* 八卦) of the *Yì Jīng* and five steps (*wǔ bù,* 五步) that are believed to be related to the five phases (*wǔ xíng,* 五行).

Qi Gong

Qi gong is a method of physical and mental regulation created by the Chinese out of a desire for a long life, to help maintain health, and fight against disease.

By regulating their bodies, training their respiration, and concentrating and conducting their minds, qi gong practitioners reach a high level of integration of mind, qi, spirit, and body. Qi gong practice can help maximize the efficiency and effectiveness of how we store, move, and use qi to enhance health and wellbeing. It is effective in regulating and strengthening bodily functions, inducing and developing internal potentials, preventing and curing diseases, maintaining and strengthening health, increasing intelligence, and prolonging life. Qi gong is different from general physical exercise, since it is psychosomatic, and works to ease, smooth, and regulate breathing to store up or accumulate energy in the body.

Just like there are various physical exercises with specific purpose, qi gong can be divided into internal qi gong, which is practiced by individuals to preserve and promote health by regulating qi and harmonizing the internal energy of the body, and external qi gong, which is performed by a qi gong master to another person for healing purposes. The internal qi gong also can be classified into the still and the moving. Qi gong practice, whether still or moving, share the common principles that underpin the theories and therapies of Chinese medicine -- reinforcing what is depleted and clearing what is blocked or in excess. Moving qi gong is practiced by coordinating body movements with breath and mind. Static qi gong focuses mostly on control and coordination of breath and mind, which is more difficult for beginners. Moving qi gong, which is often mistaken for tai ji, is what most people have seen before. Qi gong is not magic, nor is it mere exercise. For centuries it has been an important element of Chinese medicine. During the Spring and Autumn period (770-476 B.C.) or Warring States era (475-221 B.C.), a monograph on qi gong entitled *Inscription on Moving Qi on a Jade Pendant* (*Xíng Qì Yù Pèi Míng*, 行气玉佩铭) appeared. This text, possibly over 2,500 years old, was the first written reference to qi gong.

However, it is more difficult to locate a real qi gong practitioner than to find a tai ji practitioner because qi gong is not easy to learn, practice, or evaluate. Scientists are still exploring specific methods to study qi gong and some are showing prospects.

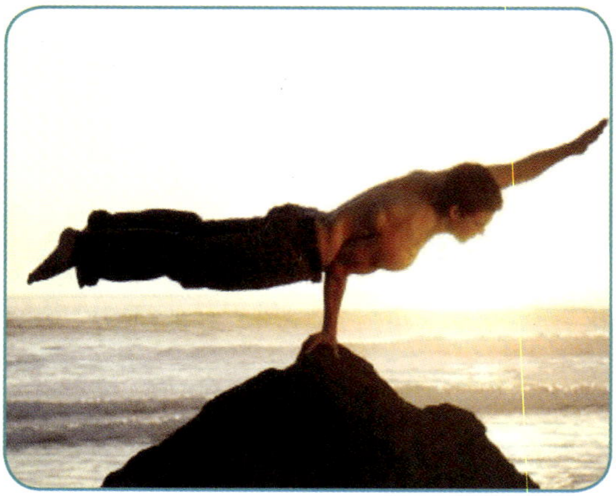

No matter when sitting still, standing upright, or lying on the back or side, qi gong can be practiced through incorporating posture, movement, breathing, meditation, visualization, and conscious intent. The basic requirement is to stay comfortable and relaxed. The key to practicing qi gong is the regulation and coordination of body, mind, and breath. You also must choose a style suitable for your condition. In most cases you will need an instructor.

Obsessive practicing may do more harm than good. A practice is meant to relax the body and mind, so it must be performed in a relaxed manner.

From the perspective of Chinese medical theory and practice, qi gong can supplement qi, strengthen the body, harmonize yin and yang, regulate qi and blood, smooth the flow in the channels, and calm the mind. Modern research has proven that qi gong can help cure various illnesses and maintain health.

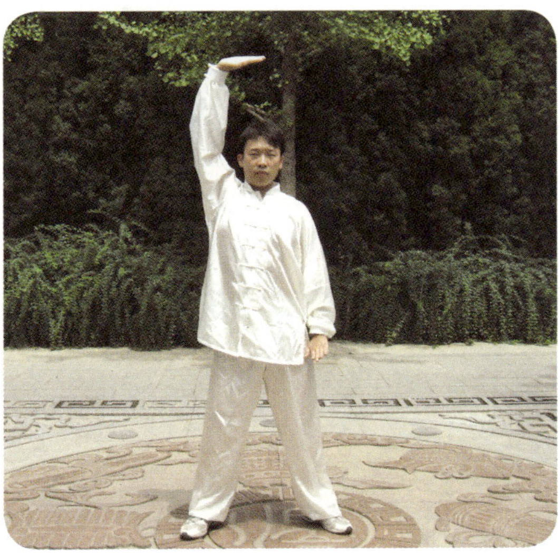

Five Animal Exercises

In addition to the methods mentioned above, there are many other forms of exercises, such as *The Classical Exercises of Changing the Muscles and Tendons* (*Yì Jīn Jīng*, 易筋经), *The Turtle Longevity Qi Gong* (*Guī Xíng Gōng*, 龟形功), *Peng Zu Health Exercise* (*Péng Zǔ Yǎng Shēng*, 彭祖养生), *Five Animal Exercises* (*Wǔ Qín Xì*, 五禽戏, a.k.a. "Five Animal Frolics"), and the *Eight Pieces of Brocade* (*Bā Duàn Jǐn*, 八段锦). Practicing any of these forms of exercise will greatly benefit health and are not only for those with depression. *Five Animal Exercises*, for instance, was introduced by Hua Tuo (110-207 A.D.), a famous doctor in China. It is an ancient exercise based on the natural movements and postures of five different animals: crane, bear, monkey, deer, and tiger. It is easy to learn, and we can learn how to move and position our bodies to increase our balance and well being, and how to meditate through control of the breath to be relaxed and accomplished. We can also use these exercises to stretch, warm up and, prepare ourselves to learn other more complex exercises.

The traditional *Five Animal Exercises*, imitating the movements of Tiger, Deer, Bear, Monkey and Crane, is also known as *Hua Tuo Frolics of Five Animals*, which includes 54 movements in all. The Five Animal Exercises popular in China today were simplified and rearranged by the General Administration of Sport in China, and every exercise has two movements, namely: tiger raising, tiger pouncing, deer colliding, deer running, bear moving, bear shaking, monkey lifting, monkey picking, crane stretching, and crane flying. Each movement needs to be done once bilaterally and symmetrically with the combination of breath regulation. Each exercise function is helpful for the human well-being but in different ways. Specifically speaking, the bear exercise helps develop rooted power, create greater leg strength, fortify the bones, and develop energy in the kidneys, which is the fundamental source of vitality. The tiger tends to develop muscular power, strengthen the waist, sinews, and kidneys, and build internal power. The monkey aims to help you develop agility, be alert, and be nimble. The deer is to develop grace and relaxation, give a long stretch to the legs and spine, and create open and expansive movement with very flexible sinew and bones. Last but not the least, the crane exercise helps to develop balance, lightness, and agility; relax your whole body; balance the heart-spirit; and gently stretch your ligaments and release your spine.

To practice Five Animal Exercises requires the relaxation of whole body, concentration of mind on the *dān tián* (elixer field), even breathing, natural practice, and, unification of body and spirit. There are some tips for the practice: the movement of bear should be steady, nimble and gentle for manifesting its fierce and brave characteristics. The movement of tiger should be practiced firmly and softly with powerful and courageous facial expression. The movement of monkey should be modeled after a monkey's agile and flexible nature. The movement of deer should be practiced with a deer's tranquil and calm attitude. The movement of crane should be practiced with a posture of spreading wings so as to realize the unification of body and spirit. Regular practice can relax the waist and limb joints, strengthen the waist and kidneys, soothe the liver and invigorate the spleen, tonify the heart and nourish the lung, and accordingly attain the goal of enjoying a happy and healthy life, curing diseases, and prolonging life.

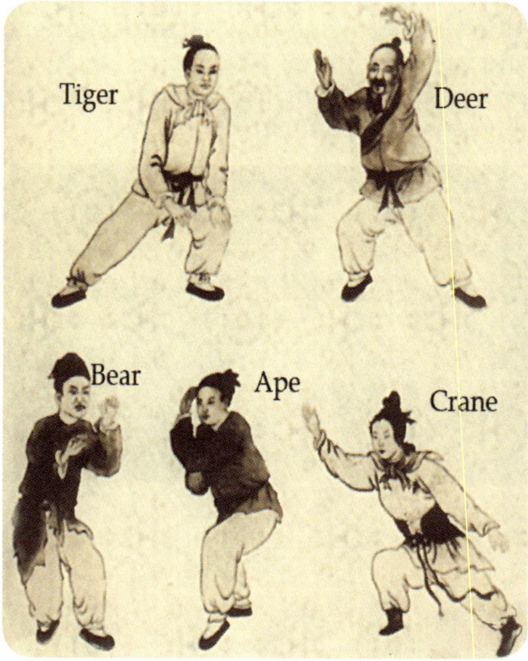

Eight Pieces of Brocade

Eight Pieces of Brocade, originated during the Northern Song Dynasty (960-1,127 A.D.) and has had a time-honored history of over 800 years, is a complete set of independent exercises for health preservation and is one of the commonest forms of Chinese qi gong used as exercise. It was compared to "brocade" by the ancient Chinese, due to its fluent and graceful movement, the silken flow of energy it brought to the body, the delicate arrangement of movements, as well as significant effect on curing diseases and promoting health.

The Eight Pieces of Brocade as a whole is broken down into eight separate exercises, each focusing on a different physical area, channel, and collateral:

➡ Holding up the Sky with Two Hands: regulates the *sanjiao* channel. It includes a pressing upward movement of the palms when the fingers are loosely interlocked while raising the heel. If you are in the right position, there is numbness in both little and ring fingers when raising both hands with palms facing upward.

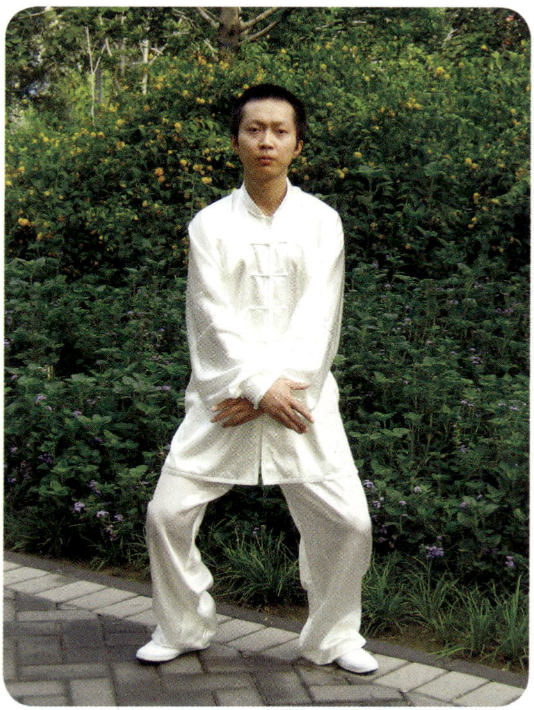

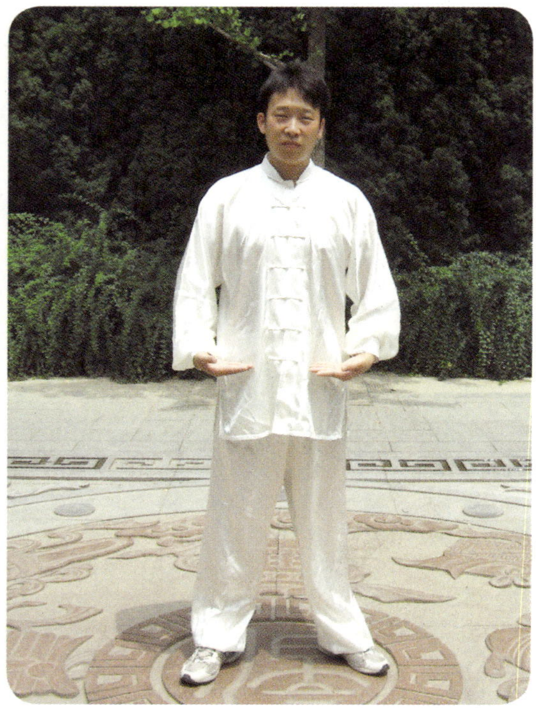

➡ Drawing the Bow like Shooting a Hawk: exercises the waist area, focusing on the kidneys and spleen. With a lower horse stance, the practitioner imitates the action of drawing a bow across the chest to either side. The index finger of the forward hand points upwards while the thumb inclines upwards; there is numbness and distention when practiced correctly.

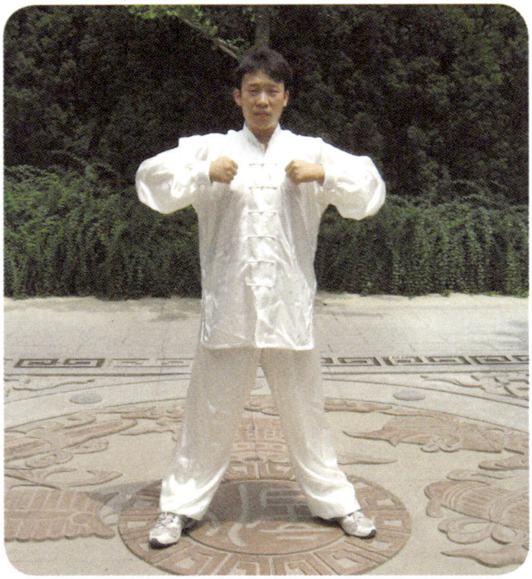

➡ Alternatively raising one arm to regulate the spleen and stomach: resembles a variation of the first movement with one hand pressing upward with the fingers pointing to the opposite side of the body, while another palm presses downward at the side with the fingers pointing forward; one palm up, and one palm down. Switching hand positions over the abdomen and chest in a fluid motion is the main focus.

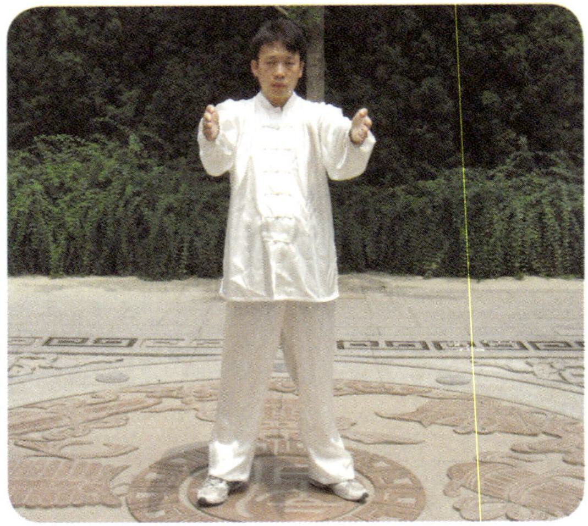

➡ Turning the head backwards or looking back to treat injuries and consumptive diseases: stretches the neck to the left and the right in an alternating fashion. There is no occurrence of diseases with unblocked *ren mai* and *du mai*, which is kept free by turning one's head while pressing one's hands downward.

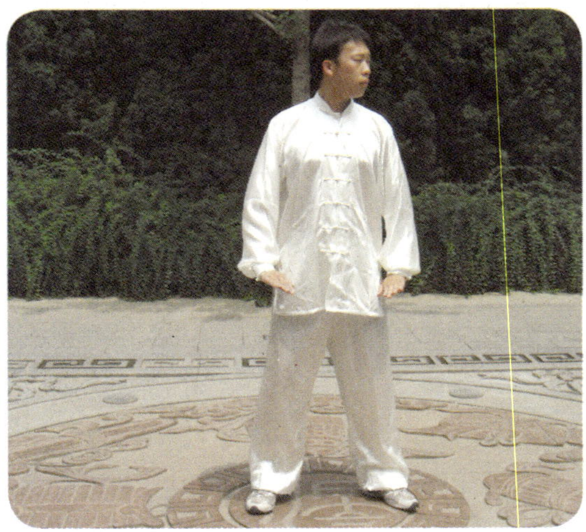

➡ Swaying the head and swinging the buttocks to eliminate the heart-fire: regulates the function of the heart and lungs, with the primary aim of removing excess heat from the heart. The practitioner is suppose to squat in a low horse stance with the hands on the thighs with the elbows facing out and twist to glance backwards on each side.

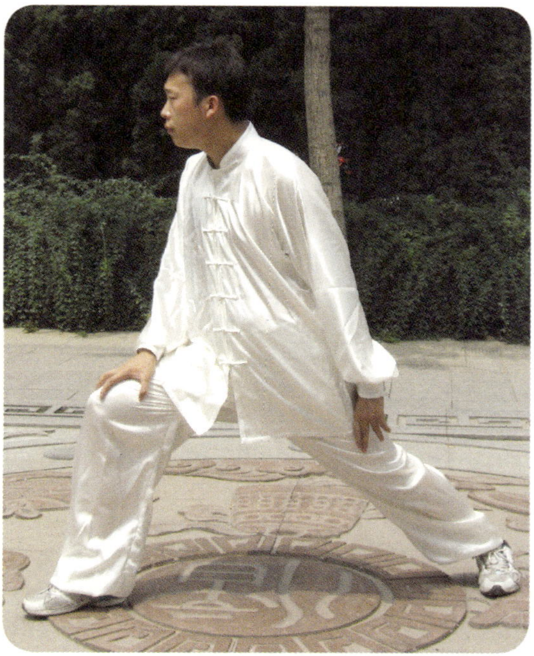

➡ Holding the feet with two hands to reinforce the waist and kidneys: it involves a stretch upwards followed by a forward bend and a holding of the toes. Moving the body forwards and backwards and placing the hands on the life gate (*mìng mén*) to strengthen the kidney.

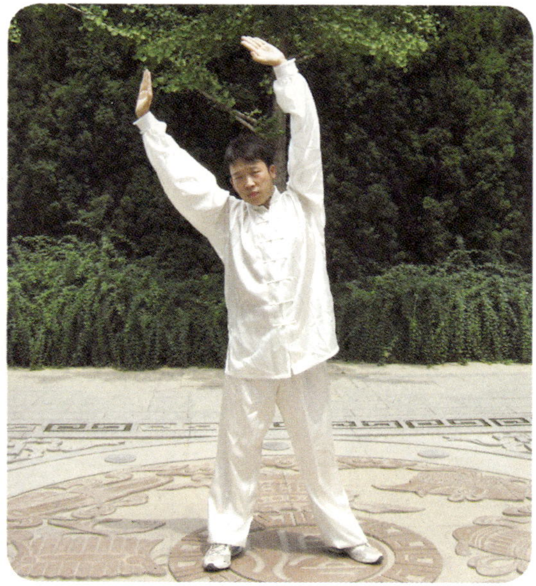

➡ Clenching the fists and glaring angrily to increase power: increases general vitality and muscular strength. It is largely a punching movement either to the sides or forward while in a horse stance.

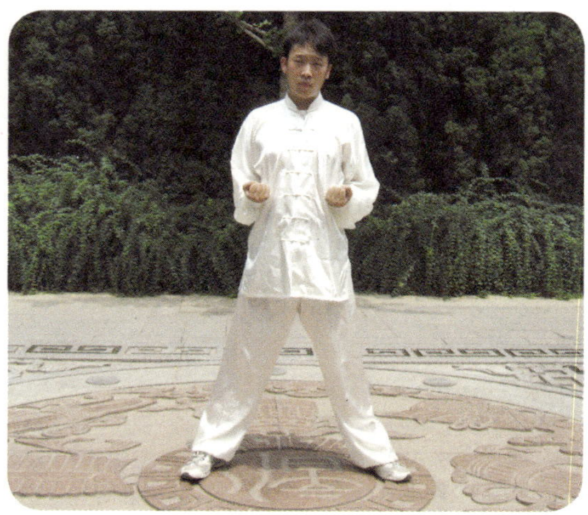

➡ Bouncing on the toes to prevent diseases: the gentle shaking vibration of this movement is to smooth out qi after practicing the previous seven segments. This is a push upward from the toes with a small rocking motion on landing.

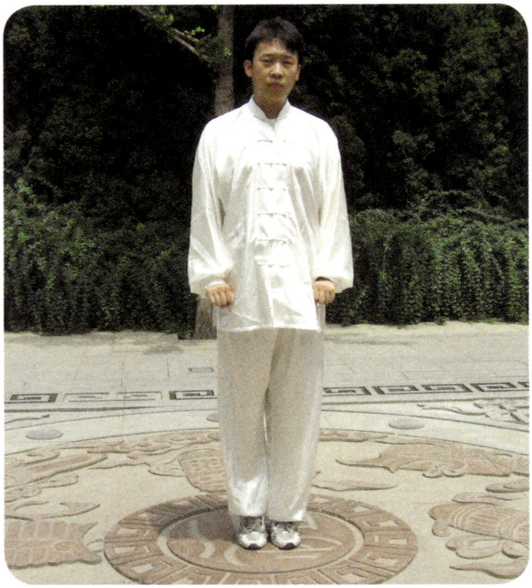

To gain the full benefits of any exercise regimen and reduce the risk of injury, one should learn the correct way to perform the postures and movements. During practice, you should breathe evenly, concentrate the mind on elixir field, and combine softness with hardness. Strict attention to your body position and breathing are critical, so it's best to study directly under a teacher rather than with a book or DVD. The instructor can give you personal guidance and correct any errors in your approach before they become habitual. Appendix 4 lists some information on finding a class near you. For people with depression, it is very hard to get up and moving. Digging yourself out of that dark room is a big challenge, and it may seem impossible at the very beginning, but please at least try to do some exercise step-by-step, and you will be paid back with some immediate relief.

Sound Sleep

We are aware that a good night's sleep can recharge us and make us more effective the next day, and poor sleep can negatively influence all aspects of our lives. Unfortunately, today witnesses an increasing popularity of sleep problems, which may result from stress, physical illnesses, an uncomfortable bed, working different shifts, jet lag, side-effects from some medicines, etc. In addition, depression also commonly causes sleep disturbance, which will cause a great deal of stress for people. Sleep problems can both cause and prolong depression. It is reported that probably more than 80 per cent of people suffering from depression have problems with their sleep -- difficulty falling asleep or staying asleep. Hence restoring healthy sleep patterns is fundamental to your overall wellbeing. Chinese medical diagnosis seeks to identify the root imbalance that leads to the symptom of insomnia.

The Classic of Difficult Issues stated that, "when man is in a peaceful sleep, the spirit goes back to the heart; the ethereal soul returns to the liver; the corporeal soul returns to the lung; the desire returns to the spleen; and the will goes back to the kidney. Only when everything falls into its proper place can sound sleep be possible." That is to say, most chronic insomnia is caused by the disturbance of spirit, ethereal soul, corporeal soul, desire, and will. The reason lies in excessive emotional expression, just like the saying in *The Yellow Emperor's Inner Classic* that "excessive joy impairs the spirit, anger damages the ethereal soul, sorrow hinders the corporeal soul, thought hampers the desire, and fear is harmful to the will." The following therapies are recommended for the treatment of insomnia induced by emotional upset[21]. Some patients respond well to treatment and enjoy a deep sleep 10 days after receiving treatment.

Therapy for Insomnia Caused by Over-Thinking Impairing Spleen

Medicine: *Guī Pí Wán*
Acupoint: RN 8 (*shén què*, 神阙) (navel)
Methods: Mince one pill of *Guī Pí Wán* (Spleen-Restoring Pill, 归脾丸), pour the minced pill into the navel and fix with medicinal gauze and adhesive tape. Apply at night and discard the next morning.

Guī Pí Wán is a famous Chinese medicine formula for replenishing qi and tonifying blood, invigorating spleen, and nourishing the heart is most suitable for treating various symptoms of spleen and heart impairment as a result of excessive contemplation.

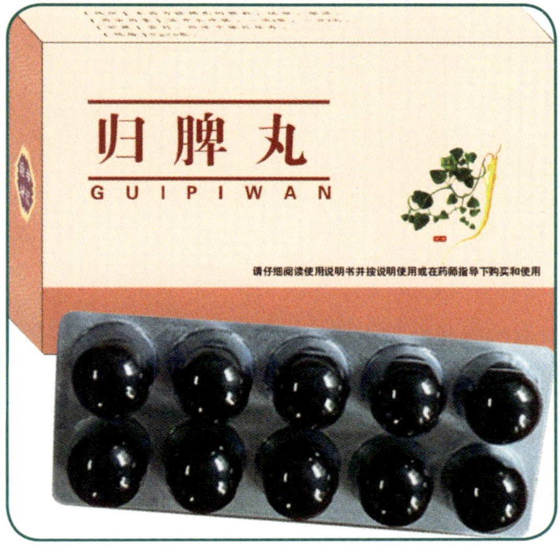

The navel, RN 8 (*shén què*), is a point located on the *ren mai*. RN 8 (*shén què*) is the place where the prenatal life force is received from the mother before birth. The *ren mai* controls all other yin meridians after birth. It runs alone in the midline of the chest and abdomen, connect upwards to the heart and lung, passes through the spleen and stomach, and reaches downwards to the liver and kidney. RN 8 (*shén què*) is both the sea of meridian qi of the *ren mai* and the root of *zang-fu* organs, and has the function of regulating the qi and blood of the whole body. That is to say, the medicine applied externally on RN 8 (*shén què*) can act on the whole body. Meanwhile, RN 8 (*shén què*) is located next to the spleen and stomach, so *Guī Pí Wán* applied on the navel can regulate the spleen and stomach qi promptly and further help patients sleep well. The patients who do not get used to the navel application can also take *Guī Pí Wán* orally. Besides this, taking a walk around a park routinely to breathe in the clear and fresh fragrance from trees and grasses is also helpful for sleep in that the fragrance of grasses and trees tends to be wood in nature and can restrict the thoughts and anxieties that are associated with earth in nature.

Therapy for Insomnia Caused by Over-Sorrow Impairing Lung

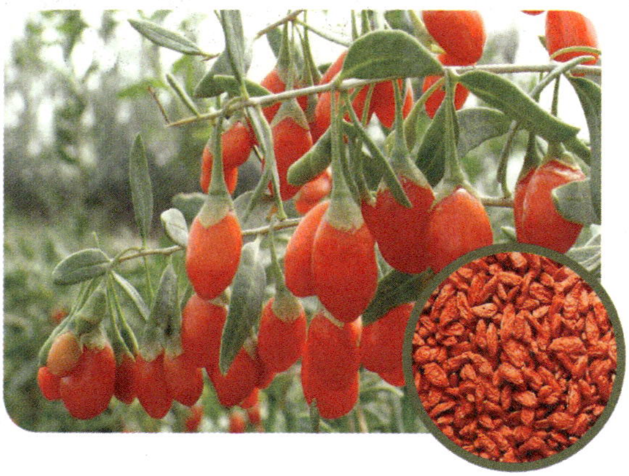

Medicine: *gǒu qǐ zǐ* (Fructus Lycii, 枸杞子)
Acupoint: left LU 9 (*tài yuān*, 太渊)
Methods: Grind few pieces of *gǒu qǐ zǐ*, apply it externally on left LU 9 (*tài yuān*), then fix with adhesive tape. Apply at night and discard the next morning.

Excessive sadness will impair the lung at first. LU 9 (*tài yuān*) is the source point of the lung meridian, in which most original lung qi gathered and from which lung qi runs incessantly to the body as a whole. Therefore, applying medicine to this point can maximize the effect of tonifying the deficiency of lung qi through promoting the lung qi in the channels to converge in the lung. *Gǒu qǐ zǐ*, sweet in flavor, neutral in property, and fresh red in color, corresponds to *Duì* (兑, lake) in *the Book of Changes* (*Yì Jīng*, 易经) and is the optimum acupoint for tonifying and moistening the lung. When being applied on LU 9 (*tài yuān*), the effectiveness of *gǒu qǐ zǐ* lies in its entry an impaired lung along the pathway of the lung channel. Sleep disturbance is relieved when the lung can store the corporeal soul.

Therapy for Insomnia Caused by Over-anger Impairing Liver

Medicine: Mulberry
Acupoint: left LV 3 (*tài chōng*, 太冲)
Methods: Grind one black ripe mulberry, apply it to the left LV 3 (*tài chōng*), then fix it with medicinal gauze and adhesive tape.

Anger impairing liver causes insomnia induced by the smoldering anger, so the liver should be tonified as the first step in treatment. Chinese medicine believes mulberry, sweet in flavor and cold in property, has the function of enriching blood, nourishing yin, and tonifying liver and kidney. It has been widely applied for regulating liver qi since ancient times. LV 3 (*tài chōng*) is the source point of the liver channel in which the original liver qi gathered and remained. Therefore, applying mulberry on LV 3 (*tài chōng*) can tonify liver qi, repair the liver, and get the ethereal soul to return to the liver.

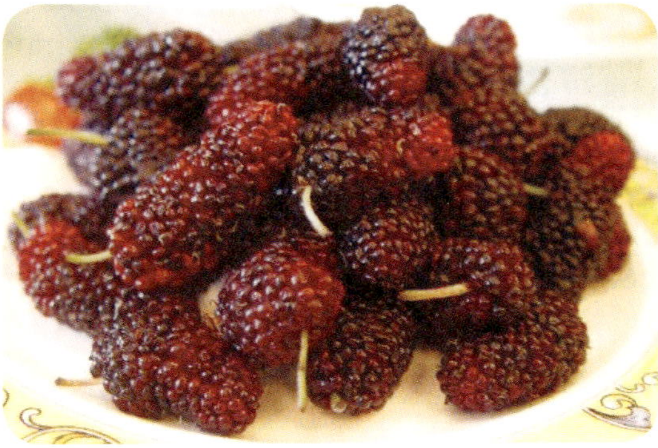

Therapy for Insomnia Caused by Over-fear Impairing Kidney

Medicine: white ginseng slice
Acupoint: left KI 3 (*tài xī*, 太溪)
Methods: Apply one small slice of white ginseng on the left KI 3 (*tài xī*), and fix it with adhesive tape. Apply before sleep at night, and discard the next morning.

When frightened, you may have nightmares or even fail to fall asleep. The reason is that over-fear impairs the kidney will which fails to return to the kidney.

KI 3 (*Tài xī*) is the source point of the kidney channel and plays the role of nourishing kidney yin, tonifying kidney qi, and invigorating kidney yang. Ginseng is most suitable for tonifying original qi, and is beneficial to all the *zang-fu* organs. Hence, the combination of white ginseng and KI 3 (*tài xī*) is applicable for insomnia induced by fear impairing the kidney.

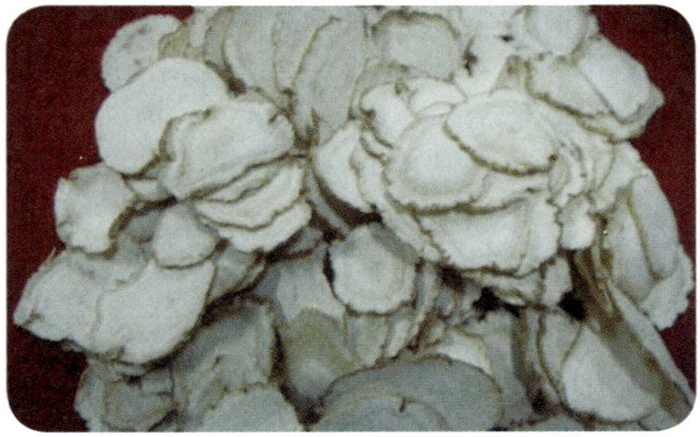

Therapy for Insomnia Caused by Over-anxiety Impairing Stomach

Medicine: *mài dōng* (Radix Ophiopogonis, dwarf lilyturf tuber; ophiopogon tuber, 麦冬) and *mài yá* (Fructus Hordei Germinatus, germinated barley, 麦芽)
Acupoints: left PC 6 (*nèi guān*, 内关) and HT 7 (*shén mén*, 神门)
Methods: Remove the wheat husk of *mài yá*, grind the sprouts and apply on the left PC 6 (*nèi guān*), then pound *mài dōng* into pieces and apply on left HT 7 (*shén mén*). Apply before sleep at night and discard the next morning.

The Yellow Emperor's Inner Classic states, "There is sleep disturbance when the stomach is in disharmony." Hangover, irregular diet, and the taking of cold raw food impair your stomach qi impairment, which may further cause you to toss and turn, and have trouble falling asleep.

PC 6 (*nèi guān*) is the connecting point of the pericardium channel, which is primarily responsible for the movement of wind-qi around the spleen and stomach. As stomach disharmony is mostly caused by wind invasion, the problems can be solved by means of externally transferring the wind-qi through PC 6 (*nèi guān*). *Mài yá* is effective in fortifying the spleen and increasing appetite. The combination of them is helpful to recover stomach qi harmony.

Mài dōng has the function of nourishing the heart yin, while HT 7 (*shén mén*) is the source point of the heart meridian. With the same role as *Tiān Wáng Bǔ Xīn Dān* (Celestial Emperor Heart Supplementing Elixir, 天王补心丹), applying *mài dōng* on HT 7 (*shén mén*) can supplement vital qi to the heart immediately. Heart belongs to fire while stomach belongs to earth; fire can generate earth, so to supplement the qi of the heart actually tonifies the stomach.

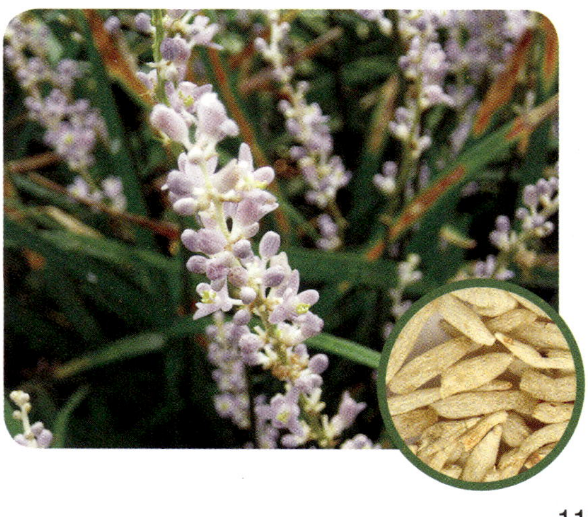

Therapy for Insomnia Caused by Disrupted Heart Spirit

Medicine: dry lotus leaf (Folium Nelumbinis, *hé yè*, 荷叶) and *mài dōng* (Radix Ophiopogonis, dwarf lilyturf tuber; ophiopogon tuber, 麦冬)
Acupoints: right GB 38 (*yáng fǔ*, 阳辅) and left HT 7 (*shén mén*, 神门)
Methods: Crumble lotus leaf into pieces and apply it on the right GB 38 (*yáng fǔ*), then grind *mài dōng* and apply it on left HT 7 (*shén mén*), fix with adhesive tape. Apply before sleep at night, and discard the next morning.

Insomnia of this the kind is due to the invasion of fire into heart channel that normally should circulate within the gallbladder channel and *sanjiao* channel. Therefore, attention should not only be paid constraining fire and guiding it back to the gallbladder and *sanjiao* channels, but also regulating imbalanced heart qi.

GB 38 (*yáng fǔ*) is the river point of the gallbladder channel, and the fire-qi within it is the major reason for insomnia. With the function of dissipating fire, lotus leaf can dredge the aggressive excessfire when being applied on the right GB 38 (*yáng fǔ*).

As mentioned above, applying *mài dōng* on HT 7 (*shén mén*) can tonify heart qi. Spirit can be governed by the heart if there is sufficient heart qi, and insomnia can be cured accordingly.

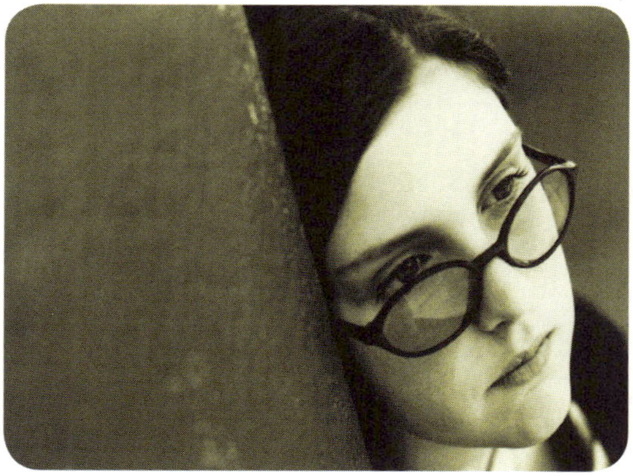

Therapy for Insomnia Caused by Common Cold

The common cold can also lead to poor sleep. For patients suffering from insomnia of this kind, the formula *Guì Zhī Tāng* (Cinnamon Twig Decoction, 桂枝汤) is useful. Typically, insomnia of this kind is accompanied with the symptom of sweating, headache, runny nose, floating pulse, etc.

Sleep disturbances and depression are closely related. The longitudinal studies of sleep researcher Michael Perlis, Ph.D. shows that insomnia appears to precede episodes of depression by about five weeks, indicating that insomnia may be an early harbinger of depression if he is right. In Chinese medicine, depression is caused by emotional expression either excessive or lengthy, which also triggers the sleep disturbance. And the symptomatic treatment mentioned above should be utilized in accordance with your own condition.

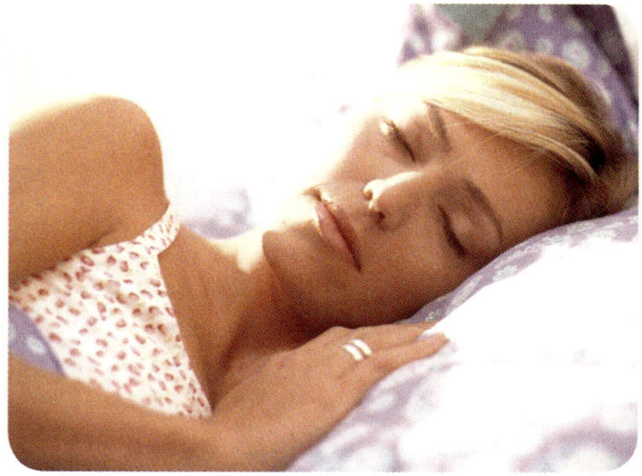

Maintain Interpersonal Relationships and Say What You Think

Experts say it is difficult for a patient to overcome depression without the help from the outside. Whenever faced with a depressing task or situation, patients should tell their best friends or family members instead of holding those bad feelings back and addressing them alone. Maintaining this kind of interpersonal relationship can effectively prevent and treat depressive syndrome. As a specialist in depression, Dr. Edington points out there are many social groups providing support for patients with depression in the United States. People can talk about their stress and problems without fear of discrimination. This is very helpful for the treatment of depression. Dr. Li Chang-min also emphasizes the importance of communication. For instance, the topics of suicide and death, which are taboo in Chinese society, should be discussed more openly. When being asked whether the patient has ever considered suicide, the patient will discuss his feelings concerning his anguish, and would be more willing to tell what is giving him trouble at the present. Thus, an extreme reaction, like suicide, can be prevented.

In Chinese medicine, the seven emotions directly affect the corresponding *zang-fu* organs, "excessive anger impairs the liver, excessive joy harms the heart, excessive contemplation impairs the spleen, excessive grief or melancholy impairs the lung, and excessive fright or fear hurts the kidney." Furthermore, the relationship between and among those *zang-fu* organs are complicated, the impairment of one *zang-fu* organ will eventually lead to the abnormality of other organs. For instance, depression and anger impair the liver, and the subsequent adverse flow of liver qi frequently attacks the spleen and stomach, resulting in the imbalance between the liver and the spleen as well as the disharmony between the liver and the stomach. The abnormal emotions also influence qi activity of the *zang-fu* organs and lead to the dysfunction in ascending, descending, going out, and coming in of qi. Specifically speaking, over-joy makes the qi of the heart sluggish, over-anger causes the qi of the liver to move upwards, over-thinking causes the the qi of the spleen to be depressed and stagnated, over-sorrow makes the qi of the lung exhausted, over-fear induces the qi of the kidney to dissipate and descend, and over-fright causes the disturbance of qi.

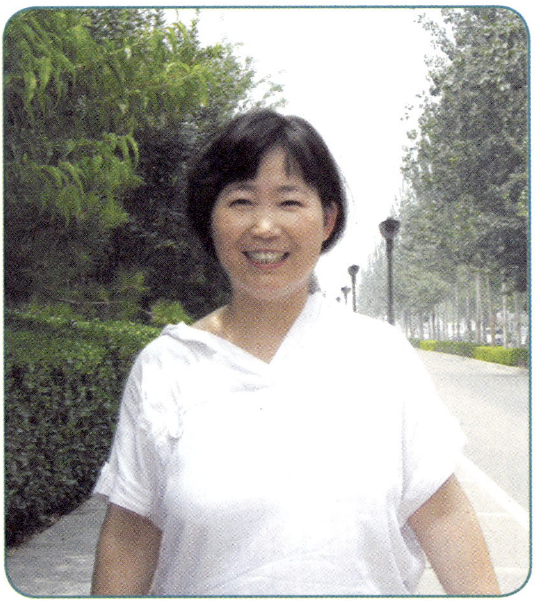

Hence, Chinese medicine encourages people to prevent the seven emotions causing harm, achieve mental peace, and relieve qi stagnation through regulating and controlling feelings and giving expression to the accumulated depression. Doctors are expected to use words to persuade, encourage, comfort, delight, and direct the patient, and switch the concentration or attention of a patient from one thing to another. The psychology of Chinese medicine stresses the understanding of emotions and their relationship to the internal organ systems and their influence on health. Meanwhile, the five-phase theory plays an important part in treating such emotional disturbance as depression and anxiety.

Preserving Health Based on Midday-midnight Law

Midday-midnight law is a well-known empirical law in Chinese medicine stating that the circadian rhythm of the internal organs influences their paired organs according to the time of day. M.S. Lee, et al.,[22] used a digital readout instrument to measure electrical conduction properties at 12 acupoints corresponding to the 12 meridians at four times: 12:00, 14:00, 22:00, and 24:00. The result displayed the mean current values of 12 acupoints changed significantly over time ($P<0.0001$), suggesting the existence of some type of daily variability in electrical current.

➡ The period from 5 AM to 7 AM (*mǎo shí*, 卯时), qi and blood move to the large intestine channel. The normal function of the large intestine is to defecate. During these hours, it will be beneficial to defecate normally. Undefecated stool can become retained stool and its toxin stays in the body longer. With the function of transporting secreted waste, the large intestine may get diseases if there are dietary irregularities, eating unclean food, or disharmony of other organs. Frequent problems of the large intestine can easily cause dry mouth and tongue, abdominal distention and pain, or gastroenteritis, typhlitis, intestinal function disorder, habitual constipation, and so on. Therefore, the habit of defecation every morning is beneficial for avoiding the formation of retained stool.

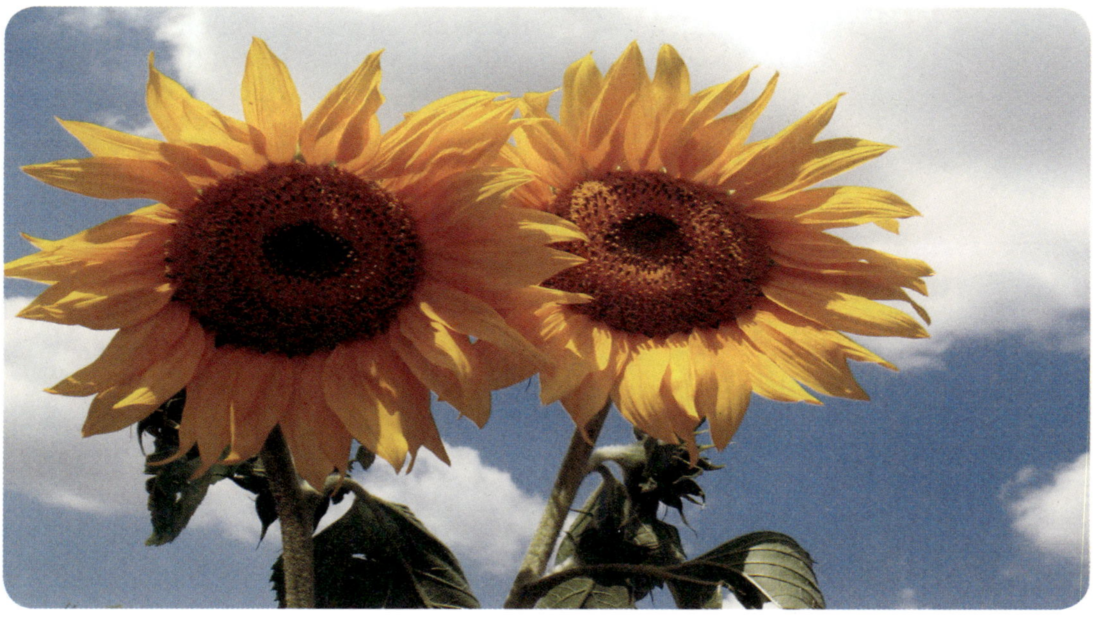

➡ The period from 7 AM to 9 AM (*chén shí*, 辰时), qi and blood move to the stomach channel. The normal function of the stomach meridian is to help in digestion. Food taken in during this period is most easily digested, absorbed, metabolized, and utilized, and thereby supplies the necessary calories for the whole day. There may be symptoms present such as distention and pain, vomiting and regurgitation, bad breath, and dyspepsia when the intestine and stomach get impaired. Having a regular breakfast early every morning is most beneficial to the health.

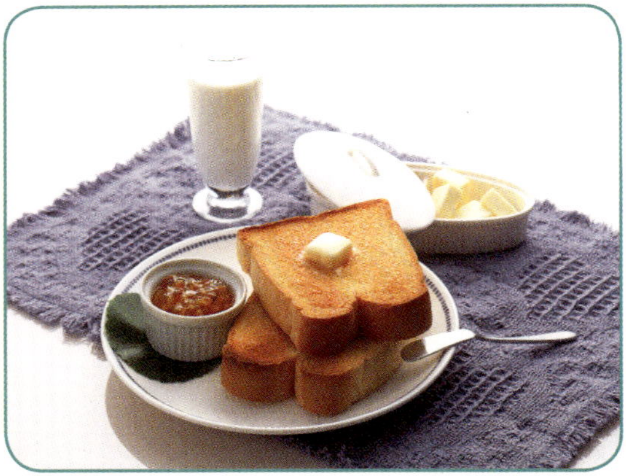

➡ The period from 9 AM to 11 AM (*sì shí*, 巳时), qi and blood move to the spleen channel. The normal function of the spleen meridian is to help both the absorption of nutrition and hematosis. Deficiency of spleen is often manifested as poor appetite, lassitude of extremities, dizziness, sallow complexion, abdominal distention, hiccup easily, etc. It is inadvisable to take drier and hotter food during this period.

➡ The period from 11 AM to 1 PM (*wǔ shí*, 午时), qi and blood fill in the heart channel. The normal function of the heart meridian is to help blood circulate throughout the whole body, and heart-fire generating stomach-earth will help digestion. In light of the heart governing blood-vessels and spirit, maintenance and rest should be stressed. If there is an obstacle to blood movement, such disorders as irritation, insomnia, and sores in the mouth will occur.

➡ The period from 1 PM to 3 PM (*wèi shí*, 未时), qi and blood move to the small intestine channel. The normal function of the small intestine is to help in food absorption. The small intestine has the function of separating the clear and the turbid, and absorption. Deficiency of the small intestine is often manifested as vexation, thirst, abdominal distention and pain, diarrhea, disturbance of nutrition, weight loss, poor appetite, enteritis, etc.

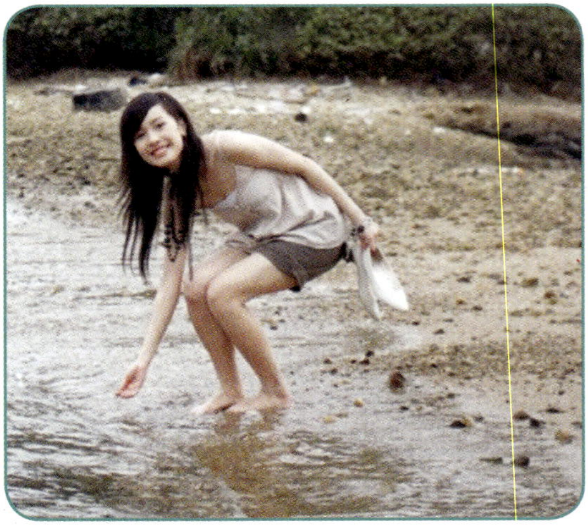

➡ The period of the day from 3 PM to 5 PM (*shēn shí*, 申时), qi and blood move to the bladder channel. The normal function of the bladder channel is to discharge fluid downflow from the small intestine and dredge fire from all over the body. The bladder is the main organ in the urinary system, and can store and discharge urine; symptoms may include: inhibited, frequent, or turbid urine when the bladder is deficient.

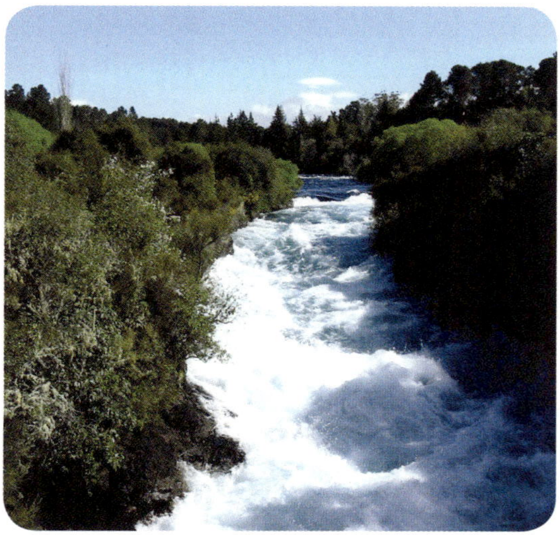

➡ The period from 5 PM to 7 PM (*yǒu shí*, 酉时), qi and blood move to the kidney channel. The normal function of the kidney is to help store the essence of the *zang-fu* organs for a whole day. The kidney meridian is responsible for coordinating two basic life energies, yin and yang, and is closely connected with the heart, liver, spleen, and lung. If the kidney is deficient, there will present symptoms such as cold extremities, apathetic spirit, soreness and weakness of waist and knees, dizziness, tinnitus, insomnia, poor memory, menopause, etc.

➡ The period from 7 PM to 9 PM (*xū shí*, 戌时), qi and blood abound in the pericardium channel. The normal function of the pericardium meridian can enhance the power of the heart once again, which is to help digestion because heart fire generates stomach earth. The pericardium refers to the surrounding tissue next to the heart, which can protect the heart from external attack. But there may be symptoms present such as hot palms, swelling of the armpit or chest and hypochondrium, palpitation and restlessness, and a sallow complexion when illness strikes.

➡ The period from 9 PM to 11 PM (*hài shí*, 亥时), qi and blood move to the *sanjiao* channel. The *sanjiao* passes through all vessels which get recharged after the person falls asleep. The *sanjiao* meridian is mainly responsible for governing the various forms of qi which are all transported and spread to each organ through the *sanjiao*. If there is a disorder in the meridian, there are often symptoms present such as auditory masking, swelling of the throat, sore throat or eyes pain, tinnitus, pain of both posterior and lateral parts of the shoulder, and elbow and forearm pain. The period from the beginning of *hài* (亥) time at 9 PM to the ending of *yín* (寅) time the following day's 5 AM is the right time for body cells to get rehabilitated and metabolized, so one can only have a good physical state with enough rest. People go to sleep late for all sorts of reasons, doing work and taking rest according to one's own biological clock, but it is advisable to fall asleep no later than 11 o'clock at night.

➡ The period from 11 PM to 1 AM (*zǐ shí*, 子时), qi and blood move to the gallbladder channel. The normal function of the gallbladder meridian is to help produce bile and bring forth the new through the old. The physiological function of the gallbladder is storing bile interiorly, and assisting the digestion and metabolism of food. Irregular sleep exerts an influence on recirculating qi and blood to the gallbladder meridian, which can easily cause dizziness, blurred vision, tinnitus, rough skin, chest and hypochondrium pain, insomnia and dreaminess, aversion to fear, anxiety, neurosis, etc. Adults should go to sleep before *zǐ* (子) time every night, otherwise they will grow old faster than normal.

➡ The period from 1 AM to 3 AM (*chǒu shí*, 丑时), is the exact time when qi and blood is abounding in the liver channel. Liver blood will bring forth the new during this period. The liver has the function of storing, distributing, and regulating the blood all over the body, and soothing functional activities of the whole body, which maintains harmony between qi and blood. Additionally, liver is related to the eyes. When the liver meridian is in disorder, there will be symptoms such as hypochondrium distending pain, chest distention, poor appetite, a bitter taste in the mouth, abdominal distention and pain, black specks in the peripheral vision, eyelid pouches, black eyes, and so on.

➡ The period from 3 AM to 5 AM (*yín shí*, 寅时), the lung channel functions most strongly. During this period, qi and blood begin to transfer from yin to yang, while the lung meridian transports fresh blood stored in the liver to all vessels. So attention should be paid to the maintenance of the lung meridian, regulation of air temperature, and especially, the use of an air conditioner in summer. Impairment of the lung meridian will cause fever and aversion to coldness, nasal blockage with secretion, headache, asthma, chest distress, chronic bronchitis, and emphysema. A person with a deficient lung meridian is liable to cough during this period.

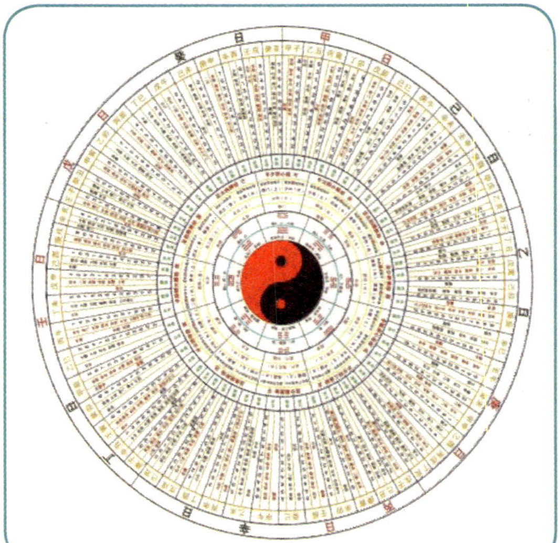

3. Research and References

➡ **Irwin MR** et al.[23] designed a randomized controlled trial with 16 weeks of teaching followed by practice and assessment 9 weeks later in order to determine the efficacy of a novel behavioral intervention, Tai Chi Chih (太极智), to promote sleep quality in older adults with moderate sleep complaints. Design: The main outcome measure was sleep quality, as assessed by the Pittsburgh Sleep Quality Index (PSQI). Setting: General community at two sites in the US between 2001 and 2005. Participants: Volunteer sample of 112 healthy older adults, aged 59 to 86 years. Intervention: Random allocation to Tai Chi Chih or health education for 25 weeks. Results: Among adults with moderate sleep complaints, as defined by PSQI global score of five or greater, subjects in the Tai Chi Chih group were more likely to achieve a positive response, as defined by PSQI less than five, compared to those in health education ($P<0.05$). Subjects in the Tai Chi Chih condition with poor sleep quality also showed significant improvements in PSQI global score ($P<0.001$) as well as in the sleep parameters of rated sleep quality ($P<0.05$), habitual sleep efficiency ($P<0.05$), sleep duration ($P<0.01$), and sleep disturbance ($P<0.01$). This study concluded that Tai Chi Chih can be considered a useful nonpharmacologic approach to improve sleep quality in older adults with moderate complaints and, thereby, has the potential to ameliorate sleep complaints possibly before syndromal insomnia develops.

➡ **Kerr CE** et al.[24] conducted research on the relation between Tai Chi (TC) and enhanced tactile acuity. Experienced adult TC practitioners were recruited and compared to age-gender matched controls. A blinded assessor used a validated method Van Boven et al. in Neurology 54 (12): 2230-2236, 2000 to compare TC practitioners' and controls' ability to discriminate between two different orientations (parallel and horizontal) across different grating widths at the fingertip. Study results showed that TC practitioners' tactile spatial acuity was superior to that of the matched controls ($P<0.04$). There was a trend showing TC may have an enhanced effect on older practitioners ($P<0.066$), suggesting that TC may slow age-related decline in this measure. The author stated that to the best of his knowledge, this was the first study to evaluate a long-term attentional practice's effects on a perceptual measure. Longitudinal studies are needed to examine whether TC initiates or is merely correlated with perceptual changes and whether it elicits long-term plasticity in primary sensory cortical maps. Further studies should also assess whether related somatosensory attentional practices such as yoga, meditation, and qi gong achieve similar effects.

➡ **Mustian KM** et al.[25] randomized women who completed treatment for breast cancer to receive T'ai Chi Ch'uan (TCC) or psychosocial support therapy for 12 weeks (one hour, three times weekly). The results showed that TCC group demonstrated significant improvements in functional capacity, including aerobic capacity, muscular strength, and flexibility, as well as quality of life (QOL); the psychosocial support therapy group showed significant improvements only in flexibility, with declines in aerobic capacity, muscular strength, and QOL. It concluded that the TCC group exhibited significant improvements in functional capacity and QOL. This data suggest that TCC may enhance functional capacity and QOL among breast cancer survivors.

➡ **Wang Y**[26] conducted a study to examine the effects of Tai Chi exercise on college students' perceptions of their physical and mental health. A three month Tai Chi intervention (one hour, twice/week) was administrated to 30 college students. The SF-36v2 health survey questionnaire was employed to evaluate the mental health dimension (MHD) and physical health dimension (PHD) before and after the intervention by means of a paired T test ($p<0.05$). PHD including physical functioning, role physical, bodily pain, general health, and MHD including social functioning, role mental/emotional function, vitality, and perceptions of mental health were assessed. Results: Physical measures of bodily pain and general health, and mental measures of role mental/emotion function, vitality, and mental health were significantly improved after Tai Chi intervention. When the overall PHD or MHD scores were evaluated, the MHD increased significantly. This study concluded that Tai Chi exercise had positive effects on the self-assessed physical and mental health of college students. Scores on the MHD appeared to be particularly sensitive to change. Colleges/universities might consider offering Tai Chi as a component of their ongoing physical activity programs available to students.

➡ **Tsang HW** et al.[27] released findings of a randomized controlled trial conducted in Hong Kong to further the understanding of the psychosocial effects of qi gong on elderly persons with depression. Eighty-two participants with a diagnosis of depression or obvious features of depression were recruited and randomly assigned into the intervention and comparison group. The intervention group was given a 16-week period of qi gong practice while the comparison group participated in a newspaper reading group with the same duration and frequency. After eight weeks of qi gong practice, the intervention group participants outstripped themselves in improvement in mood, self-efficacy, and personal well being, as well as self-esteem when compared with comparison subjects. After 16 weeks of practice, the improvement began to effect all aspects of their lives. This report showed that regular qi gong practice could relieve depression, improve self-efficacy and personal well being among elderly persons with chronic physical illness and depression.

➡ **Kim SD** et al.[28] performed a study to investigate the effects of a relaxation breathing exercise on anxiety, depression, and leukocyte count in patients who underwent allogenic hemopoietic stem cell transplantation. Thirty-five patients were randomly selected, with 18 assigned to an exercise group and 17 assigned to a control group. The exercise intervention was applied to the exercise group for 30 minutes every day for 6 weeks. It consisted of physical exercises combined with relaxation breathing. Anxiety was measured by the State-Trait Anxiety Inventory and depression was measured by the Beck Depression Inventory. The total number of leukocytes was calculated from total and differential counts of peripheral white blood cells. The exercise group had a greater decrease in anxiety and depression than the control group did, but the total number of leukocytes did not significantly differ between the two groups. These findings indicate that a relaxation breathing exercise would improve anxiety and depression levels in patients who undergo allogenic hemopoietic stem cell transplantation, but would not affect the number of leukocytes.

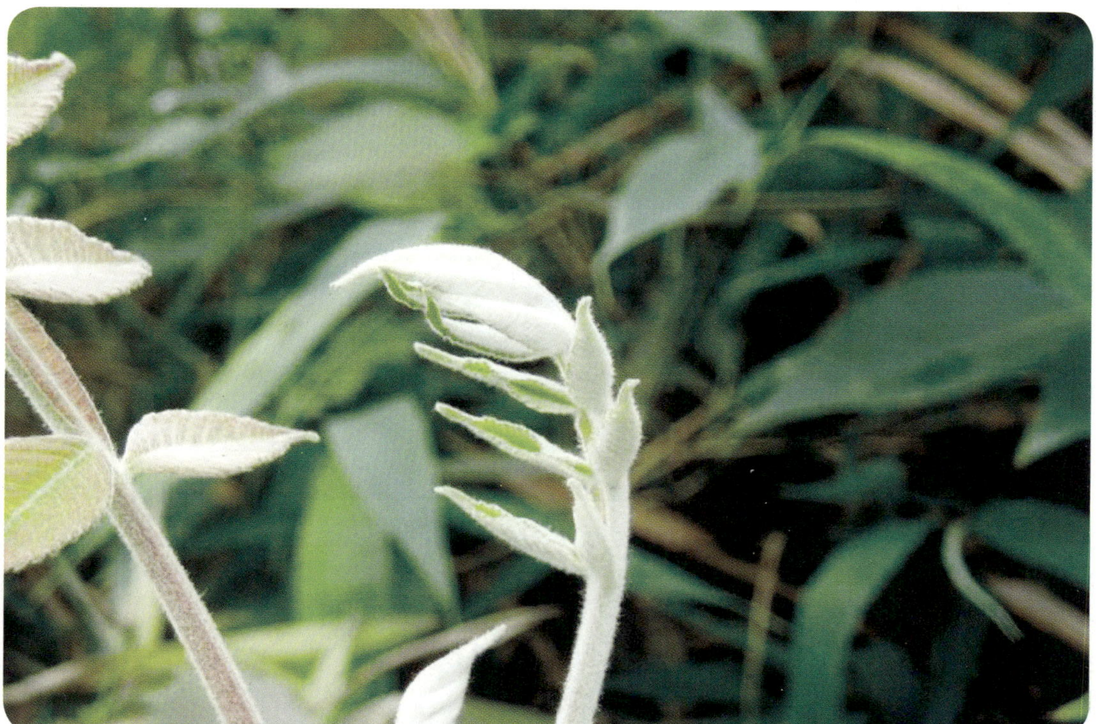

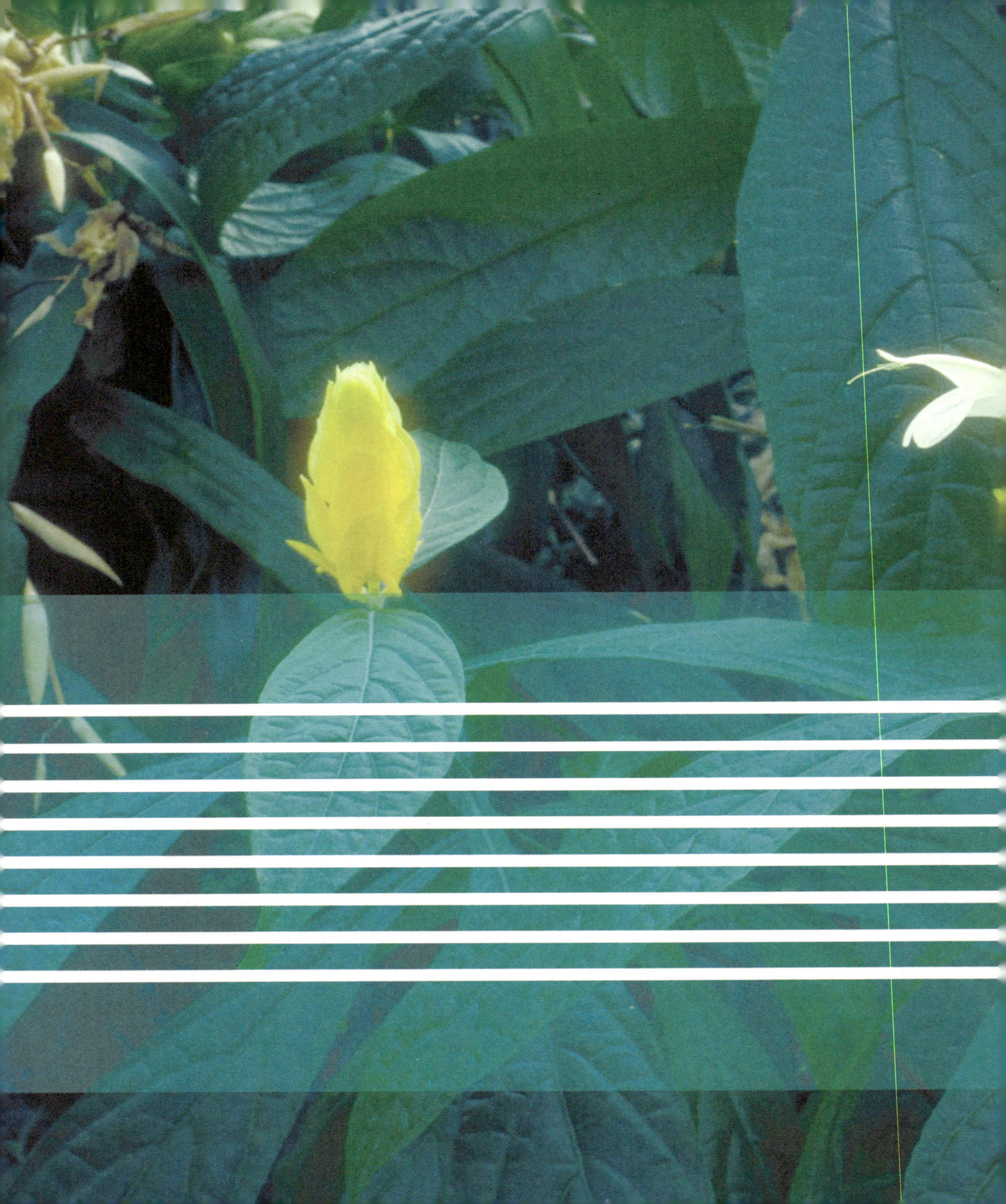

Chapter 4

How Is Depression Treated with Chinese Medicine?

Acupuncture and Moxibustion

1. What Is Acupuncture and Moxibustion?

Acupuncture is among the oldest healing practices in the world and the most commonly practiced form of Chinese medicine. As an important pillar of Chinese medicine, acupunture aims to restore balance and maintain wellbeing by using very fine needles at specific points, which are believed to be situated on energy channels called *jīng luò* (channels and collaterals).

Zhēn Jiǔ (针灸) is the Chinese term that refers to acupuncture and moxibustion, the treatment methods that have been characteristic of Chinese medicine for thousands of years. Acupuncture involves the insertion of very thin sterile needles into certain points on the body in order to influence the flow of qi. Today, this time-tested therapy continues to be validated and treats a wide range of health problems, though the way in which acupuncture works may seem mysterious.

Acupuncture began to become better known in the United States in 1971, when New York Times reporter James Reston wrote about how doctors in China used needles to ease his pain after surgery.[29] These days, acupuncture is everywhere. Searching online, one can read hundreds of reports of research involving the scientific exploration of this ancient art. Acupuncture has been proven effective in cases from cardiology to psychology. As the most studied treatment of Chinese medicine, acupuncture has become accepted as a therapy for certain conditions in the United States. Promising results have been found for the use of acupuncture in treating nausea and vomiting related to chemotherapy, postsurgery pain, and pregnancy.[30] The report from a Consensus Development Conference on Acupuncture held at the National Institutes of Health (NIH) in 1997 stated that acupuncture is being "widely" practiced, by thousands of physicians, dentists, acupuncturists, and other practitioners, for relief or prevention of pain and for various other health conditions. According to the 2007 National Health Interview Survey (NHIS), which included a comprehensive survey of CAM use by Americans, an estimated 3.1 million U.S. adults and 150,000 children had used acupuncture in the previous year. Between the 2002 and 2007 NHIS, acupuncture use among adults increased by three-tenths of 1% (approximately one million people).[31] One reason these techniques are so popular is that they are absolutely safe when properly administered by a trained acupuncturist, even though the thought of

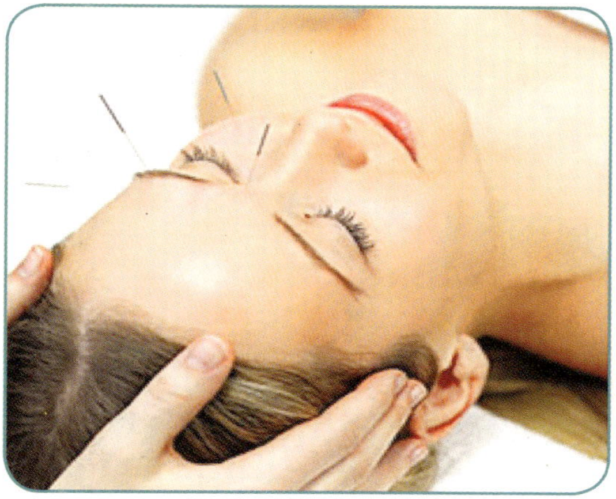

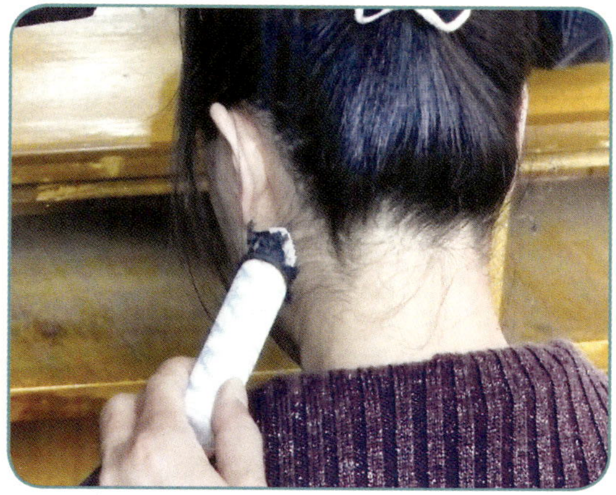

being needled can be unsettling to many first-time patients. For most people in the West, it is difficult to understand how a fine needle inserted into the foot can relieve a headache, why moxibustion to a toe can reverse a fetus' position, or how puncturing a spot on the wrist can manage insomnia. All of these actions are easily explained in the language of Chinese medicine, but there are still many theories on what exactly is at work in modern scientific terms.

Moxibustion is the application of heat using a small bundle of tightly bound medicinals (dry moxa leaves) that are ignited and held about an inch above the skin over targeted acupoints. By applying heat stimulation to certain points the practitioner can regulate the yin-yang balance of the internal organs to prevent disease and preserve health. Based on the same theories as acupuncture, it is another type of external treatment method. The material used in moxibustion is usually made of artemisia leaves, commonly called mugwort. The Chinese medicinal medical classic *Miscellaneous Records of Famous Physicians* (*Míng Yī Bié Lù*, 名医别录), based on the legendary *Shen Nong's Classic of the Materia Medica* (*Shén Nóng Běn Cǎo Jīng*, 神农本草经), states that artemisia leaves are bitter, slightly warm, without any toxicity, and should be used in moxibustion to manage various types of diseases. Artemisia leaves, warm in nature, can promote the flow of qi and blood, remove dampness and cold, and dissolve masses and accumulations in order to cure illness, prevent disease and maintain health. In general, moxa is available in a loose form which either can be used for making moxa cones, or can be packed and rolled in a long stick like a cigar 15-20 cms. in length and 1-2 cms. in diameter. Moxibustion, the ancient precursors to modern acupuncture needles, has been used for thousands of years, even longer than stone needles. In the language of Chinese medicine, the major actions of moxibustion are to regulate yin and yang by supplementing yang, improve the circulation of qi and blood in the channels, help the body fight invading pathogens, supplement qi and blood, and regulate the internal organs. These functions illustrate how moxibustion can prevent disease and delay aging. A single treatment of moxibustion usually lasts 10-15 minutes. Attaching a moxa stub (about 2 cms. long) to an inserted needle, known as needle-warming moxibustion, is usually used for expelling cold and damp, tonifying qi and blood, or enhancing the effects of needling. Like acupuncture, much research has been done on the effects of moxibustion on the body. Presently, it is widely used as an effective supplement to acupuncture treatment.

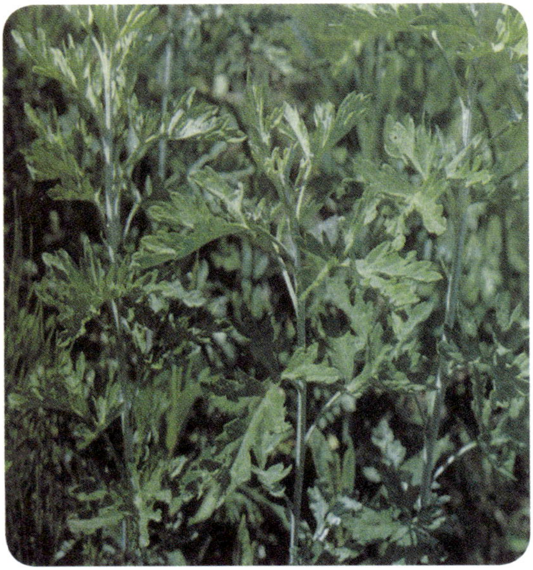

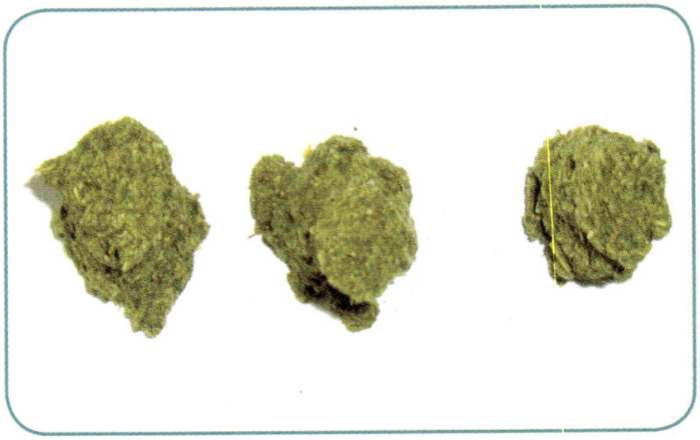

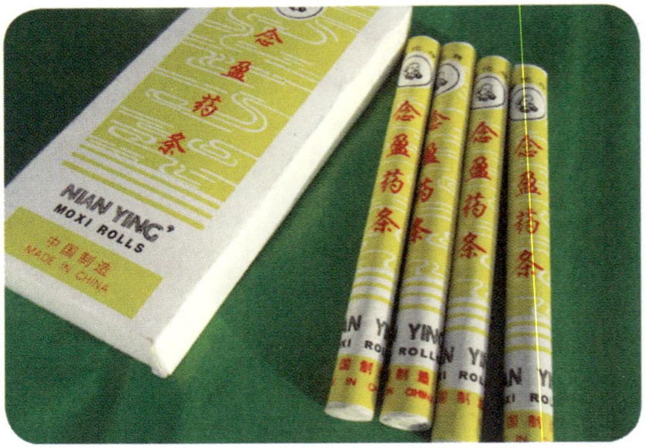

What Is *Jīng Luò* and *Shù Xué?*

In order to understand acupuncture and moxibustion better, an understanding of *jīng luò* (channels and collaterals) and *shù xué* (acupoints) based on Chinese medical theory is necessary. According to the NIH consensus statement on acupuncture, these traditional Chinese medical concepts "are difficult to reconcile with contemporary biomedical information but continue to play an important role in the evaluation of patients and the formulation of treatment in acupuncture."

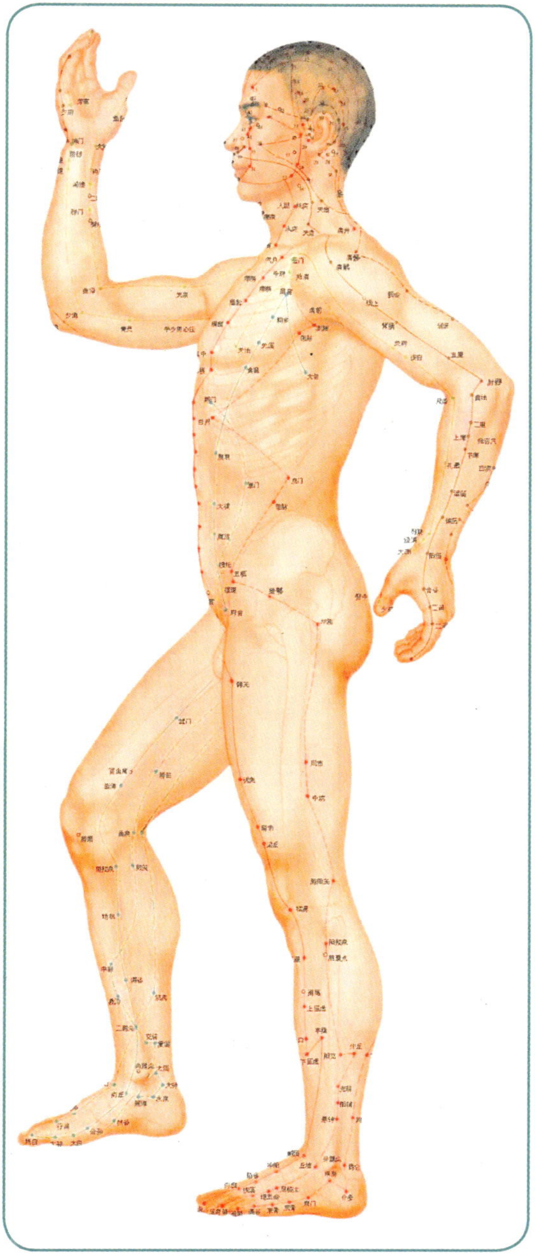

In Chinese medicine theory, the human body is an organic whole and the internal organs, external surface, and extremities are connected to each other by a network called the *jīng luò* (channels and collaterals). According to this theory, the channels and collaterals connect the internal organs with the external surface and extremities by transporting qi and blood. Chinese medicine states that "as long as qi runs freely through the channels and collaterals and the organs work in harmony, the body can avoid disease." Channels and collaterals are invisible pathways through which qi flows and forms an energy network that connects all body structures and the body in an organic whole with the universe. Like the system of highways and roads that connects the different parts of the city, the channels and collaterals is the network that connects the different parts of the body. When the streets in a city are blocked with traffic, this will bring troubles to the city. This metaphor offers an approach to understand how blockages in meridians can cause problems in organs. An acupuncturist may perform treatment along tiers of pathways, commonly the twelve primary channels that circulate throughout the body. Other pathways include the eight extraordinary vessels, the collaterals, the divergent collaterals, and the twelve sinew channels. An analogy can be made between this network and the earth's water system, with big rivers as the main thoroughfares, and the tributaries as smaller branches, so the land is closely connected. Acupuncture and moxibustion are applied according to this system. Most of the main acupoints (*xué wèi,* 穴位) are on the twelve primary channels and two of the eight extraordinary vessels (*du mai* and *ren mai*). There are also "extra points" not belonging to any channel and tender points known as *ashi* points which are generally used for treatment of local pain. By stimulating the points, or the gates of this network, the human body will be influenced, moving naturally towards healing. Acupoints are the openings of these channels and collaterals. Inserting needles into these points will stimulate or block the flow of qi and blood. When properly administered, the flow of qi and blood will be smoothed and organ functions will be restored. Weakness is strengthened while excess is reduced. Therefore balance is restored and health is regained. More than three hundred acupoints are identified by Chinese medicine, each of which has its own therapeutic action. For instance, the point LI 4 (*hé gǔ,* 合谷), located on the dorsum of the hand between the first and second metacarpal bones, can relieve constipation, control irregular menstruation, improve facial paralysis, and reduce pain in the head and mouth. The point HT 7 (*shén mén,* 神门), located on the medial end of the transverse crease of the wrist, can relieve angina pectoris, improve palpitation and dysphoria, and induce relaxation.

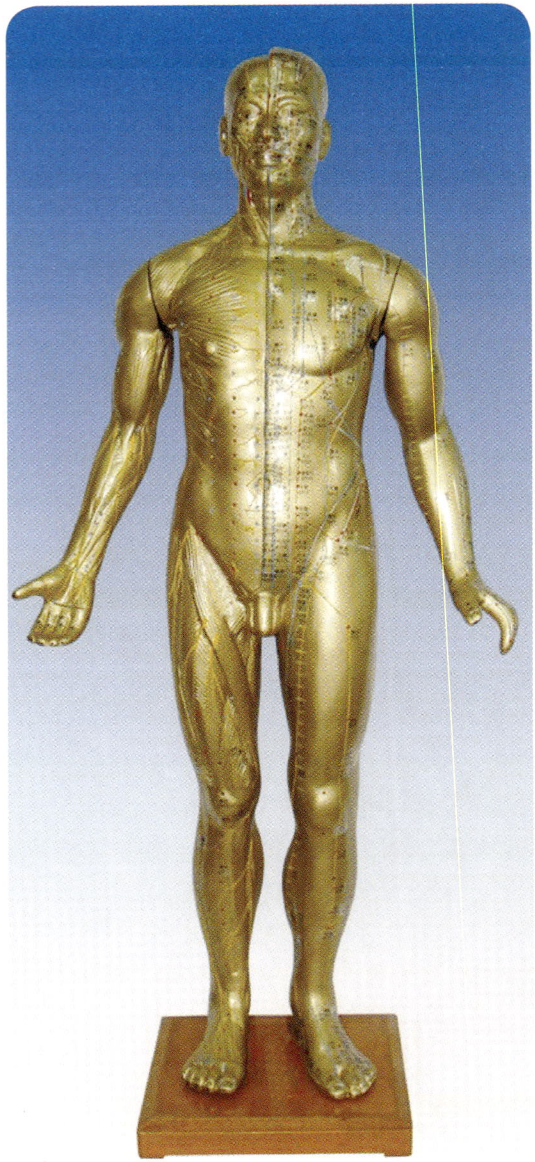

System of Channels and Collaterals

- System of Channels and Collaterals
  - Channels
    - Twelve Primary Channels
      - Three yin channels of hand
        - Hand lung taiyin channel
        - Hand pericardium *jueyin* channel
        - Hand heart *shaoyin* channel
      - Three yang channels of hand
        - Hand large intestine *yangming* channel
        - Hand *sanjiao shaoyang* channel
        - Hand small intestine *taiyang* channel
      - Three yin channels of foot
        - Foot spleen *taiyin* channel
        - Foot liver *jueyin* channel
        - Foot kidney *shaoyin* channel
      - Three yang channels of foot
        - Foot stomach *yangming* channel
        - Foot gallbladder *shaoyang* channel
        - Foot bladder *taiyang* channel
      - Appendix
        - Twelve divergent channels
        - Twelve sinew channels
        - Twelve cutaneous regions
    - The Eight Extraordinary Vessels
      - *Du mai*
      - *Ren mai*
      - *Chong mai*
      - *Dai mai*
      - *Yangqiao mai*
      - *Yinqiao mai*
      - *Yangwei mai*
      - *Yinwei mai*
  - Collaterals
    - Divergent collateral
    - Superficial collateral
    - Minute collateral

Amazingly, channels and collaterals are sensitive to time and place. They reflect and respond to the changing energy of the seasons, the time of day, and the climate of a particular place.[32]

Types of Acupuncture Needles

Currently, the most common acupuncture needles are called filiform needles, which are normally between 0.5 and 1.5 inches long (1.5-4.5 cms.), but can be up to 5 inches (15 cms.) depending on the location of the point to be needled and the size of the patient. Although gold and silver needles are sometimes used, needles are usually made of stainless steel. The needles are used on one patient and then disposed of in a medical "sharps" container. Other types of acupuncture needles including three-edged needle, plum-blossom needle, and intradermal needle are still popular with clinics in China. A three-edged needle looks like a lance and is used to prick blood vessels for the therapeutic purpose of blood letting. A plum-blossom needle, also known as seven star needles, is a group of seven filiform needles arranged together in the form of a flower and attached like a hammer head to a long handle. It can be used to tap the skin along a channel or at specific points lightly and swiftly. Intradermal needles are very thin and very short, which is often used to treat chronic disease. Inserted to a very shallow depth in the skin, it is left in place and covered with waterproof tape. The press needle is inserted more deeply than the intradermal needle, its insertion is perpendicular to the skin's surface rather than angled like the insertion of the intradermal needle. Both intradermal needles and press needles can be used for auricular (ear) acupuncture.

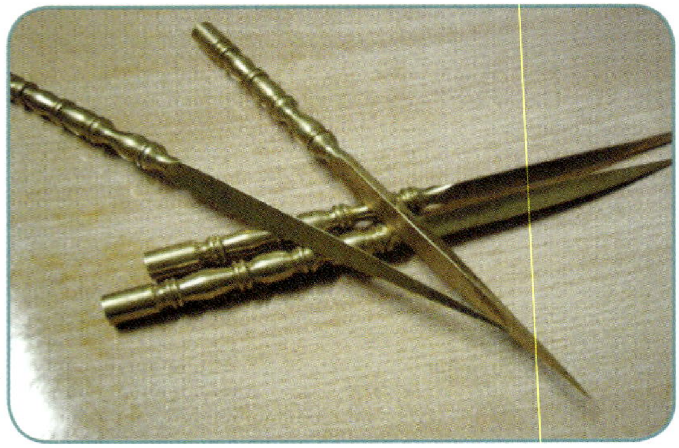

Three-edged Needle

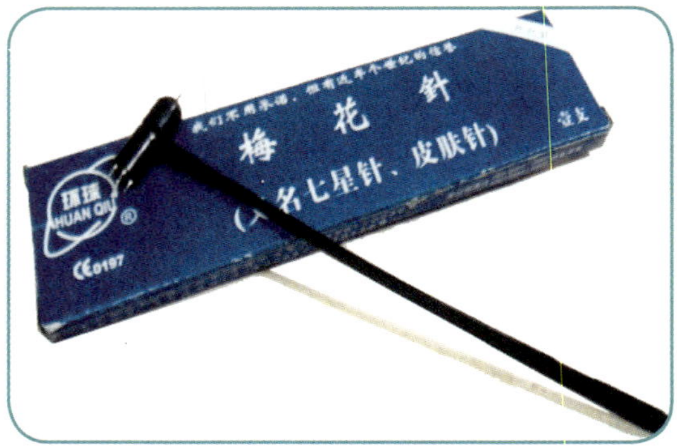

Plum-blossom Needle

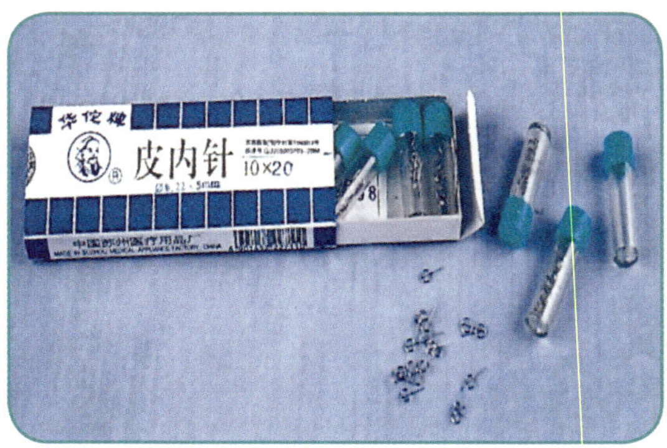

Intradermal Needle

Acupunture Positions and Clean Needling Practice

Different positions are used based on the points selected. As long as the patient feels comfortable, any position is suitable.

Acupuncturists are required to take a course called the "Clean Needle Technique" to train them how to handle, insert, and remove needles so both patient and practitioner are protected from any kind of contamination. The acupuncurist will wash his or her hands thoroughly with soap and water before and after treatment, and the points to be needled will be disinfected by swabbing the point with a cotton swab dipped in 70% alcohol. Anything that punctures the skin will be sterile, and any other implements used in treatment will be thoroughly sanitized between patients. The needles must be sterile, nontoxic, and labeled for single use by qualified practitioners only.[33] So far, relatively few complications from the use of acupuncture have been reported to the FDA, in light of the millions of people treated each year and the number of acupuncture needles used.[34] It is still worth noting that acupuncture may also result in such serious adverse effects as infections and pneumothorax due to inadequate sterilization and improper delivery of treatments.

Types of Moxibustion

> Direct moxibustion

Direct moxibustion uses what are called moxa cones. These are usually shaped to roughly half an inch (1.5 cms.) high, placed directly on acupoints, lit, and left in place until the cone is burnt out or until the sensation becomes painful. This is a strong form of treatment and can produce pain, blisters, and even scarring. Some Chinese traditions still deliberately induce scarring, which is believed to have the strongest effect. This form of treatment is usually reserved for serious cases being managed by experienced practitioners. It should not be used nearby sensory organs such as the eyes, mouth, nose, or anus, on the face and breast, on the place where large blood vessels are located or on major creases such as elbows and knees. Additional care must be paid when burning moxa on areas of numbness or when the patient is in coma.

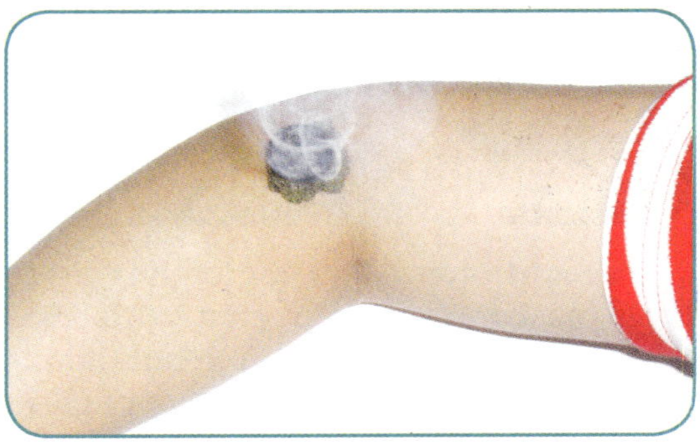

> Indirect moxibustion

The second, more common form of moxibustion is indirect moxibustion. It involves either the use a cigar-shaped moxa pole, or the burning of moxa cones on top of a layer of ginger, garlic, or salt. With a moxa pole, a practitioner holds the stick roughly 1.5 inches (3 cms.) above the skin and holds it in place until the skin becomes red or appears congested. When garlic, ginger, or salt is used with moxibustion, they provide a buffer from the heat of the moxa as well as adding their own properties to the therapeutic effect. These forms of treatment do not usually cause severe pain or leave any blisters or scars, though the skin may remain red for a while.

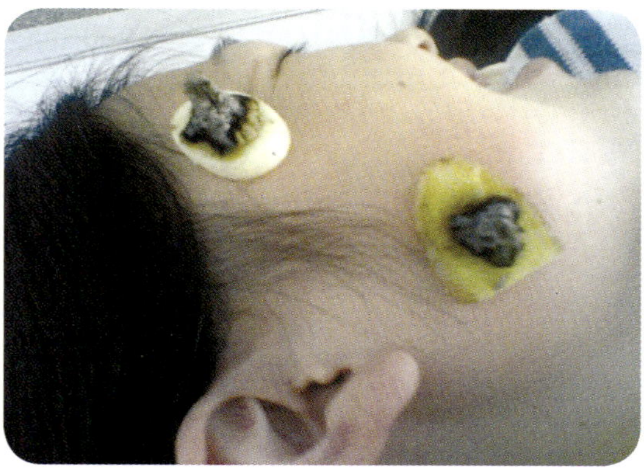

Practitioners also sometimes place the moxa cone on top of an acupuncture needle and burn it. If good ventilation is not available, heat can also be applied to points from an electrical source designed for the purpose as well.

Moxibustion is not for everyone. It is indicated mainly for patients suffering from cold, dampness, or stagnation. It is not used regularly on anyone diagnosed with too much heat (e.g. fever), nor on the back or lower abdomen of pregnant women. But if there are isolated problems such as pain, injury, or digestive problems, moxa may be used.

How Does Acupuncture and Moxibustion Work?

There have been recent studies on acupuncture and whether it works for certain health conditions such as depression, headache, and paralysis; what happens in the brain or in the body during acupuncture; and what is the better way to identify the potential neurological properties of the channels and collaterals and the acupoints. The underlying mechanism is still being researched. There exist many theories as to how acupuncture may affect the human body, and each one can explain part of the picture. In studies of its pain-relief effect, researchers found that acupuncture blocks the impulse transmissions between the spinal cord and brain, stopping pain by closing the nerve fibers that carry impulses. This is a common theory and often referred to as the gate control theory. Various other theories also attempt to answer the question from different angles. The theory of boosting immunity involves levels of important substances such as white blood cells, antibodies, triglycerides, and gamma blovulins are raised during treatment and this stimulates the immune response. Another theory involves endorphins, which act to both stop pain and promote a sense of wellbeing, are stimulated through acupuncture. Neurotransmitter studies indicate that levels of seratonin and noradrenaline are altered during treatment. The circulatory theory states that the release of vasodilators, which cause blood vessels to constrict and dilate. According to the World Health Organization (WHO), acupuncture is an effective treatment for mental-emotional conditions such as anxiety, depression, stress, and insomnia. Besides this, in general acupuncture has few to no side-effects, it is very safe when done by a certified acupuncturist, and can be used safely in combination with drug therapy and psychotherapy. Futhermore, it helps integrate the therapeutic components of psychotherapy.[35]

NIH has established the National Center for Complementary and Alternative Medicine which funds research studies in holistic treatments. In 1998, researchers used acupuncture to treat a sample of women with depression and found after a total of 12 sessions, 70% of the women experienced at least a 50% reduction of symptoms. This research marked the first U.S. randomized, controlled, double-blind study of acupuncture's effectiveness in treating depression. The NIH-funded study concludes, "Acupuncture may alter brain chemistry by changing the release of neurotransmitters and neurohormones in a good way". Researchers found that moxibustion at acupoint Ren 4 (*guān yuán*) on sarcoma S180 ascitic mice increased the decreased erythrocytic C3b receptor rosette-forming rate, decreased the raised immunocomplex rosette-forming rate, and increased activity of erythrocytic immunosuppressive factor in tumor-bearing mice, initiating moxibustion strengthens erythrocytic immunity.[36]

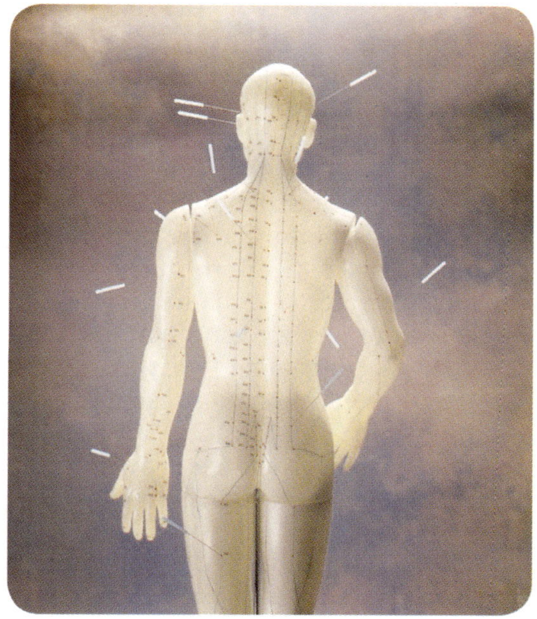

What we can conclude from these theories is that acupuncture acts on many targets. A synthesized drug has a definite target and expected effects together with expected side-effects as well. The function of acupuncture is done in reverse by stimulating the body's power to regulate its own function and relieving localized symptoms. The relief of symptoms are only "side-effects" of the general changes going on at the root level. And the effectiveness of an acupuncture treatment is strongly dependent on an accurate Chinese medical pattern differenciation, sufficient stimulation of properly selected acupoints, as well as sophisticated needling skills and techniques of the practitioner. Psychological support is also an important factor in all healing experiences.

2. What Can I Expect?

During your first visit, you may be asked at length about your health condition, lifestyle, and behavior. After collecting detailed information (symptoms, signs, tongue inspection, pulse taking, and environment) and obtaining the whole picture of your condition, the Chinese medical practitioner will identify the pattern of disharmonies present. Based on this pattern identification, an optimal treatment protocol will be drawn up according to theories of Chinese medicine.

The practitioner will then decide which modality (needles, moxa, cupping, etc.) to use during the present treatment. Usually needling is performed and often one or more additional treatment modalities are used. The number and location of the needles is decided by the acupuncturist and will probably vary from treatment to treatment, though some points will remain the same and begin to feel familiar. The points that remain the same are usually for your underlying root condition, while the points that change frequently are often to deal with whatever symptoms are most serious at the time of treatment. An acupuncture needle is metallic, solid, and hair-thin. The number of needles is not set and can be as few as two or three or as many as 30, but usually is around 5 to 15. Needles are mainly placed on the abdomen, back and limbs, with points on the scalp and face also used from time to time. The depth of the needles is determined by the specific points since the amount of flesh is different throughout the body. The length of needles is also decided by the acupuncturist and normally is between 0.5 and 1.5 inches (1–3 cms.).

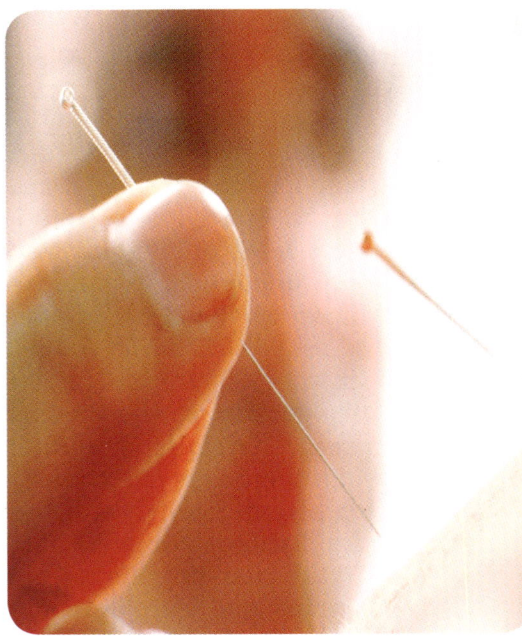

The needles are inserted quickly at an angle of 15 to 90 degrees in relation to the skin's surface. When an experienced acupuncturist inserts the needles, there is not usually any pain. The sensation is at most like being bitten by an ant. Acupuncture needles are much finer than the hypodermic needles used in hospitals. But most importantly, trained acupuncturists can insert the needles quickly and correctly without causing unnecessary discomfort. Once the needle has been inserted, if the point is correctly located and the required depth reached, the patient is supposed to get a specific sensation called "*dé qì*." *Dé qì* is a sensation specific to acupuncture treatment and literally means "obtaining the qi." The exact feeling varies with each individual patient. It is usually not pain but a unique sensation of soreness, heaviness, distension, or radiation in some direction. While the acupuncturist will simultaneously feel that the needle is tightened. It is generally believed that the stronger the *dé qì* sensation is, the more effective the acupuncture treatment will be. By acupunture treatment, some people feel energized and refreshed, others feel relaxed. However, improper needle insertion, movement of the patient, or a defect in the needle can cause soreness and pain during treatment. So it is important to seek treatment from a qualified acupuncturist.

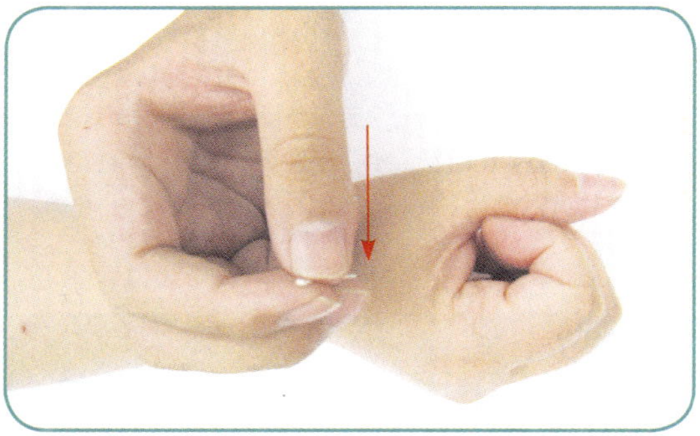

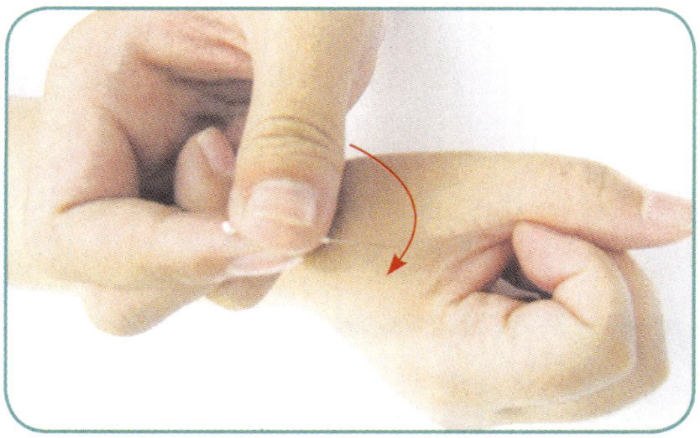

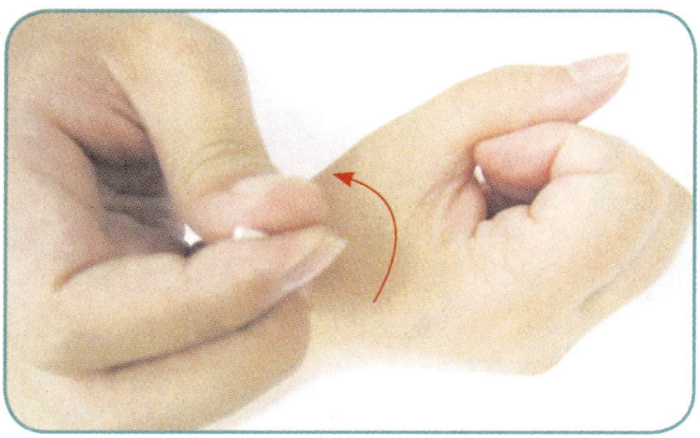

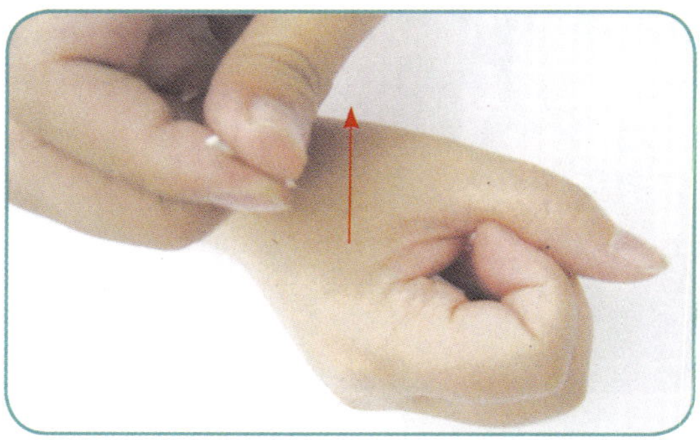

The needles are usually left in for 20-30 minutes. During this time the needles may be manipulated to achieve better therapeutic effect. According to treatment specification for the health issue, there are a variety of techniques like raising, thrusting, twirling, plucking, and scraping, which strengthen the stimulation and sensation. The technique used will depend on the disease that is being managed. After a few treatments, patients usually start to enjoy this sensation because it is both pleasant and they know the good results it brings. During manipulation, it is best to relax and move as little as possible, unless the practitioner asks you to. Too much movement might cause the needles to bend, get stuck, or even break. These accidents are very rare, but if anything happens, stay calm and let the practitioner remove the needles immediately.

After the needles are inserted, the patient is usually left to relax for about 20-30 minutes. During the process, needling may also be activated by electrical stimulation, a procedure usually called electroacupuncture, in which manipulations are obtained through changing frequencies and voltages. Currently, it is possible for an electrical impulse to be sent through the acupuncture needles that mimics constant manipulation. Practitioners are trained to operate the machines in the safest way and the amount of power sent through the needles is usually only a few microamperes. Electroacupuncture is commonly used for problems that require constant needle stimulation. The machine will allow the practitioner to do other work while the point is receiving stimulation. Originally from China, this technique is commonly used in many countries. The frequency and the amount of power used in electroacupuncture tend to vary to a great degree depending on the patient's condition and the practitioner's decision.

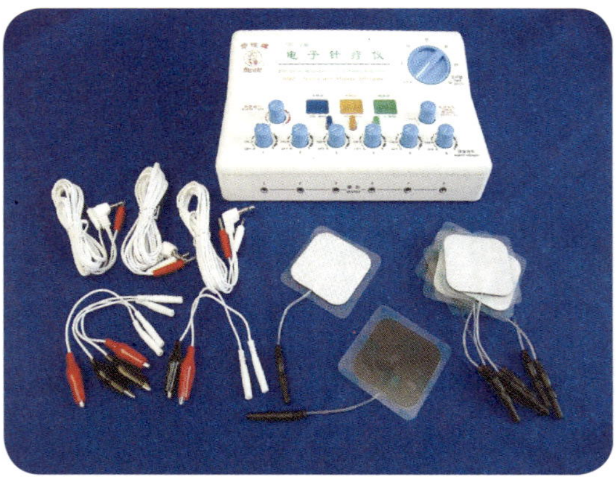

Electric Acupuncture Instrument

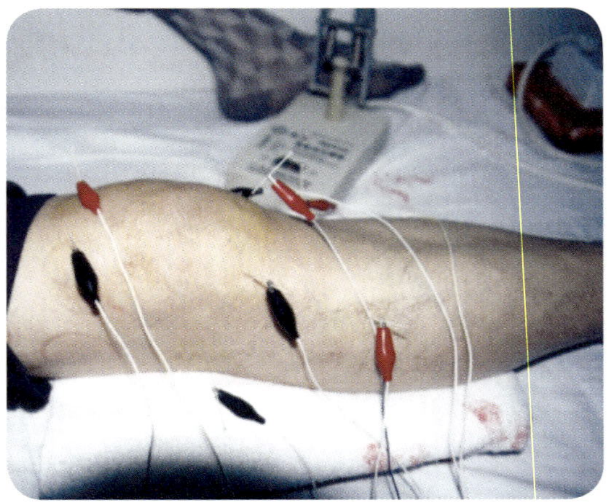

Other techniques such as moxa or cupping can be performed before or after needling, depending on the practitioner. After the needles are removed, get up slowly and carefully. There is normally no bleeding during or after acupuncture treatments. If bleeding occurs, it will only be a few drops due to the breakage of small capillaries. Bruising is also very rare, but sometimes happens due to subcutaneous bleeding also from broken capillaries.

After treatment, you will probably feel relaxed and energized. Some of your symptoms may disappear instantly. You may sleep better, have a more regulated appetite, feel less pain, or experience less anxiety. Even though most patients begin to feel some relief after the first several treatments, acupuncture works on a very deep level, and to effect lasting change, ample time must be given. In some cases, people with chronic disease use acupuncture as their last option because they urgently want to get better, but the journey to health with Chinese medicine is like everything else in the natural world, there will be ups and downs, times of rapid growth and times of hibernation. With commitment and good communication between practitioner and patient, the journey can be life changing.

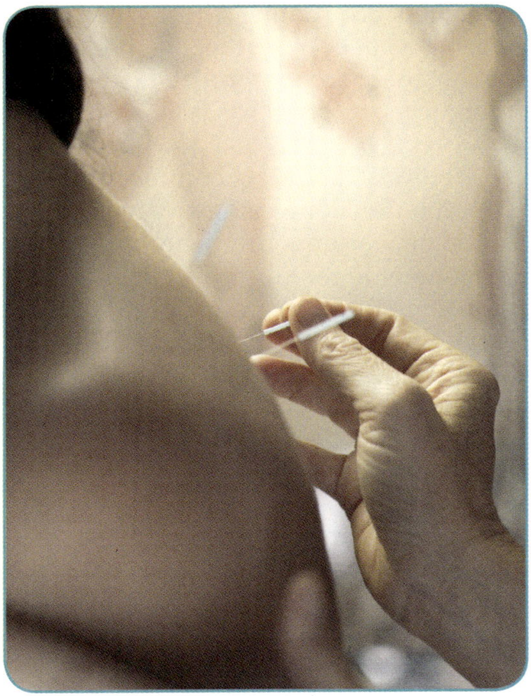

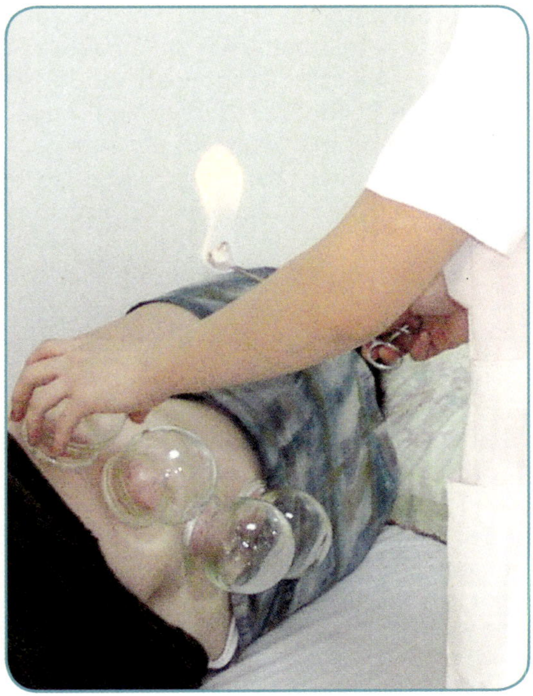

In rare cases a patient will be over responsive to the treatment. This usually occurs when a patient is extremely hungry, weak, nervous, or the stimulation and *dé qì* sensation is too strong. The patient might experience nausea, possibly vomiting, develop a very pale complexion, feel weak, sweat excessively, or even faint. If this happens, the acupuncturist will remove all the needles and allow the patient to lie down and rest for a while. Normally the patient will recover quickly. If the patient still feels unwell, a few points may be needled that will help relieve the patient's symptoms.

It is advised to be in the best condition possible when you have your acupuncture treatments. Don't come for your acupuncture treatment when you are very hungry or just after a big meal, and try to be rested. Get the most out of your treatment by being extra careful of your general health the day before and after treatment. Help Chinese medicine help you!

Before you start treatment, ask the practitioner about the expected number of treatments needed, how much each treatment will cost, whether acupuncture is covered by your insurer, and if yes, to what extent. A typical treatment course for depression will be once every other day for about seven days. After this the practitioner and patient will reevaluate and decide on future treatment. Since depression is a chronic disease, treatment will often take no less than one month.

Commonly Used Acupoints

There are hundreds of acupoints on the human body, most of which are situated along 14 main channels. Some of the points are more commonly used than others. The points selected in the treatment of certain disease can vary greatly, according to the patterns, the patient, and the practitioner's experience. The final prescription of point selection depends on your specific condition and the practitioner's judgment. The action of every point is to regulate yin and yang, the difference is in what way each point works exactly. Some points work on the qi aspect, while others may work on the blood; some are warming, and others are cooling. Most point functions have not been verified by modern research, but for some of the more important points, some research has been done.

Below is a list of commonly used acupoints for depression treatment.[37] Of course all patients are different, so not everyone will get all of these points. But since some of these are major points, everyone is likely to experience at least a couple of these points during the course of treatment.

> DU 20 (*bǎi huì*, 百会)

DU 20 is an important point to open the orifices, tranquilize mind, calm the liver to relieve interior wind, and fortify qi to restore prolapse.

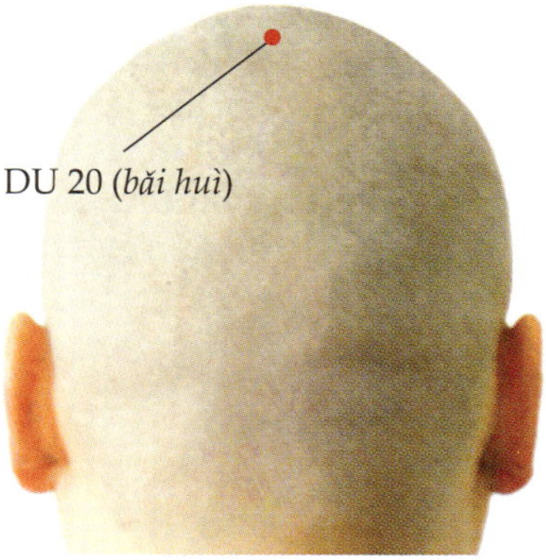

DU 20 is located on the *du mai*, seven cun directly above the posterior hairline, approximately on the midpoint of the line connecting the apexes of both ears.

> *Sì shén cōng* (四神聪)

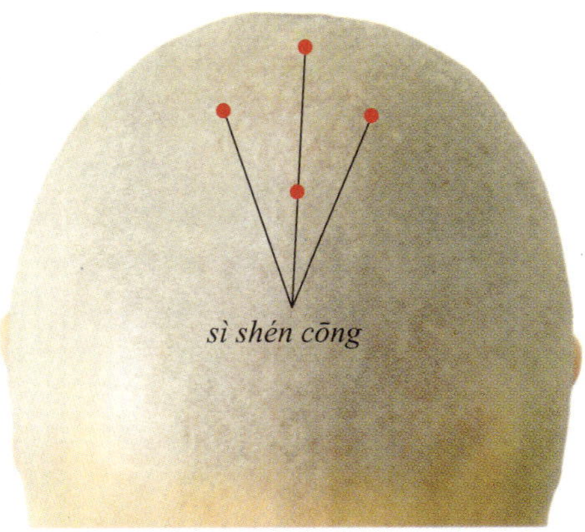

Sì shén cōng, a group of four points, can refresh the brain, and cheer spirit up.

Sì shén cōng are located at the vertex, one cun respectively posterior, anterior, and lateral to DU 20 (*bǎi huì*).

> DU 24 (*shén tíng*, 神庭)

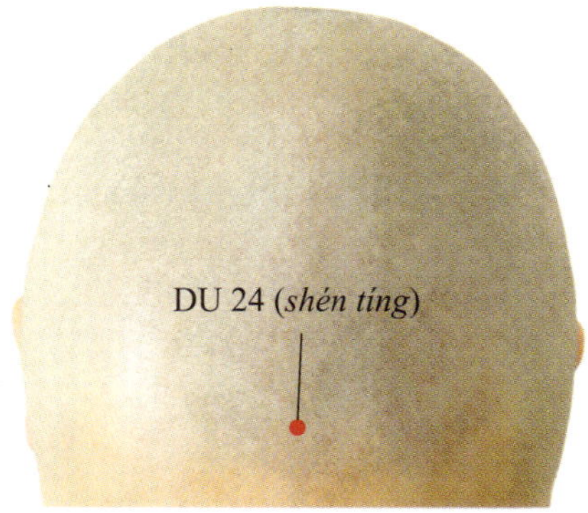

DU 24 can refresh the brain, tranquilize mind, remove obstacles in the channels, and relieve pain.

DU 24 is located on the DU channel, 0.5 *cun* directly above the midpoint of the anterior hairline.

> *Yìn táng* (印堂)

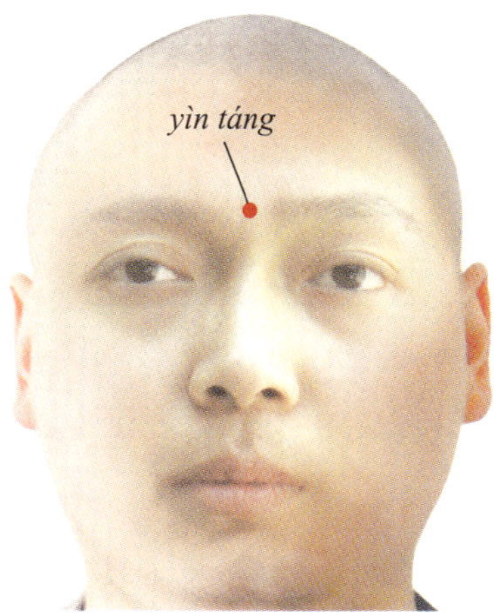

Yìn táng can refresh the brain, relieve pain, and tranquilize the mind.

Yìn táng is located midpoint between the medial ends of the two eyebrows.

> GB 20 (*fēng chí*, 风池)

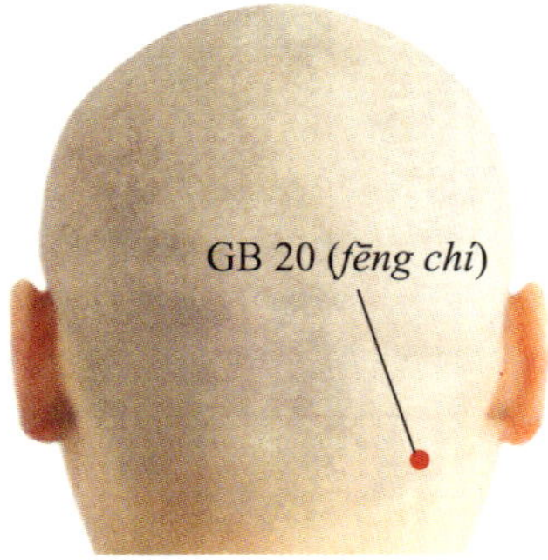

GB 20 can calm the liver to pacify endogenous wind, resolve depression, smooth the mind, and clear wind and heat.

GB 20 is located on the gallbladder channel, in the depression between the upper sternocleidomastoid muscle and trapezius muscle.

> DU 14 (*dà zhuī*, 大椎)

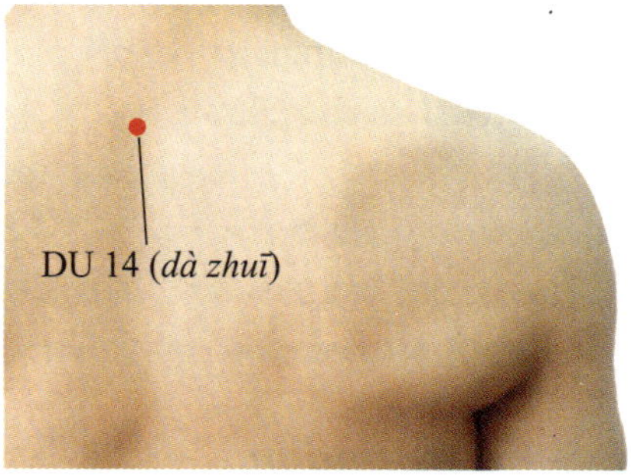

DU 14 can activate yang to relieve exterior pattern, refresh the brain, and smooth mental disturbance.

DU 14 is located on the *du mai*, in the depression below the spinous process of the 7th cervical vertebra.

> BL 15 (*xīn shù*, 心俞)

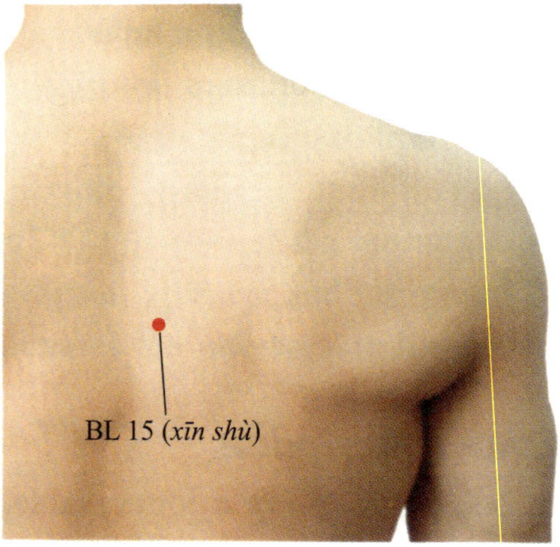

BL 15 can activate heart qi and smooth heart *shén*.

BL 15 is located on the bladder channel, on the back line, 1.5 *cun* lateral to the lower border of the spinous process of the 5th thoracic vertebra.

> BL 18 (*gān shù*, 肝俞)

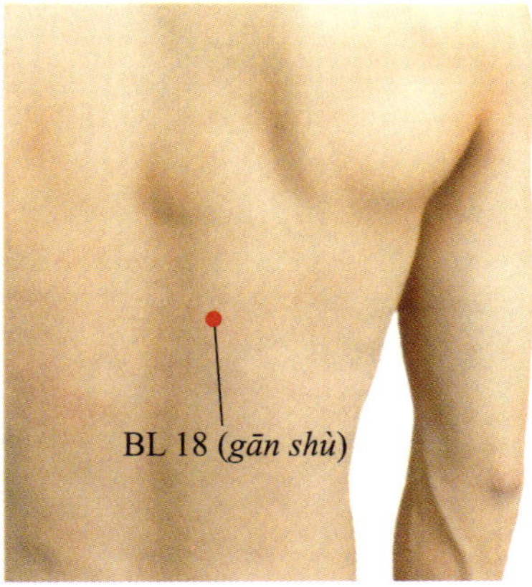

BL 18 can smooth liver qi stagnation and nourish liver blood.

BL 18 is located on the bladder channel, on the back line, 1.5 *cun* lateral to the lower border of the spinous process of the 9th thoracic vertebra.

> BL 20 (*pí shù*, 脾俞)

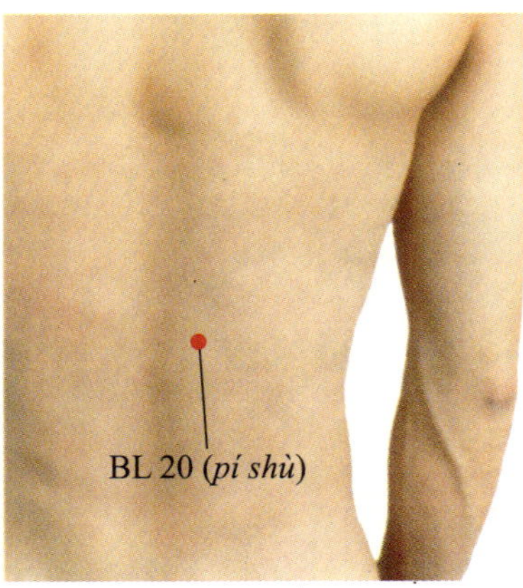

BL 20 can strengthen the spleen and stomach, and tonify qi and blood.

BL 20 is located on the bladder channel, on the back line, and 1.5 *cun* lateral to the lower border of the spinous process of the 11th thoracic vertebra.

> PC 6 (*nèi guān*, 内关)

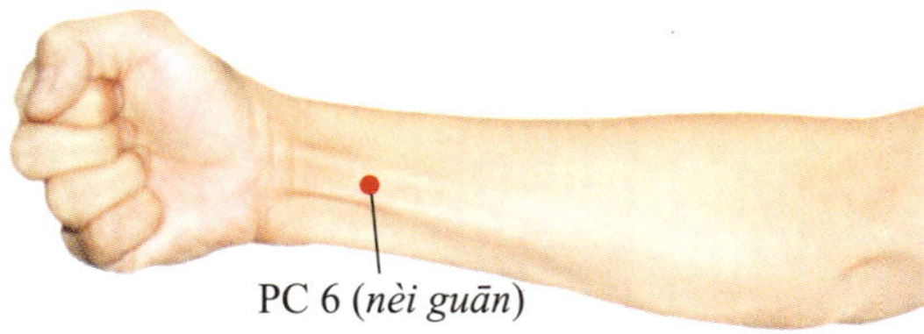

PC 6 can clear heat in the heart, harmonize the stomach, regulate the flow of qi in the chest, and regulate qi.

PC 6 is located on the pericardium channel, at two *cun* above the transverse crease of the wrist, between the tendons of palmaris longus muscle and flexor radialis muscle.

> HT 7 (*shén mén*, 神门)

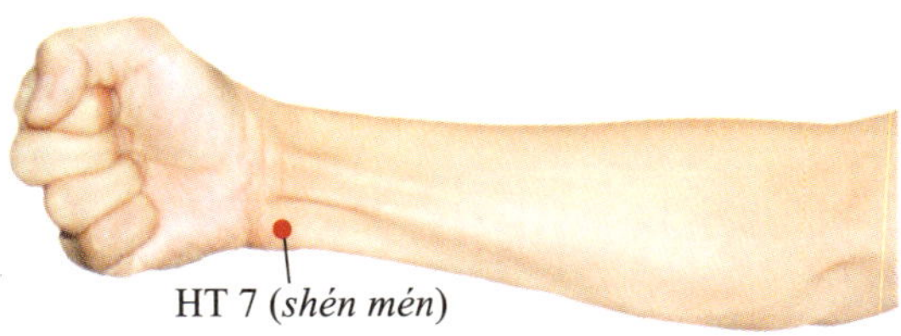

HT 7 can tonify the heart, nourish the blood, tranquilize the mind, and calm emotional disturbance.

HT 7 is located on the heart channel, at the ulnar end of the transverse crease of the wrist, and in the depression on the radial side of the tendon of flexor carpi ulnaris muscle.

> PC 8 (*láo gōng*, 劳宫)

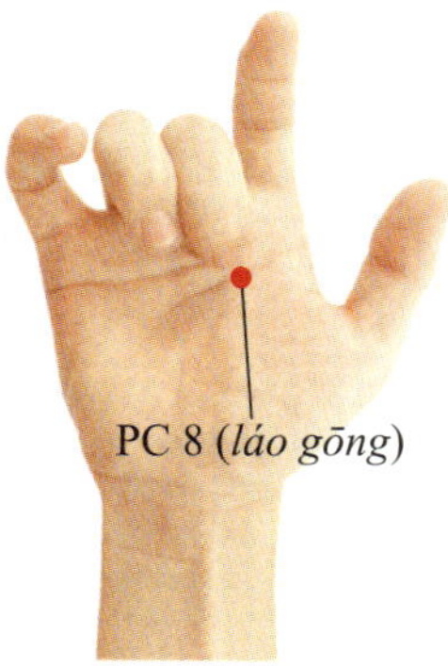

PC 8 can clear heart fire and tranquilize the heart *shén*.

PC 8 is located on the pericardium channel at the wrist crease.

> RN 17 (*dàn zhōng*, 膻中)

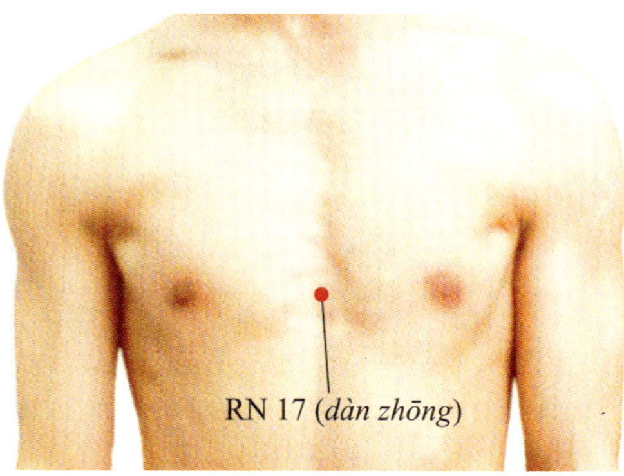

RN 17 can regulate qi activities and regulate the flow of qi in the chest.

RN 17 is located on the *ren mai*, on the anterior midline in females, at the level with the 4th intercostals space, and midway between the nipples in males.

> LV 14 (*qī mén*, 期门)

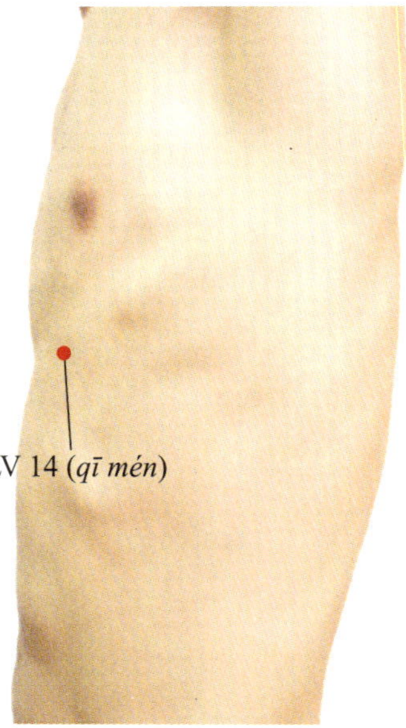

LV 14 can smooth the liver, relieve depression, tonify the spleen, and harmonize the stomach.

LV 14 is located on the liver channel, on the chest, directly below the nipple, in the sixth intercostal space, and 4 *cun* lateral to the front medium line.

> ST 40 (*fēng lóng*, 丰隆)

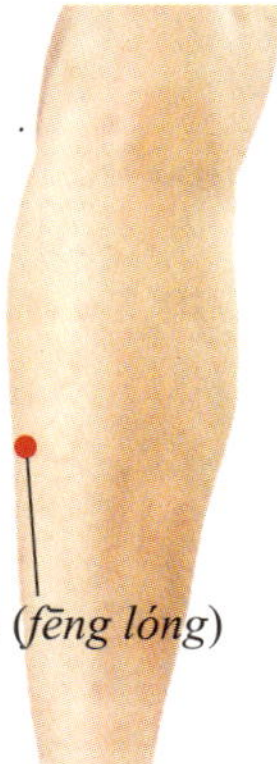

ST 40 can strengthen the spleen, relieve phlegm, dispel turbidity, and refresh *shén*.

ST 40 is located on the stomach channel, on the lateral side of the shank, 8 *cun* above the tip of external malleolus, and two finger-breadth (mid-finger) from the anterior crest of the tibia.

> SP 6 (*sān yīn jiāo*, 三阴交)

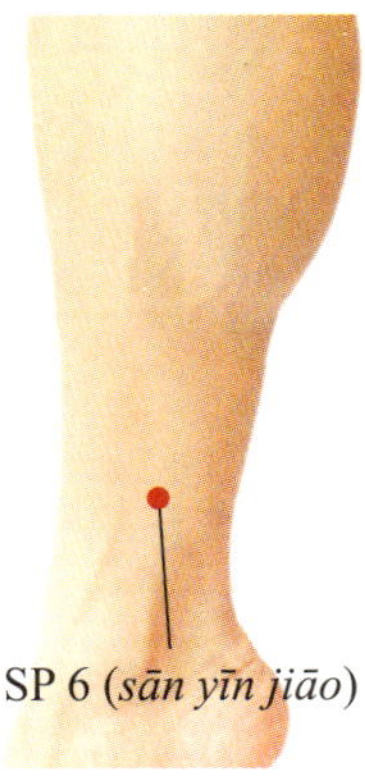

SP 6 can smooth the liver, invigorate the spleen, fortify the kidney, and regulate *shén*.

SP 6 is located on the spleen channel, on the medial side of the shank, three *cun* directly above the tip of the medial malleolus, and on the posterior border of the medial aspect of the tibia.

> KI 1 (*yǒng quán*, 涌泉)

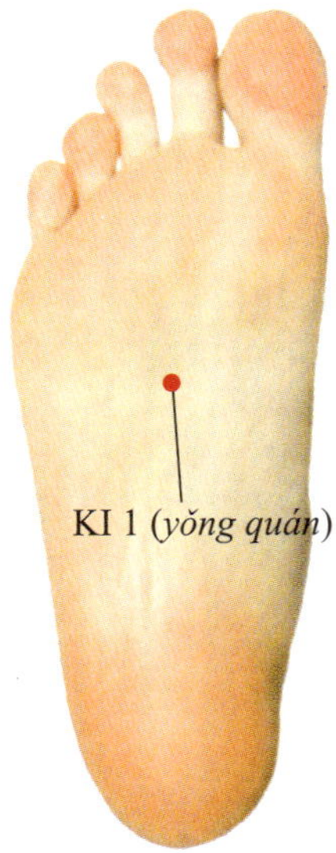

KI 1 can guide fire downwards, regulate the kidney, and tranquilize *shén*.

KI 1 is located on the kidney channel, on the sole, in the depression when the foot is in plantar flexion, in the anterior depression when the foot is fixed, and at approximately the junction of the anterior one-third and posterior two-thirds of the sole.

> KI 3 (*tài xī*, 太溪)

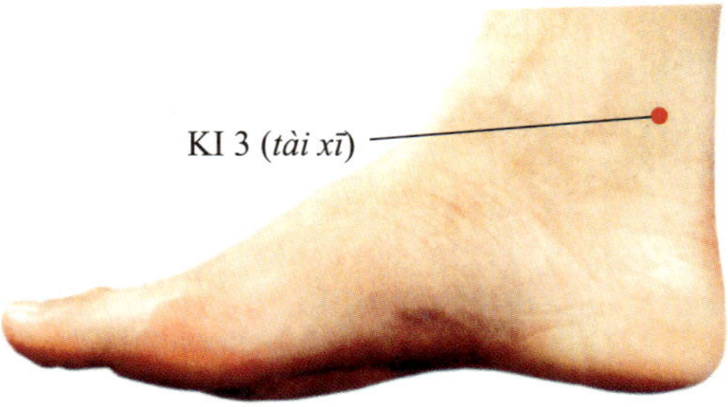

KI 3 can regulate and tonify kidney qi, enrich yin, and tranquilize *shén*.

KI 3 is located on the kidney channel, on the medial side of the foot, posterior to the medial malleolus, and in the depression between the tip of the medial malleolus and the Achilles tendon.

> LV 3 (*tài chōng*, 太冲)

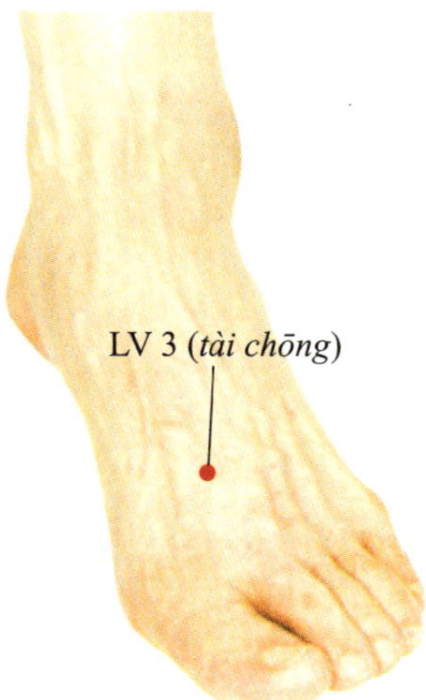

LV 3 can smooth the liver to regulate qi circulation, calm the liver, and relieve endogenous wind.

LV 3 is located on the liver channel, in the depression distal to the junction of the first and second metatarsal bones.

> LV 2 (*xíng jiān*, 行间)

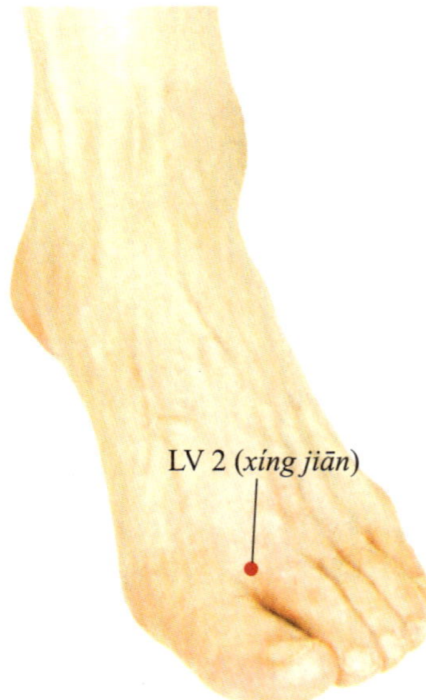

LV 2 can smooth the liver, relieve depression, as well as clear and drain liver fire.

LV 2 is located on the liver channel, on the dorsum of the foot between the 1st and 2nd toes, and proximal to the margin of the web.

> *Ashi* points (阿是)

Ashi points, literally translated as "Ah, that's it!" are not regular acupuncture channel points. There are places on your body that when pressed, you will say "Ah, that's it!" meaning that the point pressed is exactly where the pain is. Since sensitive points can appear anywhere on the body, these points have no specific names. In depression they are usually located in the region where the qi is stagnated, though sometimes they can be found in distant areas.

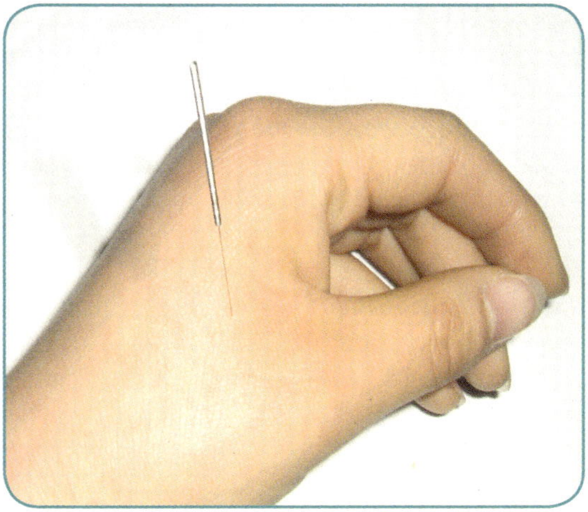

Clinically, accurate location of acupoints is of great importance for a successful outcome. The methods commonly used are anatomical landmarks measurement, proportional bone measurement, finger *cun* measurement, and natural body landmarks.

What is the *cun*? The *cun* is a measurement that is used to locate acupoints on a patient's body. Generally, one *cun* is equal to the distance between the two ends of the creases of the interphalangeal joints on the flexed middle finger. However, this *cun* can only be used on certain parts of the body, sometimes you need to use other relative landmarks. For example, the space from nipple to nipple is eight *cun* and this eight *cun* can be used to find points on the chest, etc.

Chinese medicine holds that heart governs spirit, liver governs the smooth flow of qi and regulates emotional activities, while the channels of the bladder, conceptional vessel, and governor vessel all go upwards to the brain and are closely related to emotional activities. Therefore, selecting and stimulating the acupoints located on the aforementioned channels has a potent therapeutic effect on depression. Meanwhile, other points are selected according to pattern differentiation. The manipulation of reinforcement, reduction, and even reinforcement and reduction are applicable according to the condition of deficiency and excess. The reinforcement or reduction can be realized by rotating the needle, closing or enlarging the acupuncture hole, puncturing along or adverse to the channel course, needling slowly or rapidly, or means of respiration. Wang Yu-ying[38] selected PC 6 (*nèi guān*), ST 36 (*zú sān lǐ*), and SP 6 (*sān yīn jiāo*) as chief points with psychological therapy, and the total effective rate was 91.7%. Ye

Guo-chuan[39] treated 36 depressive cases by acupuncturing HT 7 (*shén mén*), SP 6 (*sān yīn jiāo*) and ST 36 (*zú sān lǐ*), and the total effective rate was 83%. Lin Hong[40] treated 53 patients with postnatal psychogenia induced depression by stimulating the acupoints of HT 7 (*shén mén*), GB 13 (*běn shén*), BL 15 (*xīn shù*), GV 11 (*shén dào*), and SI 3 (*hòu xī*), and the total effective rate was 88.68% . Jiang Feng-liang[41] selected BL 18 (*gān shù*), BL 23 (*shèn shù*), BL 15 (*xīn shù*), HT 7 (*shén mén*), PC 6 (*nèi guān*) and GB 20 (*fēng chí*) as chief acupoints to treat 20 senile depression patient caused by liver and kidney yin deficiency or emotional stagnation, among which 18 cases improved.

Electroacupuncture

Currently, it is common for practitioners to choose to use an electrical apparatus that allows an electrical impulse to be sent through the acupuncture needles to mimic constant manipulation. In Chinese medicine, illness is caused when qi and blood do not circulate smoothly and properly, and pain occurs when qi and blood is obstructed. When there is a stagnation or accumulation of qi such as in pain pattern, or qi and blood are difficult to stimulate or it takes more time to stimulate, electroacupuncture is considered to be especially useful. During the process of electroacupuncture, the same points as traditional acupuncture are selected, needles are inserted at specific points, and then they are attached using small clips to a device that generates continuous electric pulses. It is employed as an alternative for manual manipulation to stimulate acupunture points, and pairs of needles can be stimulated simultaneously for less than 30 minutes at a time.

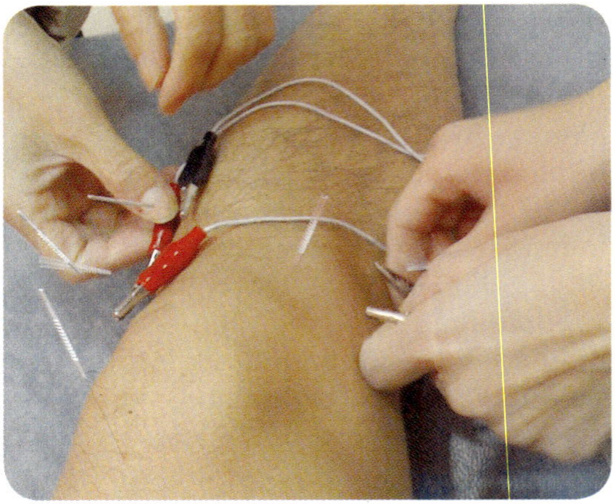

Practitioners are trained to operate the machines in the safest way and the amount of power sent through the needles is usually only a few microamperes. Electroacupuncture is commonly used for problems that require constant needle stimulation, including pain, musculoskeletal trauma, muscle dysfunction, spasms, and sprains. The machine will allow the practitioner to do other work while the point is receiving stimulation. Originating in China, this technique is commonly used in many countries. The frequency and the amount of power used in electroacupuncture tend to vary to a great degree depending on the patient's condition and the practitioner's decision. These devices are used to adjust the frequency and intensity of the impulse being delivered, depending on the condition being treated. Studies show that head point-through-point electroacupuncture can obviously increase plasma 5-HT content of the patient with PSD, and cure poststroke depression with better therapeutic effects; electroacupuncture combined with Paroxetine had better clinical efficacy than that of Paroxetine alone, with a milder adverse reaction and a quicker initiation of effect.

Electroacupuncture is pretty effective in treating depression due to a better stimulation effect. Kang Bo et al.[42] electrically needled the acupoints of DU 20 (*bǎi huì*), *yìn táng*, DU 17 (*nǎo hù*), DU 21 (*qián dǐng*), and DU 19 (*hòu dǐng*), and the total effective rate was 83%. Luo He-chun et al.[43] treated 30 patients with depression by electroacupuncturing DU 20 (*bǎi huì*) and *yìn táng*, and the total effective rate was 90%. Dong Zi-ping[44] treated 101 patients with depression by electroacupuncturing DU 20 (*bǎi huì*) and *yìn táng*, and the total effective rate was 81.2% and the biennial recurrence rate was 12.2%.

Ear Acupuncture

Ear acupuncture, also known as auriculotherapy or auriculoacupuncture, is a form of alternative medicine. Placing needles in the ear is a new addition to Chinese medicine's treatment arsenal. Similar to reflexology and iridology, the ear represents a microsystem of the entire body. The shape of the ear is described by ear specialists as looking like a curled up human figure upside down, with the head as the lobe and the legs curled up to form the top of the ear. The entire human body with all its different parts and organs has been mapped out. Diseases of the entire body are presumed to be treatable by stimulating the points in the ear. Although there are specialists who mainly use ear acupuncture, most practitioners use it as a helpful adjunct therapy. A popular technique is to place a small seed, metal pellet, or tiny needle on an ear point and keep it in place with a small piece of tape. These objects will then provide a constant stimulation to the points chosen. Usually you will be instructed to press or rub each of these points several times a day for a few minutes. This convenient form of therapy allows for around the clock treatment. Normally the tape can be taken off in three or four days.

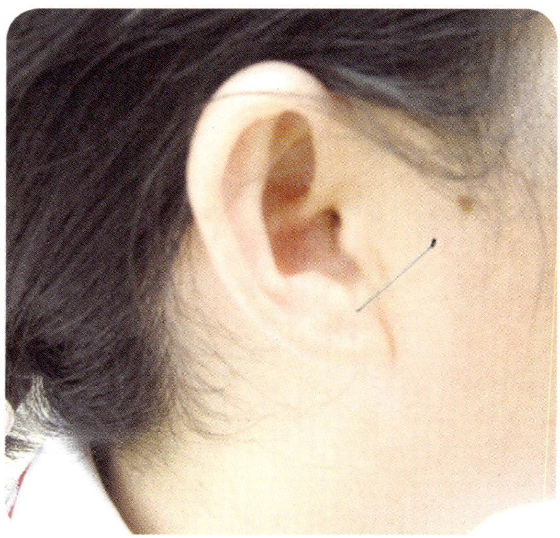

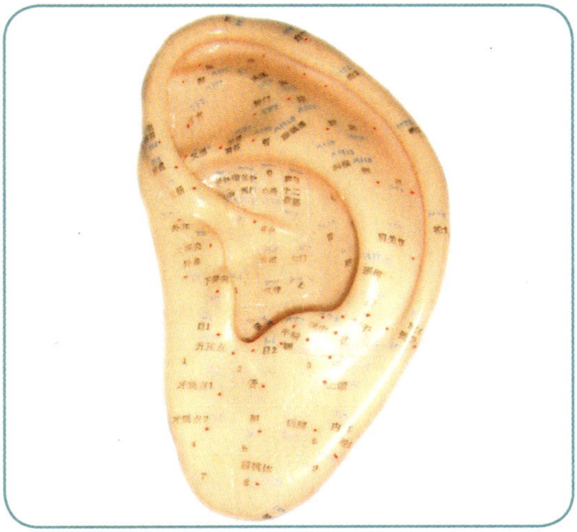

Ear acupoints stimulus can regulate the general visceral activities and brain functions as well. He Ling et al.[45] treated menopausal syndrome with ear acupuncture of *shén mén*, endocrine, sympathetic nerve, and thalamencephalon, and the total effectiveness rate was 93.75%. Ren Jianning[46] treated 50 patients suffering from depression by stimulating ear acupoints of liver, gallbladder, heart, spleen, kidney, *shén mén*, endocrine, subcortex, sympathetic nerve, small intestine, stomach, and *sanjiao*. Five to six acupoints were used each time, and the effective rate was 88%.

Scalp Acupuncture

TCM holds that the brain is the house of the original spirit and there is a close relationship between the brain and mental activities. While modern neurophysiology, neuroimageology, and neurotransmitter theory also prove that depression is closely related with the brain, a patient with depression frequently suffers from functional abnormity of neurotransmitter including serotonin, noradrenaline, and others, and also a changing volume of the hippocampus. This lays the theoretical foundation for treating depression with scalp acupuncture. Modern research denotes that scalp acupuncture has good effect in treating depression through regulating the function of the cerebral mantle, and improving glycometabolism in different encephalic regions. Song Ying et al.[47] treated 29 patients with cerebral apoplexy induced depression with scalp acupuncture on the middle line of the vertex, middle line of the forehead, lateral line one of the forehead, and lateral line three of the forehead, and the total effective rate was 86%, revealing a therapeutic efficiency much better than that of the control group treated with fluoxetine ($P<0.05$). Li Han-jun[48] treated 75 patients with neurasthenia by penetrating DU 20 towards any of the *sì shén cōng* points, and the total effective rate was 97.35%.

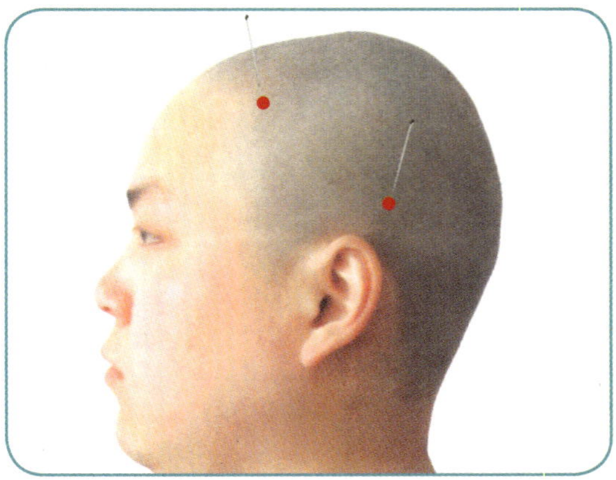

Acupuncture Point Injection

Acupuncture point injection is a procedure in which drugs, vitamins, medicinal extracts, or other fluids are injected into the body at an acupunture point using a syringe and needle.

With a stimulative and pharmaceutical effect on the point via puncture and injection, this therapy can improve physiological functions, correct the pathological state, and raise the therapeutic effects. The sizes of the syringe needle and the syringe used in the treatment are different according to the dosage and the location of injection. However, great attention should be paid to the solution to be used, the tissue to be injected, and the aseptic manipulation during the treatment. Sometimes, a skin test is necessary.

Zhao Xiu-min et al.[49] treated depression by injecting vitamin-B2, *dāng guī,* and *huáng qí* into bilateral back-*shu* points, and had satisfying therapeutic efficiency.

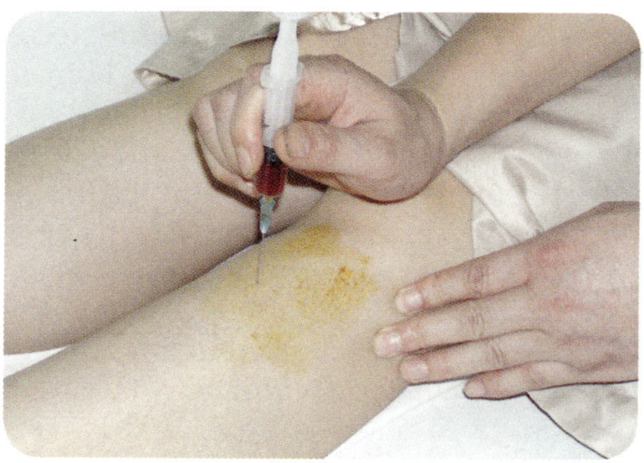

Other Techniques

Though acupuncture and moxibustion are the main techniques used by practitioners of Chinese medicine, there are a variety of other techniques that may be used. These include, but are not limited to, cupping, *gua sha*, plum-blossom needling, dermal needling, and burning-rush moxibustion. These techniques may cause slight damage to the skin and tissues, but in turn, they stimulate the points much stronger with a lasting effect. If applied properly, these techniques can sometimes be more effective than conventional acupuncture for pain relief. As for managing depression, these techniques can either be applied alone or be used in combination. For example, cupping is often combined with acupunture needling. The technique involves stimulating specific acupoints with needles and applying cups over areas to draw out the stagnation, dampness, and coldness.

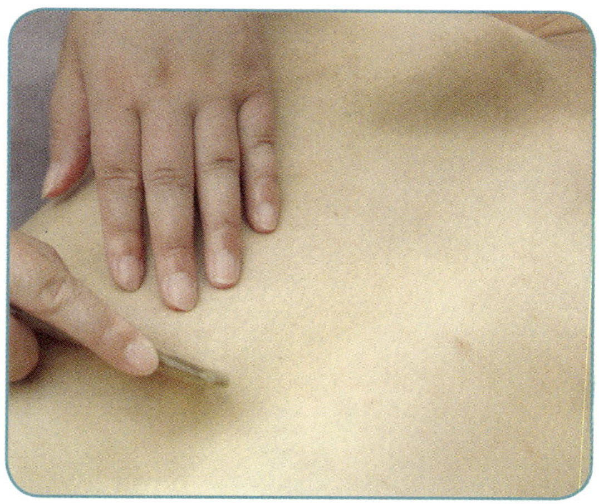

Cupping involves the application of suctions cups to the skin either near the painful area or on a related channel. Air is removed from the cups by using a burning cotton ball soaked in alcohol (modern cups using air suction are also used). There is usually no pain involved in cupping, though the sensation of suction is sometimes strange the first time.

Cupping therapy was called horning method in ancient times. The mechanical stimulation from slide cupping can be transmitted to central nervous system through the reflex pathway of cutaneous receptors and blood receptors, which can regulate the process of excitation and inhibition and keep them in balance. Qian Jie et al.[50] treated depression with slide cupping on the *du mai* and bilateral bladder channels, and the total effective rate was 96.8%. Wang Wei-hong et al.[51] treated female menopause depression by acupuncture combined with assistant therapy of slide cupping on back-*shu* points, and had significant therapeutic effects.

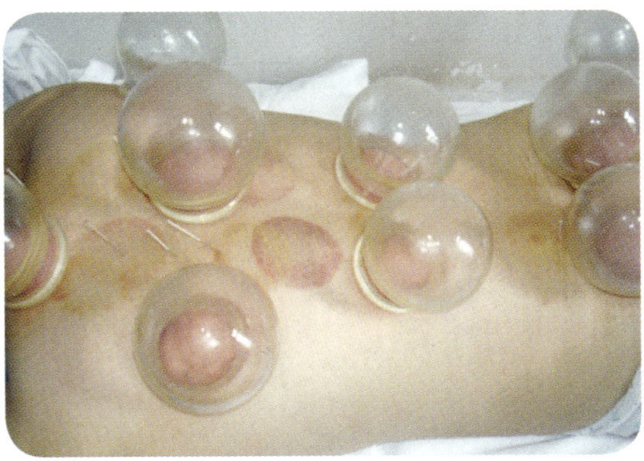

A plum-blossom needle is a small hammer with several small needles and is used to stimulate the skin and remove stagnation. The tapping is very light, but because the needles are numerous, the sensation is a little sharp, though not intense. Small drops of blood sometimes emerge from the area being tapped, helping to remove stagnation and heat.

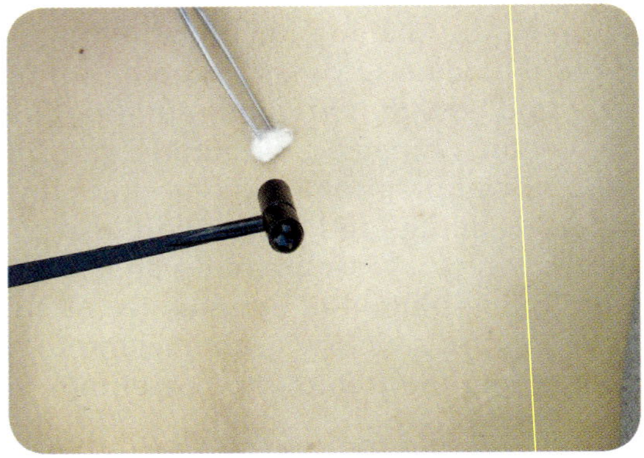

As a therapeutic method valuable in the prevention and treatment of acute and chronic disorders, *gua sha* literally means to scrape disease away in Chinese by allowing the disease to pass as sand-like objects through the skin. It is a healing technique used in clinical settings or in homes. It involves rubbing and cutaneously stimulating the selected skin by a round-edged instrument, which leads to the appearance of small red bruises called "*sha*." These bruises are very superficial and not painful and are a sign that the congestion causing pain has been activated and is leaving the body. It will fade within few days. *Gua sha* is used in many cultures and is usually used for pain that is recent and hasn't had time to go very deep. The rapid, light scraping techniques are not painful, but will elicit slight bruising in the area, which indicates the removal of blood stagnation, the elimination of pathogenic factors, such as in common cold, and the promotion of circulation and metabolic processes. The patient will experience immediate relief from pain, cough, stiffness, depression, and so on.

Cautions and Contraindications for Acupuncture and Moxibustion

Finding a qualified practitioner means a lot, since the effectiveness of an acupuncture treatment is strongly dependent upon an accurate Chinese medical diagnosis, sophisticated needling skills, and the correct location of the selected acupoints. So, check a practitioner's credentials before you decide to see him/her. Although a license does not ensure quality of care, it does indicate that the practitioner meets certain standards regarding the knowledge and use of acupuncture.

Acupuncture and its adjunct modalities are an incredibly safe kind of therapy. However, there are certain times when great care must be taken in treatment and even times where treatment should not be administered or when the equipment is not available for a treatment. Fortunately for the patient, the scope of techniques available to the practitioner of Chinese medicine is very wide. If one treatment avenue is blocked, there will probably be another that is open and available.

The following are some other cautions and contraindications for treatment with acupuncture, moxibustion, or other techniques.

※ Any acute metabolic disorder is contraindicated for acupuncture and moxibustion.

※ Extreme hunger, fatigue and mental stress are not indicated for acupuncture and moxibustion.

※ Pregnant women can be treated, but the practitioner must be very cautious.

※ History of fainting during acupuncture treatments.

※ Open or infected skin.

3. Research and References

➡ **Zhong ZG** *et al.*[52] assessed the effect of acupuncture combined with foot massage on sleeping quality of the patient with insomnia in terms of clinical therapeutic effects, and scores for Pittsburgh Sleep Quality Index (PSQI), Self-rating Anxiety Scale (SAS) and Self-rating Depression Scale (SDS) before and after treatment. The results revealed the effective rate was 93.75% in the observation group and 88.46% in the control group with no significant difference between the two groups; after treatment, there were significant or very significant differences in scores for various factors in the PSQI, SAS, and SDS ($P < 0.01$, $P < 0.05$), indicating abdominal acupuncture as main combined with foot massage can obviously improve sleeping quality of the patient with insomnia.

➡ **Wang H** *et al.*[53] conducted an updated meta-analysis to assess the beneficial effect of acupuncture in depression therapy through searching the following databases: MEDLINE, EMBASE, BIOSIS, Cochrane Central Register of Controlled Trials, and Chinese Scientific Journal Database in terms of acupuncture, acupressure, depression, depressive disorder, clinical trial, and randomized controlled trial. The results confirmed that acupuncture could significantly reduce the severity of depression, which was indicated by decreased scores of Hamilton rating scale for depression (HAMD) or Beck Depression Inventory (BDI). The pooled standardized mean difference of the "Improvement of depression" was -0.65 (95% CI -1.18, -0.11; P=0.02) by random effect model. However, no significant effect of active acupuncture was found on the response rate (RR 1.32, 95% CI 0.83 to 2.10; P=0.25) and remission rate (RR 1.30, 95% CI 0.57 to 2.95; P=0.53). It supported that acupuncture was an effective treatment that could significantly reduce the severity of disease in patients with depression. More full-scale randomized clinical trials with reliable designs are recommended to further warrant the effectiveness of acupuncture.

➡ **Li SJ** *et al.*[54] observed the curative effect of acupuncture following the principle of relieving depression and regulating mentality (RDRM) in treating patients with melancholia, and comparing the data with that of Western medicinal treatment. Patients in the observed group were treated with needling and electroacupuncture (EA), and those in the control group orally taken Fluoxetine or Paroxetine. The curative effect, Hamilton Depression Scale scores (HAMD), effect initiating time and sustaining time were observed and compared. The total effective rate was 87.5% and 79.1% in the observed group and the control group respectively, showing insignificant difference between them ($P>0.05$), but comparison of the initiating time and sustaining time between the two groups did show significant different ($P<0.01$). It concluded that acupuncture with following RDRM principle has a superior effect in treating melancholia, when compared to Western medicinal treatment.

➡ **Zhang C**[55] observed the therapeutic effects of the brain-resuscitation acupuncture method for post wind-stroke mental depression, 90 such cases were randomly divided into two groups, each consisting of 45 cases. For the treatment group, the brain-resuscitation acupuncture method was adopted, with PC 6 (*nèi guān*), DU 26 (*rén zhōng*), SP 6 (*sān yīn jiāo*), DU 20 (*bǎi huì*), and HT 7 (*shén mén*) selected as the main points. For the control group, oral medication of Fluoxetine was prescribed. Therapeutic effects and changes in the HAMD integrals of the two groups were observed. The total effective rate in the treatment group was 77.7%, and that in the control group was 75.1%, showing no significant difference between the two groups (P>0.05). The average effect starting time of the treatment group was 11.58 ± 4.89 days, while that of the control group was 15.96 ± 6.50 days, showing a significant difference between the two groups (*P*<0.05). It can be concluded that for the post wind-stroke mental depression, the brain-resuscitation acupuncture method may show a good and quicker therapeutic effect with no side effects as compared with pharmacotherapy.

➡ **Han C** *et al.*[56] observed the clinical therapeutic effects of electroacupuncture therapy for mental depression, 30 cases were treated by electro-acupuncture on DU 20 (*bǎi huì*), *yìn táng*, and the differential points. Maprotiline was used in the control group of 31 cases. After the treatment, the scores in HAMD for both groups were found to be obviously decreased as compared with those before the treatment (*P*<0.01), without significant between-group differences (*P*>0.05). The total effective rate in the treatment group was 96.7%, and that of the control group was 90.3%, showing no significant between-group differences (*P*>0.05). After the treatment, the two groups all showed obvious decrease in the TCM symptomatic integrals (*P*<0.01), with significant between-group differences (*P*<0.05), the integral of the treatment group showing obvious superiority to that of the control group. And the decrease of the Asberg scores testing the side effect of antidepressants of the treatment group was obviously superior to that of the control group. After the treatment, the cortisol (CORT) content and the endothelin-1 (ET-1) content of the two groups were all obviously decreased (*P*<0.01), and basically turned to normal, without significant between-group differences (*P*>0.05). This study concluded that electroacupuncture therapy can produce the same clinical therapeutic effect as that produced by the tetracycline drug, maprotiline, giving less side effect and better symptomatic improvement.

➡ **Tsay SL** *et al.*[57] conducted a study to test the effectiveness of acupressure and Transcutaneous Electrical Acupoint Stimulation (TEAS) on fatigue, sleep quality, and depression in patients who were receiving routine hemodialysis treatment. The study was a randomized controlled trial; qualified patients were randomly assigned to acupressure, TEAS, or control groups. Patients in the acupressure and TEAS groups received 15 minutes of treatment three times a week for one month, whereas patients in the control group only received routine unit care. A total of 106 patients participated in the study. Methods of measurement included the revised Piper Fatigue Scale (PFS), the Pittsburgh Sleep Quality Index, and the Beck Depression Inventory. Data were collected at baseline, during the intervention, and post-treatment. The results indicated that patients in the acupressure and TEAS groups had significantly lower levels of fatigue, a better sleep quality, and less depressed moods compared with patients in the control group based upon the adjusted baseline differences. However, there were no differences between acupressure and TEAS groups in outcome measures. This study provides an alternative method for health care providers in managing dialysis patients with symptoms of fatigue, poor sleep, or depression.

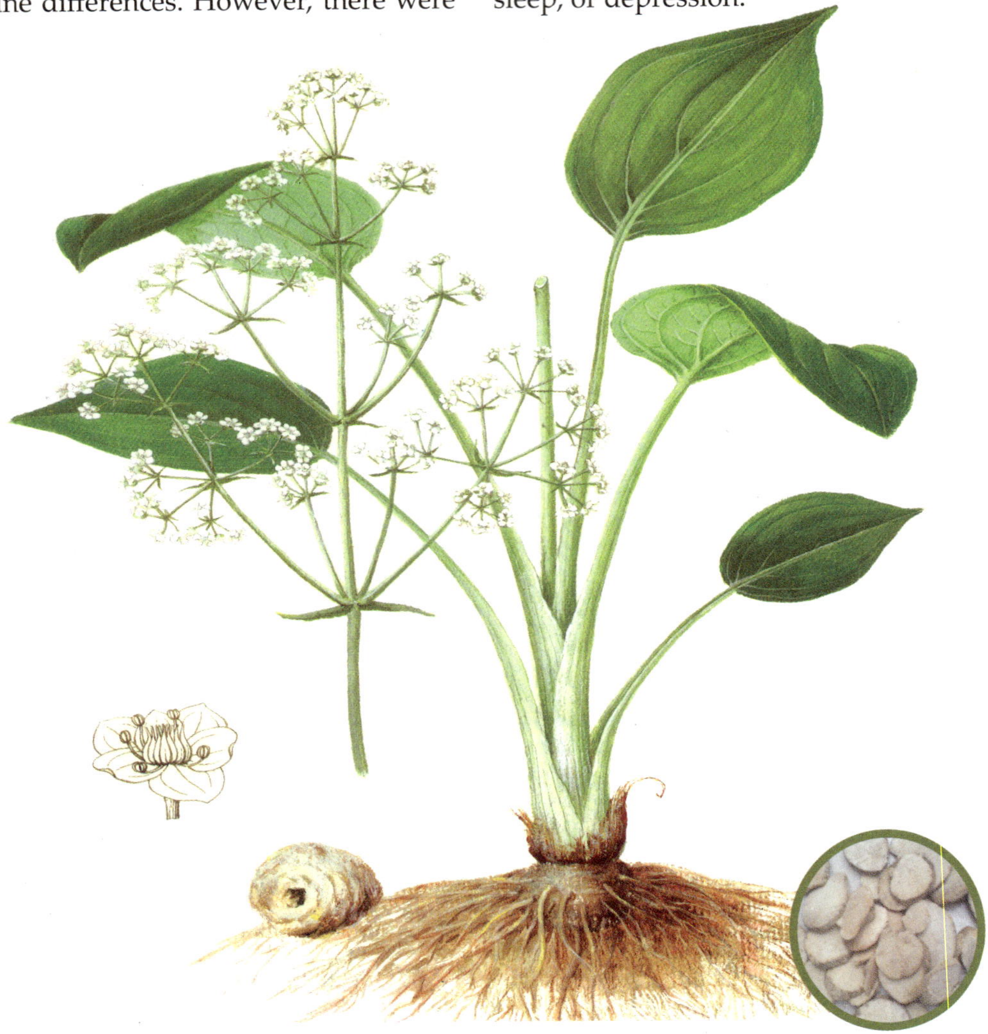

Alisma Rhizome

Chinese Medicinals

1. What Are Chinese Medicinals?

Together with acupuncture, Chinese medicinals is a major pillar of Chinese medicine. In China, using medicinals is more popular than using acupuncture to treat illness. Medicinal treatments have been documented and practiced since the 3rd century B.C. Shen Nong (2,737-2,697 B.C.) is credited with launching Chinese medicine, and identifying hundreds of medicinals by personally tasting and testing various plants and their parts to see how they would affect his body and what kind of medical value they have, which was crucial to the development of Chinese medicine. Later on in history, Emperor Huang Di (also known as the Yellow Emperor) presented *The Yellow Emperor's Inner Classic*, which is now known as the world's oldest medical textbook and the bible of Chinese medicine. Chinese medicine practitioners around the world still refer to this classic today for insight on Chinese medicine.

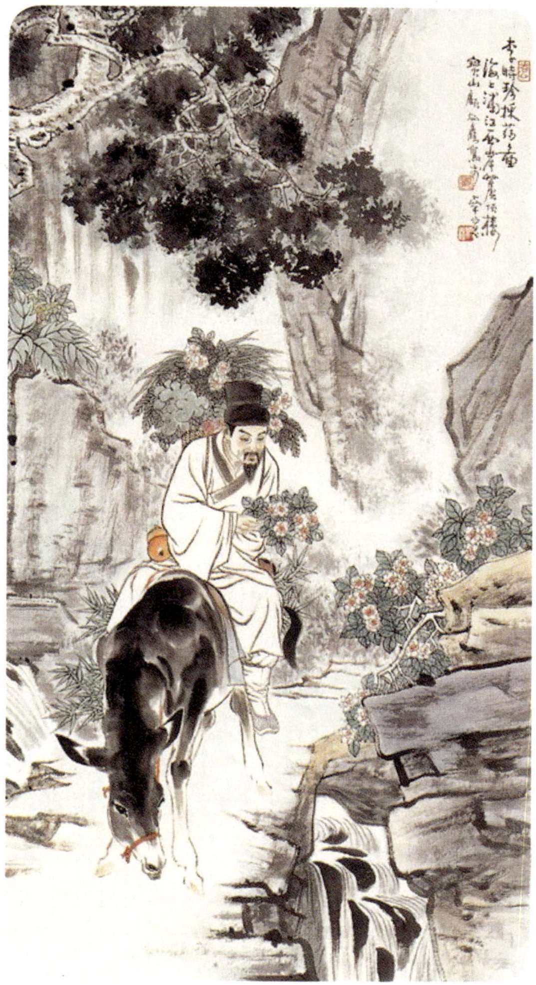

Li Shi-zhen

The phrase "Chinese medicinal" refers to substances that occur naturally in the environment and can come from plant, animal, or mineral sources. These substances can be prepared in a variety of ways so that they can be used by the body. Chinese medicinals can be drunk, eaten,

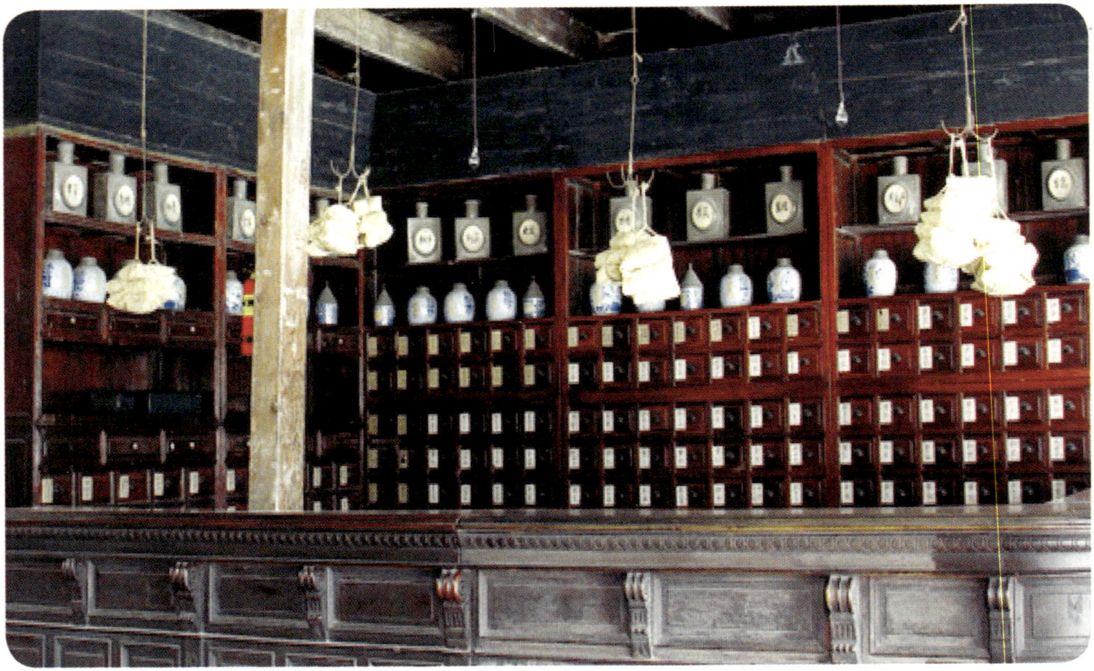

inhaled, or applied to the skin. They can regulate the body's qi, blood, yin, yang, and expel pathogens as well. An ancient Chinese pharmacopoeia lists over 3,000 different medicinal substances in terms of their source, properties, collection, processing, channel entered, actions, and the symptoms, syndromes, or diseases that they treat, though there are only about 400 or so in common use today. In general, most comprehensive medicinal pharmacies have 200-300 substances. Medicinals used in Chinese medicine are often derived from plant, animal, and mineral substances, among which plant-derived medicinals, such as leaves, roots, fruits, and barks, are the commonest, while minerals and animal substances such as oyster shells and magnetite are also prescribed. In fact, any natural substance can be used in Chinese medicine, but it will be called a Chinese medicinal only when it is used according to the theories of Chinese medicine.

Chinese medicinals recorded in ancient texts are still used today. The medical value of medicinals is different in terms of four major dimensions: property, flavor, channel entered, and actions. The property ranges from cold (cool) to neutral to hot (warm) in nature. Generally, if the nature of a pattern is hot, the prescription of cool or cold medicinals is appropriate. The flavor refers to sour, bitter, sweet, acrid, and salty, each of which has specific functions and characteristics. Sour, bitter, and salty tastes pertain to yin, whereas acrid and sweet are attributed to yang. Medicinal representing different tastes are applied to treat different conditions. Specifically, sour constricts or consolidates, and medicinals of sour taste are often prescribed in such cases as perspiration due to deficiency and chronic diarrhea; bitter possesses the function of clearing heat, purging the bowels, lowering the qi, improving appetite, and drying dampness; bitter medicinals are commonly used in heat pattern and damp-heat pattern; sweet plays the role of tonifying, improving, moistening, harmonizing, relieving pain due to the constrictive action of muscles, and is commonly used for deficiency and disharmony pattern; acrid disperses, circulates qi, vitalizes blood, and actives metabolism, which is used in the treatment of external patterns; and salty has the function of softening masses and purging the bowels, which are often indicated in sores, inflammatory masses, cysts, and connective tissue proliferation. The channels entered refer to the affinity that a medicinal has for one or multiple *zang-fu* organs. Action refers to the specific therapeutic effect that a medicinal poses. There are primarily twenty-one categories of medicinals such as: medicinals of eliminating heat and toxin, medicinals of nourishing yin, or medicinals of regulating qi circulation.

Mechanism of Chinese Medicinals

Every single Chinese medicinal has multiple active chemicals, let alone the interaction between and among different medicinals, which may constitute a formula. We are just at the initial stage of understanding how Chinese medicinals work, but the underlying idea about how Chinese medicinals work is fundamentally different than that behind biomedical pharmaceuticals. A pharmaceutical is a finely crafted and intensely focused creation, and most scientific research focuses on a single compound and mode of action by using laboratory models. Years, sometimes decades, of research goes before any drug is released on the market. Scientists strive to isolate the exact chemical or combination of chemicals that can cause a very specific change in bodily function. The change elicited by these drugs is often effective at relieving symptoms, but does not usually restore the damaged body part or function that was responsible for the symptoms in the first place. For example, antibiotics will kill invading bacteria, but will not strengthen the body against further invasions; or a pain killer may relieve the aching joints of an arthritis patient, but it will not stop or even retard the progression of the disease. In addition, it is not uncommon for a drug to cause unwanted side-effects in addition to its desired actions. Biomedical drugs may damage the nervous system, the digestive system, or most commonly, the liver or kidneys.

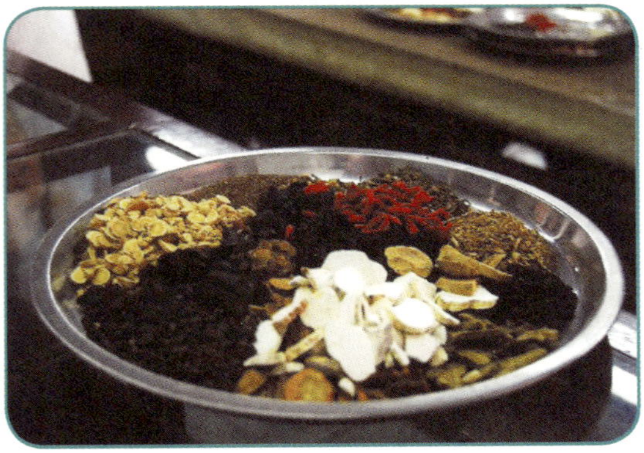

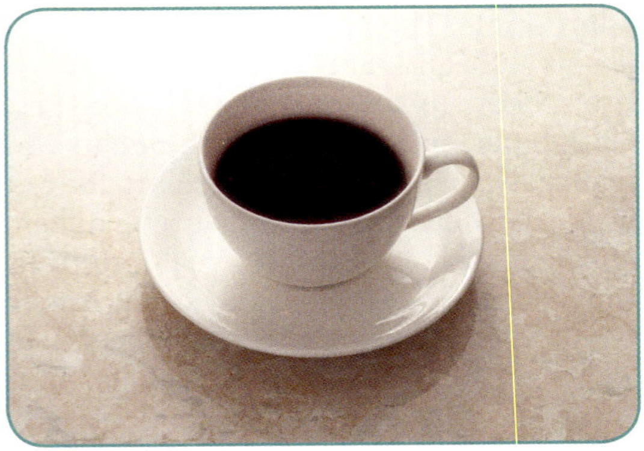

Chinese medicine practitioners specifically address the issue concerned with a formula that directly corresponds to the pattern differentiations. Each formula is commonly comprised of 5-15 Chinese medicinals and is designed to target both the root and the symptoms of the disease. In general, a formula is comprised of such elements as chief, deputy, assistant, and envoy. Specifically, the chief refers to the medicinal that exerts the strongest effect on the primary pattern being treated; the deputy is the medicinals that reinforce the actions of the chief medicinals and addresses any secondary pattern; the assistant means the medicinals that harmonizes any harsh effects of other medicinals in the formula and augments the actions of the other medicinals in the formula; and the envoy is the medicinal guiding other medicinals to specific organ systems, and helping the other medicinals absorption by aiding their digestion. This mixture enhances the therapeutic effect of each medicinal and minimizes any possible negative aspect.

In Chinese medicine, as mentioned above, the idea is to restore the body's innate ability to remain in a state of health. In severe cases, long term treatment is necessary to provide constant support to the body, but usually patients who start treatment with Chinese medicine are able to stop treatment after their symptoms have been brought under control. Treatment is able to be stopped because the medicinal used was helping to restore the body's damaged functions, not just substitute for them. These patients then gladly use the principles of Chinese medicine throughout their lives to maintain health, only visiting an acupuncturist or medicinalist to take care of any health problems that appear as a natural result of aging.

To a doctor of Chinese medicine, side effects are a sign of improper treatment, either due to faulty diagnosis, or inappropriate treatment methods. A properly constructed medicinal formula will exactly match the patient's internal patterns and will not cause any other kind of imbalance. What is weak will be strengthened, what is too strong will be reigned in, leaving no room for other problems to develop due to the ingredients of the prescription. It is commonly thought that because Chinese medicinals include the whole biological substance (as opposed to an artificially isolated biologically active constituent), the naturally occurring ingredients that make up the harmonious living organism help to buffer the body from side effects. Here is an analogy. Taking vitamin pills can help to quickly supplement nutrients you need. Yet they cannot replace food (a mixture of necessary nutrients and "unnecessary" substances) for the long-term maintenance of health. So is the case with synthesized drugs. Many of them are extracted from natural plants. They are effective and helpful. But they cannot replace natural medicinals (a mixture of effective ingredients and "ineffective" ingredients) for the long-term treatment of chronic diseases.

Another mechanism that makes Chinese medicinals safe is that they are counterbalanced within the formula. As an example, medicinals that take out excess heat from the body are considered cold, and can damage the digestive system. Therefore, in many formulas that treat excess heat, a couple of medicinals that promote and strengthen digestion may be added. If the patient has a weak digestion to begin with, even more ingredients are reserved for that purpose. This kind of treatment is much more than simply anti-symptomatic. Each prescription must be a balanced entity, which perfectly compliments the patient's condition. When used properly, Chinese medicinals are safe and effective. This takes experience and active involvement by the practitioner. Sound and individualized diagnosis is made based on the patient's present condition to ensure efficacy and safety.

Processing of Chinese Medicinals

Chinese medicinals are processed before use. Processing refers to the procedure of preparing crude Chinese medicinals under the guidance of the theories of Chinese medicine. There are several reasons for this. First, processing detoxifies medicinals and prevent poisons to remove any possible side-effect. Another reason for processing is for promoting therapeutic effects of selected medicinals. For instance, *chuān xiōng* (Sichuan lovage root) dry-fried with wine exerts a better effect on pain relief or *xiāng fù* (nutgrass galingale rhizome) prepared with wine plays a bigger role in smoothing and regulating liver qi. Processing also modifies the property and actions of Chinese medicinals so as to be in line with therapeutic requirements, for instance, *dà huáng* (rhubarb root and rhizome) in raw form has a strong purging effect, however its purgation effect is weakened after processing; it becomes a blood stopper instead after stir-baked until charcoal. In addition, processing can facilitate decoction, preparation-making, and storage of medicinals. Last but not least, processing filters out impurities such as mud and sand, takes non-pharmaceutical parts away, and can tone down a strong taste or smell.

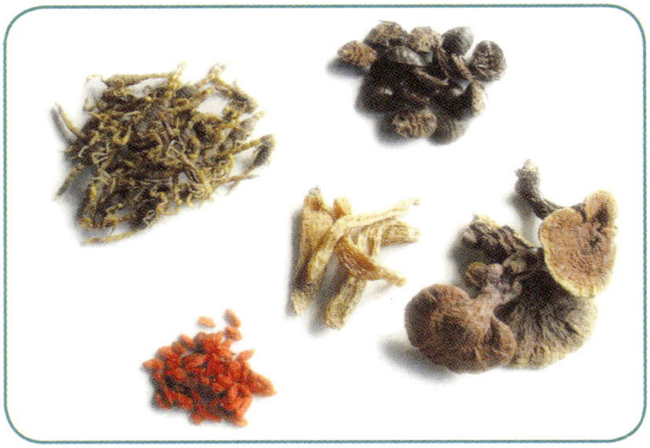

It involves such means as liquid-fried, honey-fried, wine-fried, scorch-fried, dry-fried, charred, calcined, roasted, baked, blast-fried, or other means. This kind of alchemical processing is used in everyday preparation of plant, mineral, and animal medicinals. For instance, honey-fried medicinals is believed to have better effects on moistening the lung and relieving cough, invigorating the stomach and spleen, moderating the pharmaceutical property, and detoxification; frying with wine is believed to promote the blood circulation and reduce the side-effects of certain medicinals; vinegar-fried medicinals can exert better influence on soothing the liver, relieving pain, and detoxification; frying with salt is believed to draw the Chinese medicinal actions to the kidneys, nourish yin, and lower the fire better; ginger juice-fried ones can provide more remarkable effect on relieving cold, vomiting, and detoxification. There are still other special processing methods according to different requirement, such as fermentation, frost-like powder, and germination.

Compatibility of Chinese Medicinals

Medicinals are seldom used singly. Compatibility refers to the combination of more than two medicinals with the purpose of enhanced therapeutic effect, detoxification, and moderatation or elimination of the original toxic side-effects. There are several forms of compatibility: mutual promotion, mutual enhancement, mutual restraint, counteract toxicity of another drug, antagonism, and incompatibility. This is practical information of medicinal application and the basis of making up a formula.

There are four ways to beneficially combine Chinese medicinals. Mutual promotion involves combining two or more medicinals with similar property and actions to reinforce each other's function and create a strong effect, for instance, the combination of *táo rén* (peach seed) and *hóng huā* (safflower) can enhance their respective action of invigorating blood and removing blood stagnation. Mutual enhancement is the method of using one medicinal for the dominate aspect and the other as its assistant to raise its therapeutic effects. Mutual restraint relies upon one medicinal reducing or eliminating toxicity, poison, or side effects of another medicinal in the combination. Counteracts toxicity means the elimination or removal of the toxic property or side-effects from one Chinese medicinal by the effects of the other. Two other types of combinations show why one should immerse himself/herself enough in Chinese medicine before attempting to combine them. Antagonism indicates that the decrease or even complete loss of therapeutic effect of certain Chinese medicinal after combining with another medicinal, for instance, the qi-tonification effect of *rén shēn* (ginseng) will be weakened by *lái fú zǐ* (radish seed), so it is reasonable to say there is an antagonism between those two. Incompatibility occurs when two incompatible medicinals are used with the by-product being the production of a poison or a side effect. The compatibility forms of mutual promotion and enhancements are preferred. For the medicinals with toxicity, since sometimes in Chinese medicine the toxicity is just part of its action, the medicinals with mutual restraint and mutual detoxication are recommended. And the medicinals with the relation of mutual antagonism and incompatibility should be prohibited as much as possible.

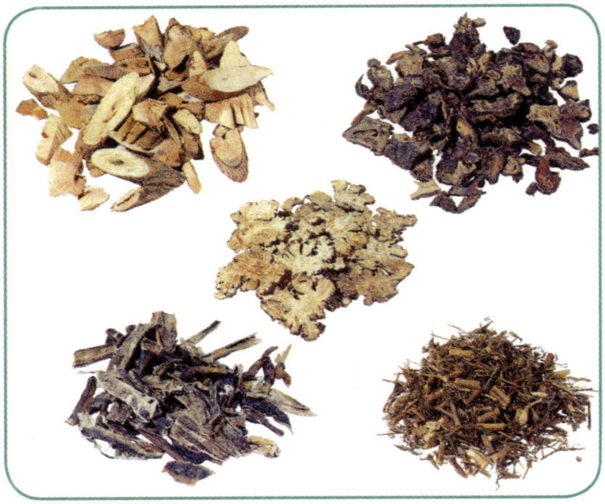

2. What Can I Expect?

Chinese medicinals are the mainstay of Chinese medicine. Although acupuncture is the best known modality here in the West, in China the great majority of patients who seek treatment from Chinese medicine get medicinal formulas. Treatment with medicinals is thought to have a wider scope than the more commonly known acupuncture, and for most diseases it works faster. Another, more practical advantage of treatment with Chinese medicinals is the frequency of office visits. Acupuncture patients are frequently seen two or three times per week, while medicinal prescriptions are usually modified once a week, with visits becoming even less frequent as the patient's condition stabilizes. Chinese medicine works holistically. During your visit to a Chinese medicine clinic, a good practitioner will get detailed information from you, analyze your condition comprehensively, then give you a complete evaluation including what kind of deficient or excess imbalance you have, which energy pathway is blocked, what foods to eat or avoid, and how these things relate to your mental disturbance. He or she will decide what is the best medicinal remedy for your depression.

Similar to the modalities that work on the points and channels like acupuncture, moxibustion, and cupping, medicinals can be administered in many different ways. The most common method is done by taking the raw medicinals, boiling them to extract their effective properties, and then drinking the resulting liquid. Chinese medicine calls this a "decoction". Taking Chinese medicinals as a decoction is the most potent and fastest working form of treatment available.

Since treatment methods vary greatly from disease to disease, and styles differ between practitioners, the exact amounts of medicinals, number of packets, and preparation instructions will likewise be very different. Described below is a typical treatment. If your practitioner gives you something that falls outside the guidelines listed here, do not be concerned.

> Preparation of the decoction

Decoction is the most traditional method of preparing medicinals. At the practitioner's office, you will most likely be given several packets of Chinese medicinals. Each packet will be for one or two days' use and will probably contain from 70-120 grams of medicinals. Take the time to examine the medicinals in the packet. Enjoy the different colors, smells, and textures. As many Chinese medicinals are common plants found around the world, you may even find something you recognize. Being able to get to know your medicine and be involved in its preparation never fails to endear a patient to Chinese medicine.

To cook the decoction, first put all the medicinals into a ceramic or glass pot (metal is not suitable) and add water until it completely covers the medicinals (your practitioner may tell you an exact amount of water to add). The mixture should be brought to a boil on high heat and then reduced to a medium flame. Usually the decoction needs to be boiled for 20-60 minutes depending on the ingredients of the formula. Strain the decoction dividing the liquid in two to be drunk twice a day in two equal portions, usually once with breakfast and once with dinner. Most often, one packet is one day's dosage. Sometimes you will be asked to save the dregs to be cooked again in the future. In this case, they should be stored in the refrigerator. There are some ingredients that have

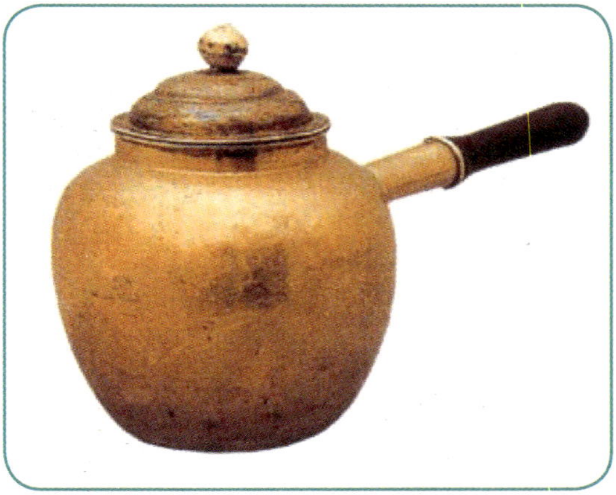

Decoction Pot

special cooking instructions such as cooking alone for 20-30 minutes before other ingredients are added (for especially dense materials), those that should be added at the last five minutes of cooking (for very delicate medicinals), or those that should be added last to the strained decoction (for materials in powder, gel, or liquid form). Medicinals have been prepared in this way for thousands of years and is not simply a combination of medicinals. During cooking, chemical reactions happen where active ingredients are released from the medicinals and components from different substances act on each other.

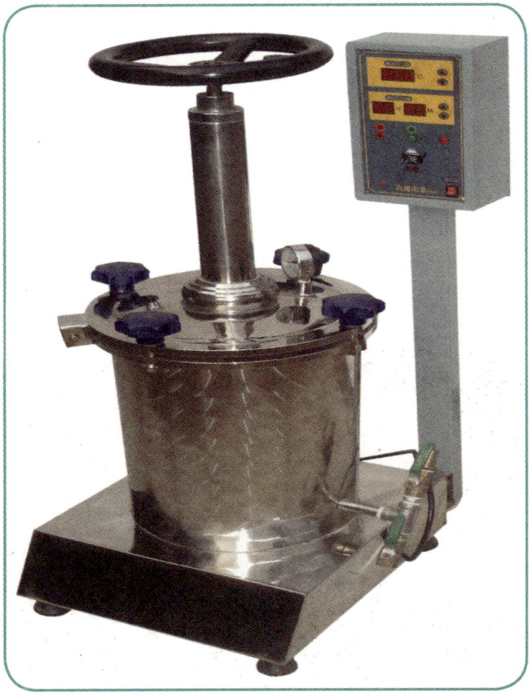

Electric Decoction Machine

Recently, some clinics have offered a decoction cooking service. The decoction will be made by a machine and sealed in plastic bags to store in the refrigerator.

No matter if you or the clinic prepares the medicinals, when you drink your decoction it should be warm. Only in special cases is room temperature acceptable.

> Treatment course

For chronic diseases, decoctions take time to have an effect. When you go to the clinic for the first time, the practitioner will usually give a prescription for 3-7 days. Each day's dose should be divided into two equal parts, usually taken in the morning and evening. You will need to come back to the clinic about once a week for the practitioner to modify the prescription. After a month or so has passed, you and your practitioner will reevaluate your condition and your treatment strategy may change allowing for gradually smaller amounts of medicinals, and more infrequent office visits. A treatment course usually lasts a few months, but may require more or less time depending on the severity of the case.

> Time and methods of taking the decoction

You are advised to take the decoction about one hour before or after meals. If a disease is related to the upper *jiao*, take it after meals; if it is related to the lower *jiao*, take it before meals; and if the decoction irritates your stomach, take it after meals. Decoctions for acute and serious diseases, take it at any time. A decoction with strengthening and purgative effect is supposed to be taken on an empty stomach; those with an action of tranquilizing the mind should be taken before falling asleep. The timing may vary with the specific prescription, but generally speaking, it is common to take the decoction once in the morning before breakfast and once at night before going to bed. Warm up the liquid before you drink it.

At first you may find the making of your decoction troublesome, and/or have a strong dislike of the unfamiliar taste. This is a common problem, especially in the West where people are accustomed to the medicine being easy to take and either tasteless or sugar coated. We can only ask that you recall the millions of people who have benefited from the decoction method of treatment and give it a chance for at least two weeks. In fact, it is the experience of many doctors and patients that if the prescription properly fits the imbalance, the initially unfamiliar or unpleasant taste will become something the patient enjoys and looks forward to.

Chinese Medicinals in Common Use

Medicinals imported into the United States must be manufactured in accordance with the stringent GMP. Chinese medicinals are very rarely used alone. But in order to construct a proper formula, the practitioner must be familiar with the properties of each individual medicinal. Since patients may present any possible combination of patterns, any one of the thousands of medicinal substances may show up in a patient's formula. But as we have seen, there are a few main patterns that are typically present in depression patients. And for each of these main patterns, there are certain medicinals that are most effective and therefore most commonly used. In addition, due to scientific research, some medicinals are known to be effective for depression treatment. Below are some brief descriptions of some of the most commonly used medicinals for depression treatment: [58]

> *Hé huān pí* (合欢皮, Cortex Albiziae)

Source: Albiziae bark
Property: Sweet and neutral, attributed to the liver and heart channels
Function: Tranquilize the mind, disperse depression, activate blood circulation, and relieve edema

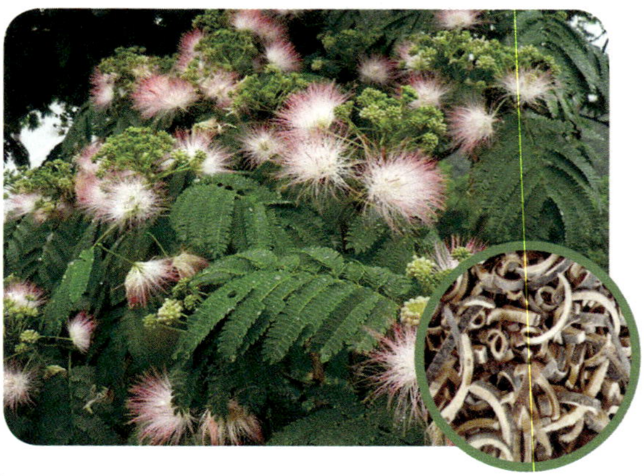

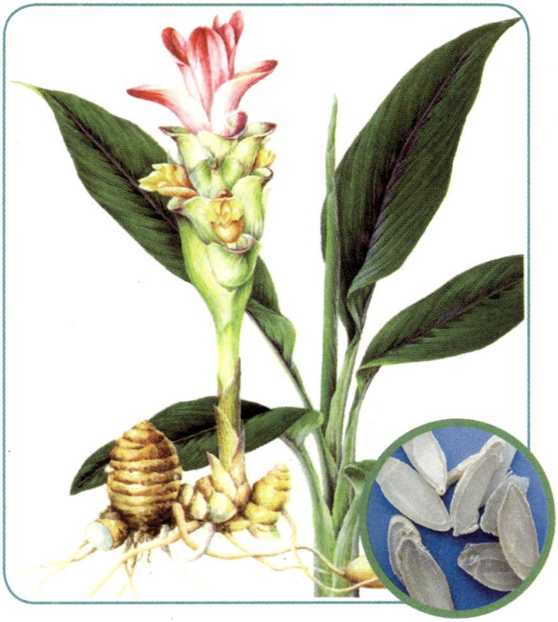

> *Yù jīn* (郁金, Radix Curcumae)

Source: Turmeric root tuber
Property: Pungent, bitter and cold, attributed to the liver, gallbladder, and heart channels
Function: Activate blood circulation to relieve pain, promote qi flow to remove depression, clear the heat of heart, cool blood, and benefit gallbladder to relieve jaundice

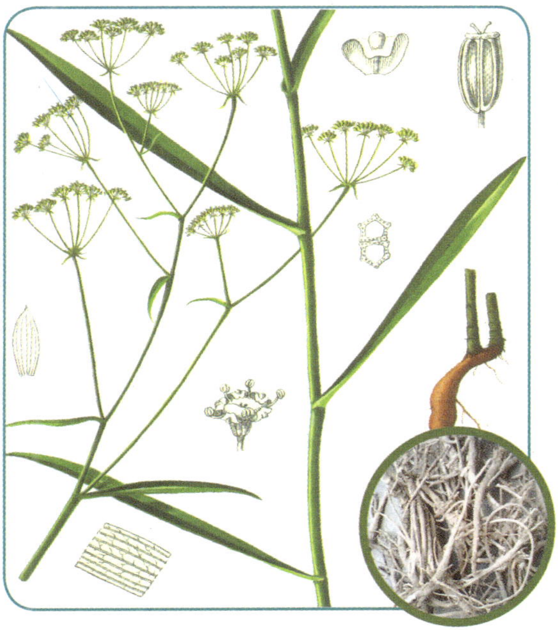

> *Chái hú* (柴胡, Radix Bupleuri)

Source: Dried bupleurum root
Property: Bitter, pungent, and slightly cold
Function: Regulate the functional relation of internal organs to relieve fever, disperse the stagnated liver qi, and uplift yang to raise the sinking

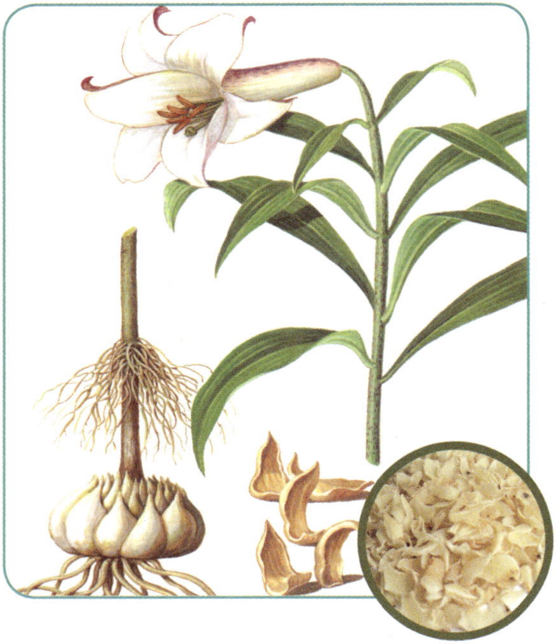

> *Bǎi hé* (百合, **Bulbus Lilii**)

Source: Lily bulb
Property: Sweet and cool, attributed to the lung, heart, and stomach channels
Function: Nourish yin to moisturize lung, and clear heart heat to tranquilize *shén*

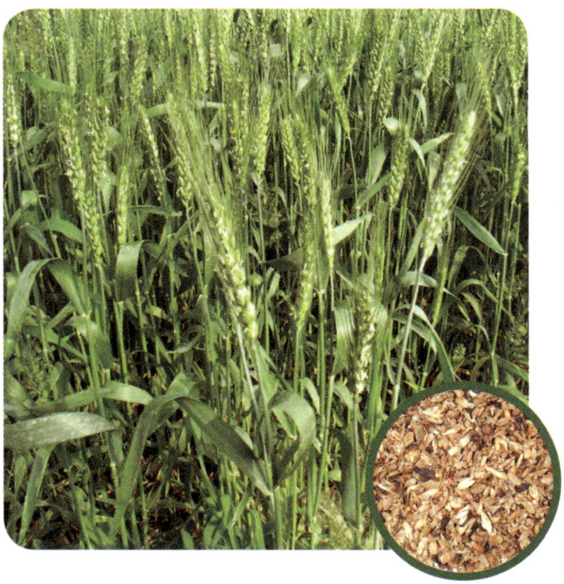

> *Fú xiǎo mài* (浮小麦, **Fructus Tritici Levis**)

Source: Blighted wheat
Property: Sweat and cool, attributed to the heart channel
Function: Enrich qi, clear heat, and relieve spontaneous and night sweating

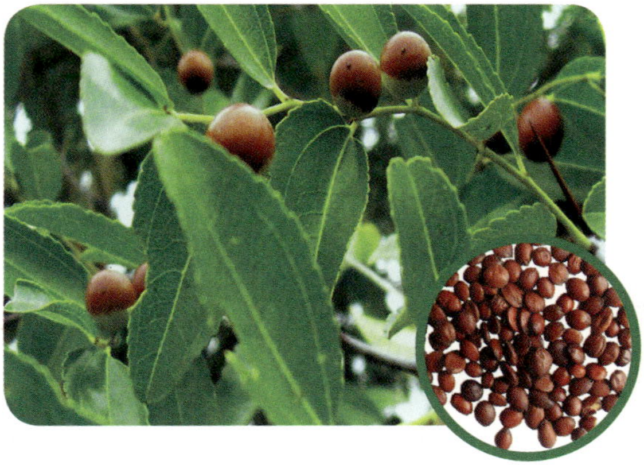

> *Suān zǎo rén* (酸枣仁, **Semen Ziziphi Spinosae)**

Source: Spiney date seed
Property: Sweet, sour, and neutral, attributed to the liver and heart channels
Function: Nourish, heart, benefit, liver, tranquilize, mind, and eliminate excessive perspiration

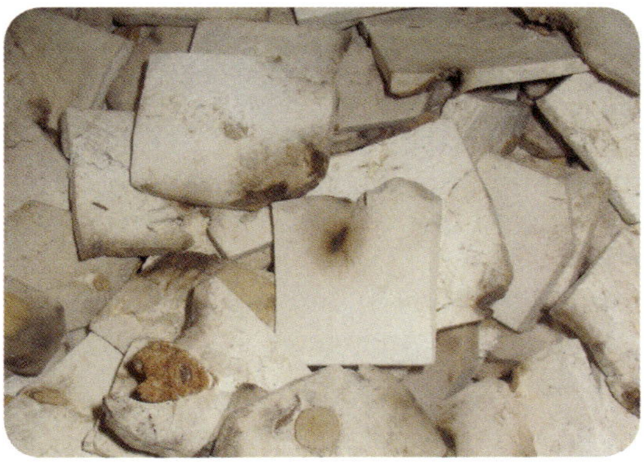

> *Fú shén* (茯神, **Sclerotium Poriae Pararadicis)**

Source: Indian bread sclerotium with hostwood
Property: Sweet, bland, and neutral, attributed to the heart, spleen, and kidney channels
Function: Tranquilize heart and benefit *shén*

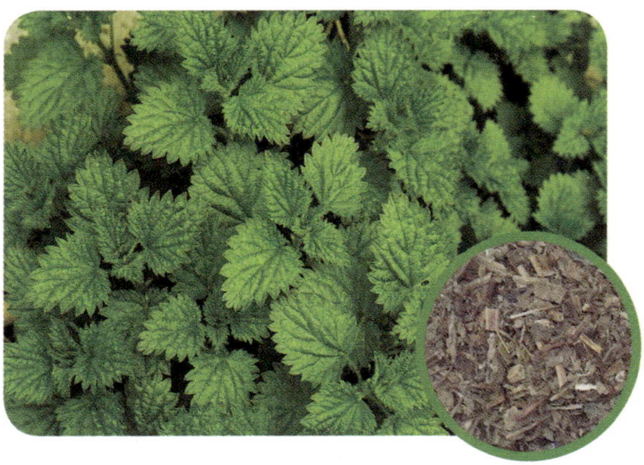

> *Bò hé* (薄荷, **Medicinala Menthae)**

Source: Field mint branch and leaf
Property: Pungent and cool, attributed to the lung and liver channels
Function: Expel wind and heat, clear head and eyes, ease the discomfort of throat, promote eruption of rash, smooth the liver, and disperse the stagnation of liver qi.

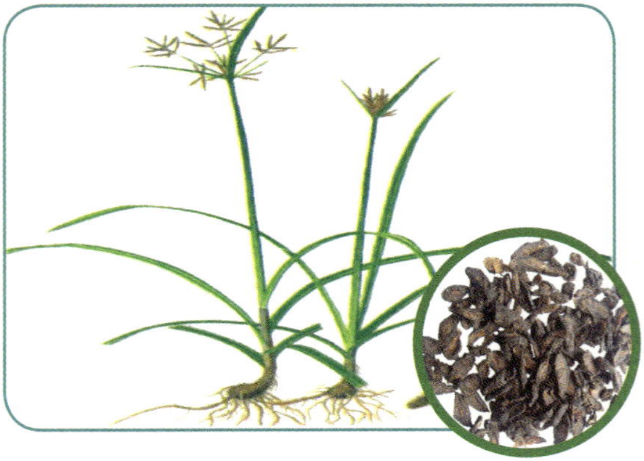

> *Xiāng fù* (香附, **Rhizoma Cyperi)**

Source: Nutgrass galingale rhizome
Property: Pungent, slightly bitter, slightly sweet and neutral, attributed to the liver, and *sanjiao* channels
Function: Smooth liver to regulate qi, and regulate menstruation to relieve pain

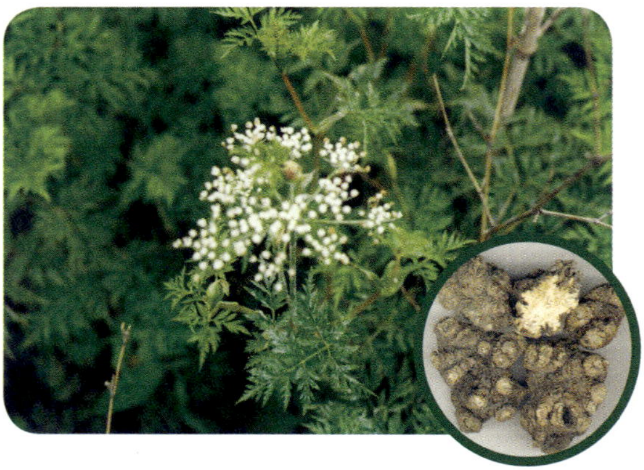

> *Chuān xiōng* (川芎, **Rhizoma Chuanxiong)**

Source: Chuanxiong root
Property: Pungent and warm, attributed to the liver, gallbladder, and pericardium channels
Function: Promote the circulation of blood and qi, expel wind, and relieve pain

Medicinal Groups in Common Use

As what we described above, medicinals are seldom used alone and medicinal combinations that mutually promote and enhance are preferred in the clinic. Some of the most common combinations used by experienced Chinese medicine physicians are below:[59]

> *Chái hú* and *bái sháo*

Chái hú has the action of opening with acridity, descending with bitterness, and regulating qi movement, while *bái sháo* is bitter and sour in flavor, and has the function of relaxing tension, relieving pain, and subduing liver yang. Both of them enter into the liver meridian, *chái hú*, acrid with dispersing property, mainly goes

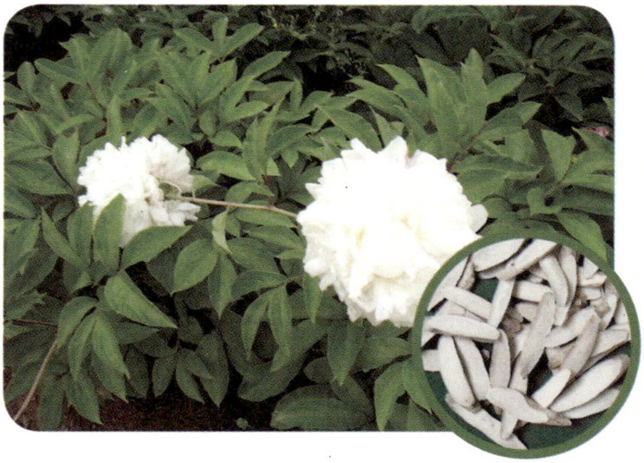

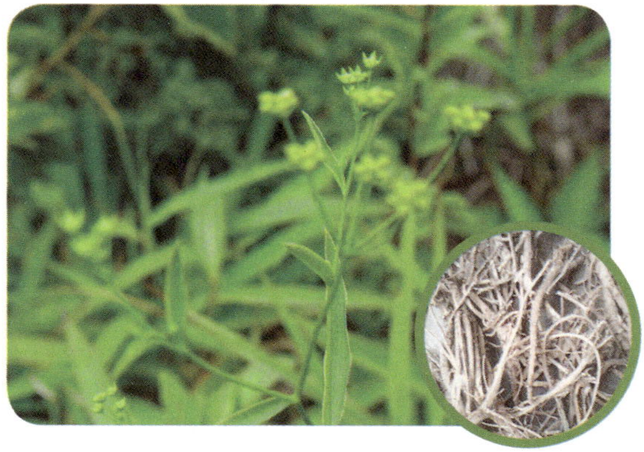

into the qi aspect, while *bái sháo*, sour with contracting property, primarily goes into the blood aspect. *Chái hú* abreacts liver qi for harmonizing liver function, whereas *bái sháo* nourishes liver blood for tonifying liver tissue. The combination of them is characterized by dispersing vs. contracting and ascending vs. descending. Assisted with contracting action of *bái sháo*, *chái hú* will not lead to consumption of liver yin due to over abreaction of liver qi; with dispersing function of *chái hú*, *bái sháo* will not block the qi movement and inhibit the liver function. They can be used together for the pattern of blood deficiency and liver hyperactivity, and liver failing to maintain the free flow of qi, which manifests as vexation, irritation, chest and hypochondrium fullness, bilateral hypochondria and breast distending pain, irregular menstruation, etc. The dosage of *chái hú* is 10 g, and that of *bái sháo* is 9-12 g.

> *Dān pí* and *shān zhī*

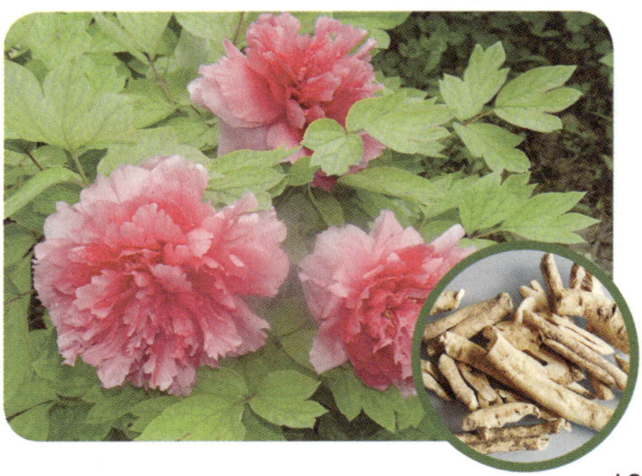

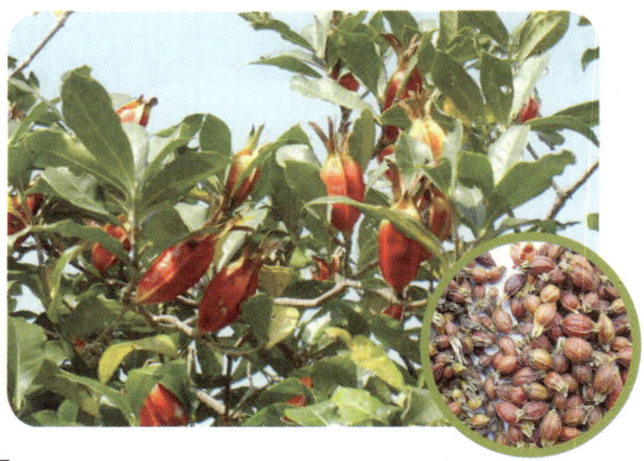

Bitter in flavor, cold in nature, and red in color, *dān pí* enters into blood, cools the blood without stasis, and activates the blood without causing frenetic movement. As described in *The Grand Compendium of Materia Medica* (*Běn Cǎo Gāng Mù*, 本草纲目), it is good for harmonizing blood, generating blood, cooling blood, clearing the hidden fire in blood, and relieving feverish dysphoria. *Shān zhī* can dredge the fire from the *sanjiao* as well as relieve restlessness. Both *dān pí* and *shān zhī* can clear heat. But *dān pí* cools blood while it clears heat, and *shān zhī* dredges fire while it clears heat; *dān pí* enters the blood aspect, and *shān zhī* enters mainly the qi aspect; *dān pí* relieves steaming bone, and *shān zhī* elimilates restlessness. The combination of them is mainly indicated for heat accumulation of the liver and gallbladder manifested as dizziness, bitter taste in the mouth, hypochondrium distention, burning heat of muscular interstices, vexation, insomnia, yellow urine, dry stool, wiry and rapid pulses, and a red tongue with greasy coating. The dosage of *dān pí* is 6-12 g, and that of *shān zhī* is 6-9 g.

> *Xiāng fù* and *chuān xiōng*

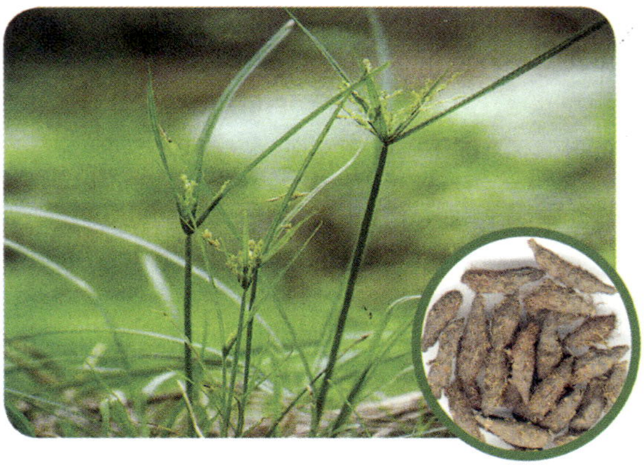

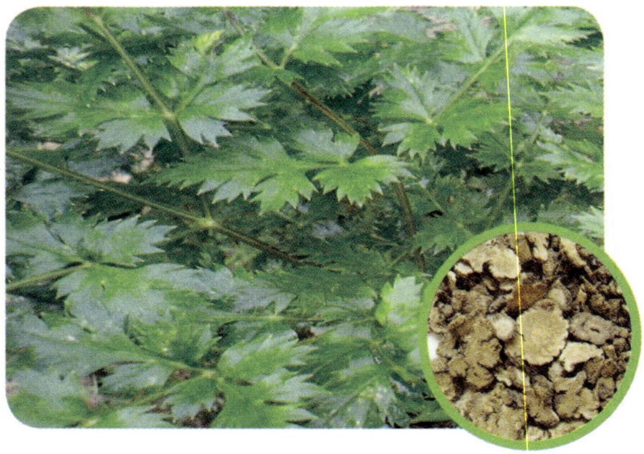

Xiāng fù has the properties of acridity, bitterness, fragrance, and dryness, and is regarded as the essential medicine for moving qi and resolving depression. It can go upwards to the chest and diaphragm, exteriorly to the skin, downwards to the liver and kidney, pass through the waist to the feet, and promote the movement of stagnant qi in the meridians. This medicinal can also enter into blood aspect to move the qi there, regulate menstruation, and relieve pain. It acts as the commander general of qi diseases and the governor in chief of gynecology. As stated in *Orthodox Interpretation of the Materia Medica* (*Běn Cǎo Zhèng Yì*, 本草正义), it is the medicinal specializing in qi stagnation. *Chuān xiōng* is acrid, warm, fragrant, penetrating, and mobile without lingering. It can go upwards to the vertex, move downwards to the sea of blood, by-pass the four limbs, and go exteriorly to the skin and hair. It is termed as the medicine for qi within blood in *The Grand Compendium of Materia Medica*. *Xiāng fù* is predominantly for qi while *chuān xiōng* is predominantly for blood; the combination of them can not only regulate qi and alleviate depression, but also activate blood and relieve pain. They are suitable for treating qi and blood stagnation characterized by hypochondrium pain, dysmenorrhea, deep and rough pulses, and a dark-purple tongue. The dosage of *xiāng fù* is 6-9 g, and that of *chuān xiōng* is 9-12 g.

> *Hé huān huā* and *yè jiāo téng*

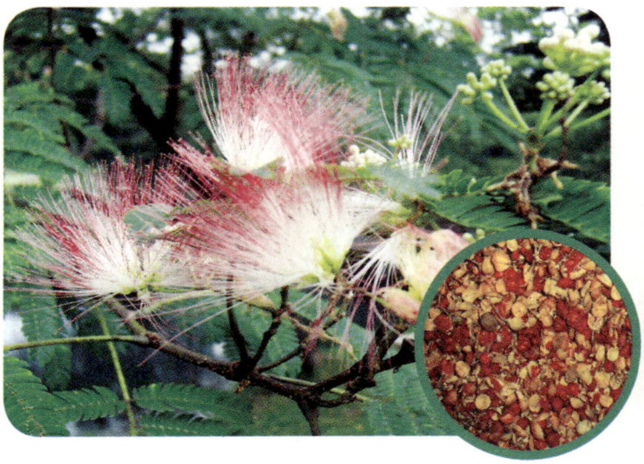

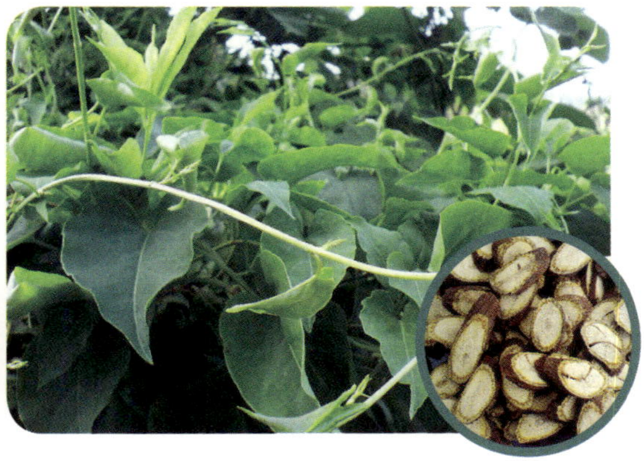

Both can calm the heart and tranquilize the spirit; *yè jiāo téng* nourishes the blood, calms the heart, and leads yang into yin to tranquilize the spirit; while *hé huān huā* alleviates depression, relieves restlessness, and tranquilizes spirit as well. It is said that *hé huān huā* can quiet the five *zang* organs, harmonize spirit, and make people happy. The combination of them can nourish blood, alleviate depression, calm the heart, tranquilize the spirit, treat emotional impairment-caused yin deficiency and blood insufficiency. Manifestation includes anger, depression, deficient restlessness, insomnia, profuse dreaming, susceptibility to fright, forgetfulness, wiry and rapid pulses, and red tongue with yellow coating. The dosage of *hé huān huā* is 10-15 g, and that of *yè jiāo téng* is 15-30 g.

> *Mài yá* and *qīng hāo*

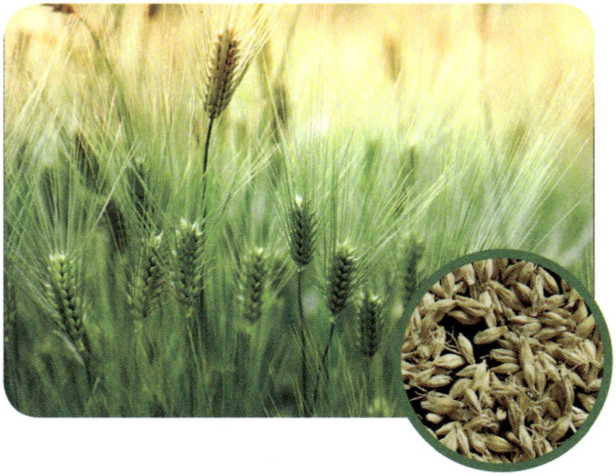

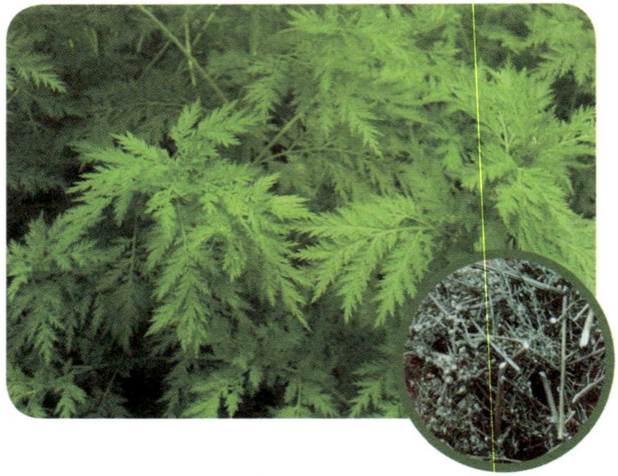

Acting as the assistant of tonifying spleen and stomach, *mài yá* is actually good at soothing the liver. *qīng hāo* is fragrant, bitter, cold in nature without stomach impairment. It goes exteriorly to penetrate the heat accumulated in the muscles, and also moves interiorly to raise spleen qi and clear heat; it enters the liver, kidney, *sanjiao*, and the blood aspect. Both *qīng hāo* and *chái hú* are indicated for malaria with alternating fever and chills; *chái hú* specializes in soothing liver and alleviating depression, has rising and dispersing properties, but impairs yin; while *qīng hāo* can clear summer heat, resolve dampness, clear deficient heat, cool blood, and relieve steaming bone without yin damage by rising and dispersing. Chinese medicine doctor sometimes combine *mài yá* with *qīng hāo* when treating depressive fire due to liver and kidney yin deficiency. *Mài yá* can not only soothe the liver and regular the spleen without yin damage, but also relieve restlessness and alleviate visceral agitation; while *qīng hāo* enters the *sanjiao* and the blood aspect, and can penetrate muscular depressive heat through moving from interior to exterior. The combination of them can soothe the liver, alleviate depression, and is good at dispersing heat accumulation in the blood aspect.

> *Bǎi hé* and *huái xiǎo mài*

Bǎi hé is sweet and a little bit cold in property, enters the heart meridian, and has the action of clearing the heart and tranquilizing the spirit. It was used as a main medicinal for treating lily disease in *Essentials from the Golden Cabinet* (*Jīn*

Guì Yào Lüè, 金匮要略). This medicinal can quiet the heart, calm the gallbladder, promote intelligence, and nourish the five *zang* organs. *Huái xiǎo mài* is sweet in flavor and cool in nature, enters the heart meridian, and has the effects of nourishing the heart and spleen, clearing deficient heat, and stopping deficient sweat. These two herbs together are effective on either visceral agitation manifested as being more susceptible to sorrow or even frequent cry, frequent sighing, being nervous all the time and insomnia, or depressive syndrome featured by general diseases and symptoms of lily disease. The dosage of *bǎi hé* is 10-30 g, and that of *huái xiǎo mài* is 30-60 g.

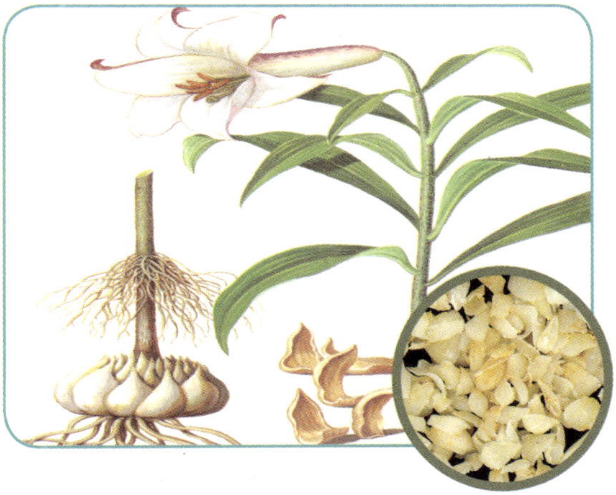

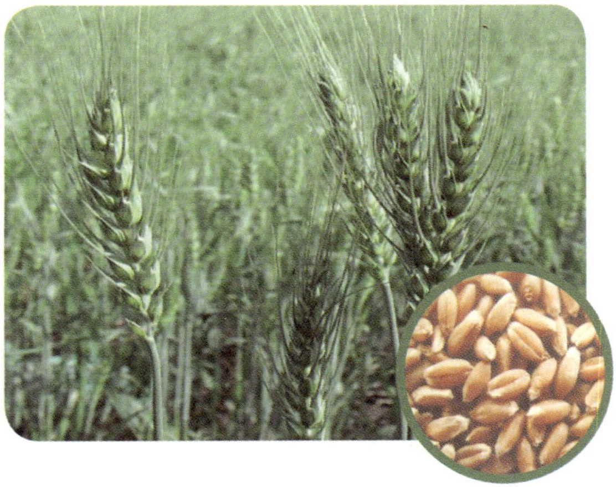

> *Zhū shā* and *cí shí*

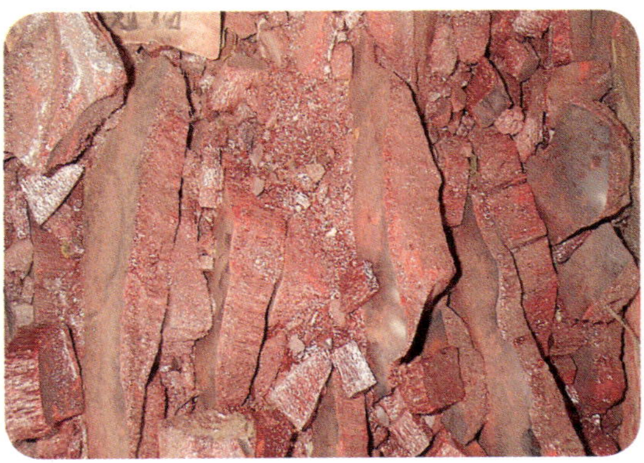

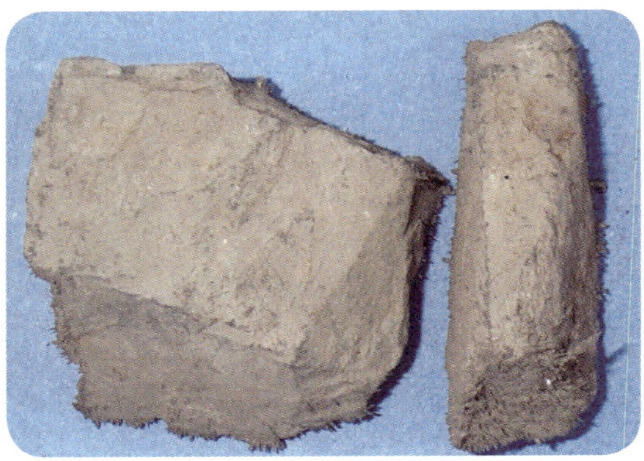

Zhū shā is cold in nature and red in color, tends to descend, enters the blood aspect, and specializes in settling the heart and tranquilizing the spirit. It can nourish the spirit, quiet the ethereal and corporeal souls, replenish qi, and brighten the eyes. *Cí shí* enters the liver and kidney, calms the liver, tonifies the kidney, calms the mind, and tranquilizes the spirit. The combination of them tranquilizes spirit with heavy property, contains floating yang, and promotes the interaction of heart and kidney. They are suitable for heart-liver effulgent fire and heart-kidney interaction disharmony manifested as palpitation, disturbed spirit, dizziness, headache, tinnitus, deafness, etc. It is worth noting that *zhū shā* as a mercury-based medicine should never be over-dosed or used for a long time so as to prevent chronic mercurialism; it is often used in pill or powder form and 0.3-0.9 g should be taken orally each time. The dosage of *cí shí* is 10-30 g.

> *Xìng rén* and *jié gěng*

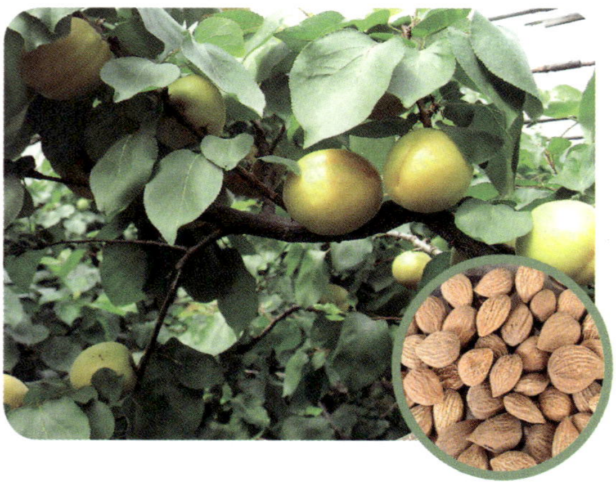

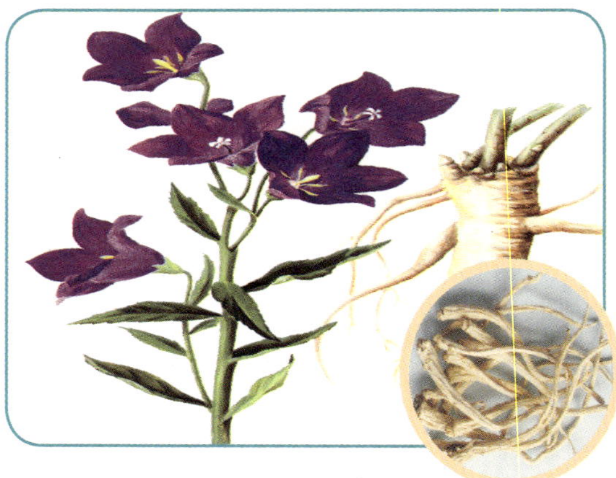

With acridity for dispersing pathogen, bitterness for descending qi, and moistness for relaxing bowels, *xìng rén* can descend qi, expel phlegm, disperse lung, relieve asthma, moisten intestine, and relax the bowels. *Jié gěng* can disperse lung qi, clear the throat, and raise and induce water. *Xìng rén* is predominant in descending while *jié gěng* is predominant in ascending. This combination, characterized by ascending and descending, can not only disperse lung and induce water for getting through the upper sources of water, but also descend qi, expel phlegm and relieve sore throat. It is therefore used for liver depression and phlegm-qi accumulation, sore throat, chest and gastric region distention, edema with fullness, and globus hystericus.

Formulae in Common Use[60]

> *Sì Nì Sǎn* (Frigid Extremities Powder, 四逆散)

From *Treatise on Cold Damage* (*Shāng Hán Lùn*, 伤寒论) written by Zhang Zhong-jing in the *Han* Dynasty, *Sì Nì Sǎn* was originally used as an ancestor formula for treating qi stagnation pattern manifested as extreme coldness of the four extremities due to stagnation of yang-qi. Gradually, it has developed into a basic formula for soothing the liver and alleviating depression. For example, *Chái Hú Shū Gān Sǎn* is the modification of it. This formula is mainly indicated for liver qi stagnation manifested as depression or sorrow, chest and hypochondrium distention and fullness or pain, fluctuation of symptoms with emotional variation, etc. The medicinal characteristics of this formula are as follows: both *chái hú* and *zhǐ shí* smooth liver qi stagnation with their bitter and acrid taste; *sháo yào* softens the liver and harmonizes the nutrient aspect with its bitter and sour taste.

> *Bàn Xià Hòu Pò Tāng* (Pinellia and Officinal Magnolia Bark Decoction, 半夏厚朴汤)

From the *Essentials from the Golden Cabinet* written by Zhang Zhong-jing in the Han Dynasty, *Bàn Xià Hòu Pò Tāng* is a famous formula for treating qi depression with phlegm stagnation. The therapeutic methods are combining qi regulation with phlegm resolution, since qi prefers free flow. Once there is qi stagnation, the fluids block, which will accumulate to form phlegm, obstruct qi movement, further aggravating phlegm stagnation, and eventually forming a vicious cycle. Thus globus hystericus occurs, a sensation of a foreign body obstructed in throat which can be neither swallowed nor ejected. In this case, *Bàn Xià Hòu Pò Tāng* is applicable, since the combination of qi regulating medicinals such as *hòu pò*, *sū yè*, etc. with phlegm resolving medicinals such as *jiāng bàn xià*, *fú líng*, etc. can act upon all concerned conditions, and enhance therapeutic efficiency. This formula is also called *Sì Qī Tāng* (Four-Seven Decoction) by subsequent generations because the four medicinals can cure the pattern of seven emotional depressions.

> *Xiāo Yáo Sǎn* (Free Wanderer Powder, 逍遥散)

From *Beneficial Formulas from the Taiping Imperial Pharmacy* (*Tài Píng Huì Mín Hé Jì Jú Fāng*, 太平惠民和剂局方) from the Song Dynasty states *Xiāo Yáo Sǎn* is the representative formula for treating depression through soothing the liver and invigorating the spleen. The Chinese call this old remedy "the happy pill" because of its well-known anti-depressant effect. Its compatibility is based on the relationship of *zang-fu* organs. Patients with liver depression caused by emotional disturbance are usually accompanied with symptoms of spleen deficiency, because both liver and spleen are in the middle *jiao*, stagnated liver qi overwhelms spleen and/or deficient spleen makes liver qi more violent. Such chronic diseases as depression accompanied with lassitude of spirit and decrease of food taking should be treated by soothing liver and regulating qi with strengthening spleen simultaneously. *chái hú*, as the liver soothing medicinals in this formula, is combined with spleen invigorating medicinals such as *fú líng* and *bái zhú*, which embodies the tenet of Zhang Zhong-jing that "if the liver is diseased, it can affect the spleen, physicians need to therefore tonify the spleen first".

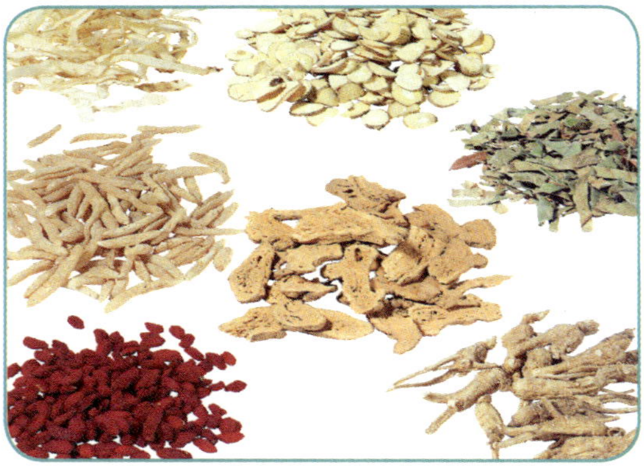

> *Guī Pí Tāng* (Spleen-Restoring Decoction, 归脾汤)

Guī Pí Tāng, from the *Formulas to Aid the Living* (*Jì Shēng Fāng*, 济生方) written by Yan Yong-he in the Song Dynasty, is the chief formula for treating chronic depression with consumption of heart and spleen blood. It treats the root aspect of the disease by invigorating the spleen with *huáng qí*, *dǎng shēn*, *bái zhú*, and *dāng guī*, and the branch aspect through nourishing blood and tranquilizing spirit with suan *suān zǎo rén*, *lóng yǎn ròu*, *fú shén*, and *yuǎn zhì*. This formula treats the root and the branch simultaneously and aims exactly at emotional symptoms such as insomnia, night fright, absent-mindedness, etc.

> *Yuè Jú Wán* (Constraint-Resolving Pill, 越鞠丸)

It derives from *Teachings of [Zhu] Dan-xi* (*Dān Xī Xīn Fǎ*, 丹溪心法) written by Zhu Dan-xi in the Jin-Yuan Period, who held that excessive joy, anger, or over-anxiety can result in qi movement problems, which further causes stagnation of qi, blood, phlegm, fire, food, and dampness. And hence *Yuè Jú Wán* was created for the treatment of six kinds of stagnation, including qi, blood, phlegm, fire, food, and dampness. Qi stagnation is regarded as the root for the others, accordingly, *xiāng fù* as the sovereign is used for soothing liver and alleviating depression, *chuān xiōng* aims to help blood, *zhī zǐ* is for fire, *shén qū* treats food accumulations, and *cāng zhú* treats dampness. This is most suitable for depression syndrome manifested as chest distress, abdominal distention, and indigestion.

> *Yī Guàn Jiān* (Effective Integration Decoction, 一贯煎)

It is from *Supplement to "Classified Case Records of Famous Physicians"* (*Xù Míng Yī Lèi Àn*, 续名医类案) written by Wei Zhixiu from the Qing Dynasty. Chronic liver depression tends to transform into fire and damage yin, and the repeated application of regulating qi and alleviating depression method may produce dryness and damage yin, thus *Yī Guàn Jiān* was created for treating depression through nourishing yin and soothing liver. This formula consists of a large amount of yin nourishing medicinals, such as *shēng dì, shā shēn, mài dōng, gǒu qǐ zǐ*, etc., which are combined with little doses of *chuān liàn zǐ* to regulate qi. The formula as a whole is capable of nourishing yin and soothing liver, it is suitable for chronic depression of yin deficiency and qi stagnation with the manifestation of hypochondrium pain, acid regurgitation and bitter tasting vomit, and red tongue with less fluid.

Formulas for the Most Commonly Seen Patterns

A typical formula consists of between 5 to 15 ingredients with each ingredient usually dosed between 6 and 30 grams. The ingredients in the formula are arranged according to a hierarchy. The chief ingredient represents the main therapeutic effect and will often have the largest dose. The assistants and deputies either support the chief, address another aspect of the imbalance, or perform a checking action against some other ingredient that may be too harsh in some way. The last soldier, the courier, serves to guide the formula to a certain body part, organ, or channel, or acts to harmonize the formula.[61]

> Liver qi stagnation

Typical manifestations: Depression, restlessness, chest stuffiness, distention and unfixed pain in hypochondriac area, epigastrium stuffiness and belching, frequently sighing, poor appetite, irregular menstruation, thin and greasy tongue coating, and wiry pulses
Therapeutic principles: Soothe liver, regulate qi flow, and relieve depression
Formula: *Chái Hú Shū Gān Sǎn* (Bupleurum Liver Soothing Powder)

Medicinal	Pinyin	Dose	Latin Name
柴胡	*chái hú*	6 g	Radix Bupleuri
陈皮	*chén pí*	6 g	Citri Reticulatae Pericarpium
川芎	*chuān xiōng*	4.5 g	Rhizoma Chuanxiong
香附	*xiāng fù*	4.5 g	Rhizoma Cyperi
枳壳	*zhǐ qiào*	4.5 g	Fructus Aurantii
白芍	*bái sháo*	4.5 g	Radix Paeoniae Alba
甘草	*gān cǎo*	1.5 g	Radix Glycyrrhizae

> Fire due to prolonged liver qi stagnation

Typical manifestations: Rashness, bad temper, distension and fullness in chest and hypochondria, gastric upset, acid regurgitation, bitter and dry mouth, constipation, headache with hot sensation, tinnitus, red and pain eyes, a red tongue with yellow coating, wiry and fast pulses
Therapeutic principles: Soothe liver, eliminate depression, and regulate stomach
Formula: *Xiāo Yáo Sǎn* (Free Wanderer Powder) with *Zuǒ Jīn Wán* (Left Metal Pill)

Medicinal	Pinyin	Dose	Latin Name
当归	*dāng guī*	9 g	Angelicae Sinensis Radix
茯苓	*fú líng*	9 g	Poria
白芍	*bái sháo*	9 g	Radix Paeoniae Alba
白术	*bái zhú*	9 g	Rhizoma Atractylodis Macrocephalae
柴胡	*chái hú*	9 g	Radix Bupleuri
甘草	*gān cǎo*	3 g	Radix Glycyrrhizae
牡丹皮	*mǔ dān pí*	6 g	Cortex Moutan
栀子	*zhī zǐ*	6 g	Fructus Gardeniae
黄连	*huáng lián*	6 g	Rhizoma Coptidis
吴茱萸	*wú zhū yú*	3 g	Fructus Evodiae

> Qi and phlegm stagnation

Typical manifestations: Depression, chest stuffiness, the sensation of a foreign body in the throat which can be neither swallowed nor expectorated, a white and greasy tongue coating, wiry and slippery pulses
Therapeutic principles: Promote qi circulation, relieve depression, and remove phlegm
Formula: *Bàn Xià Hòu Pò Tāng* (Pinellia and Officinal Magnolia Bark Decoction)

Medicinal	Pinyin	Dose	Latin Name
半夏	*bàn xià*	12 g	Pinellia Rhizoma
厚朴	*hòu pò*	9 g	Cortex Magnoliae Officinalis
茯苓	*fú líng*	12 g	Poria
生姜	*shēng jiāng*	15 g	Rhizoma Zingiberis Recens
紫苏叶	*zǐ sū yè*	6 g	Folium Perillae

> Long-term stagnation impairing spirit

Typical manifestations: Absent-mindedness, vexation, frequent sighing, palpitation, insomnia, thin and white tongue coating, wiry and thin pulses
Therapeutic principles: Nourish the heart and tranquilize the mind
Formula: *Gān Mài Dà Zǎo Tāng* (Licorice, Wheat, and Jujube Decoction)

Medicinal	Pinyin	Dose	Latin Name
甘草	*gān cǎo*	9 g	Radix Glycytthizae
小麦	*xiǎo mài*	15 g	Fructus Tritici
大枣	*dà zǎo*	10 pieces	Fructrs Jujubae

> Deficiency of spleen and heart

Typical manifestations: Over-thinking, over-suspicious, vertigo, dizziness, palpitation, timidity, lusterless complexion, fatigue, poor appetite, insomnia, forgetfulness, pale tongue, thin and white tongue coating, and thin and weak pulses
Therapeutic principles: Strengthen the spleen, nourish the heart, and tonify qi and blood
Formula: *Guī Pí Tāng* (Spleen-Restoring Decoction)

Medicinal	Pinyin	Dose	Latin Name
白术	*bái zhú*	6 g	Rhizoma Atractylodis Macrocephalae
当归	*dāng guī*	6 g	Angelicae Sinensis Radix
茯苓	*fú líng*	6 g	Poria
黄芪	*huáng qí*	6 g	Astragalus
远志	*yuǎn zhì*	6 g	Polygalae Radix
龙眼肉	*lóng yǎn ròu*	6 g	Arillus Longan
酸枣仁	*suān zǎo rén*	6 g	Semen Ziziphi Spinosae
人参	*rén shēn*	9 g	Radix Ginseng
木香	*mù xiāng*	6 g	Radix Aucklandiae
甘草	*gān cǎo*	3 g	Radix Glycyrrhizae

> Fire caused by yin deficiency

Typical manifestations: Restlessness, hypochondriac pain, dry mouth and throat; vertigo, palpitation, vexation, insomnia, forgetfulness, sore waist, spermatorrhea, irregular menstruation, red tongue with little coating, wiry, thin, and fast pulses

Therapeutic principles: Nourish yin to clear heat, calm the heart, and tranquilize the mind

Formula: *Zī Shuǐ Qīng Gān Yǐn* (Nourishing Yin and clearing Live Beverage)

Medicinal	Pinyin	Dose	Latin Name
熟地	*shú dì*	18 g	Rhizoma Rehmannia
山茱萸	*shān zhū yú*	9 g	Fructus Corni
茯苓	*fú líng*	9 g	Poria
当归	*dāng guī*	12 g	Angelicae Sinensis Radix
山药	*shān yào*	6 g	Rhizoma Dioscoreae
牡丹皮	*mǔ dān pí*	6 g	Cortex Moutan
泽泻	*zé xiè*	6 g	Rhizoma Alismatis
白芍	*bái sháo*	15 g	Radix Paeoniae Alba
柴胡	*chái hú*	3 g	Radix Bupleuri
栀子	*zhī zǐ*	6 g	Fructus Gardeniae
酸枣仁	*suān zǎo rén*	6 g	Semen Ziziphi Spinosae

> Heart yin deficiency

Typical manifestations: Restlessness, palpitation, forgetfulness, insomnia, dreaminess, burning sensation in the chest, soles, and palms, night sweating, dry mouth and throat, red tongue with little fluid, and thin and fast pulses

Therapeutic principles: Nourish the yin and blood, fortify the heart, and tranquilize the mind

Formula: *Tiān Wáng Bǔ Xīn Dān* (Celestial Emperor Heart Supplementing Elixir)

Medicinal	Pinyin	Dose	Latin Name
人参	*rén shēn*	6 g	Radix Ginseng
茯苓	*fú líng*	6 g	Poria
玄参	*xuán shēn*	6 g	Radix Scrophulariae
丹参	*dān shēn*	6 g	Salvia Miltiorrhizae Radix
桔梗	*jié gěng*	6 g	Radix Platycodonis
远志	*yuǎn zhì*	6 g	Polygalae Radix
当归	*dāng guī*	12 g	Angelicae Sinensis Radix
五味子	*wǔ wèi zǐ*	12 g	Fructus Schisandrae Chinensis
麦门冬	*mài mén dōng*	12 g	Radix Ophiopogonis

Medicinal	Pinyin	Dose	Latin Name
天门冬	*tiān mén dōng*	12 g	Radix Asparagi
酸枣仁	*suān zǎo rén*	12 g	Semen Ziziphi Spinosae
柏子仁	*bǎi zǐ rén*	12 g	Semen Platycladi
生地	*shēng dì*	36 g	Radix Rehmanniae

The above formulas are all based on prescriptions that were first put together hundreds, if not thousands of years ago. In Chinese medicine, doctors build on the experience of the past, using formulas that have been proven to be effective. However, genius lies not only in the past, and many skilled modern-day doctors and researchers have distilled their wisdom and experience into new formulas to pass on to future generations of doctors, thus Chinese medicine is continually being developed in response to modern research and changing clinical needs. This is especially true of problems that are more common now than in the past, depression being one.

Other Forms of Chinese Medicinals

Chinese medicinal formulas can be delivered in all manners of preparation. Prepared formulas are available, most of which are very convenient as they do not necessitate patient preparation time and are easily taken. However, the concentration of the Chinese medicinals in these products is low and it doesn't allow the practitioner to adjust the contents or dosages. These products are usually not as potent as the traditional preparation of decoction.

> Prepared medicines

These medicinals usually come in the form of pills or tablets, though some are given as syrups or powders. This is probably the easiest way to take Chinese medicinals as it is similar to taking a Western pharmaceutical. The practitioner gives you the bottle (or bottles) of pills, tells you how many to take and how often, and when the time comes, you simply take the proper number of pills with warm water. The advantages over decoctions are obvious as you can avoid the cooking process and the strange taste. The major disadvantage may not be as obvious, but it is significant.

In general, while prepared medicines are convenient and easy to take, they don't allow for patient-oriented and individualized medicinal formula. However, there is an increasing trend that many formulas will be available in pill or capsule form. And a patient-oriented formula can be pilled or encapsulated upon request if it is in large demand.

The reason Chinese medicine is so effective is that treatment can be tailored to exactly match the patient's individual pattern of disharmony. With Chinese medicinals, this is achieved by blending a combination of substances that correspond to the patterns presented. While formulas are helpful in that they serve as a guide to the treatment of the most common patterns, in almost all cases a formula will need to be modified to fit the patient exactly. The formula represented in a bottle of prepared medicine is unlikely to perfectly line up with a given patient's condition. Some parts of the patient's condition may remain unaddressed, and some parts of the formula may be inappropriate for the patient. This is why prepared medicines are usually used near the end of treatment, in order to consolidate the treatment effect by giving mild, long-term treatment directed at the patient's primary pattern. That being said, some practitioners combine two, three, or even more different prepared medicines to more accurately treat the patient's condition.

Take as an example a patient with severe stomach heat as well as spleen deficiency to a lesser degree. The practitioner may choose to prescribe Ledebouriella Sage-Inspired Powder which is the base formula to eliminate stomach heat and modify it to also strengthen the spleen. After a few months, when the patient's condition is brought under control, the practitioner might decide to have the patient take a small daily dose of the prepared version of Ledebouriella Sage-Inspired Powder to taper off the treatment by continuing to concentrate on the main pattern.

Another patient also has severe stomach heat and spleen deficiency. If the patient is unable to cook decoctions, the practitioner may decide to give the patient two different prepared medicines. Ledebouriella Sage-Inspired Powder could be given to treat the stomach heat, and Ginseng, Poria and Atractylodes Macrocephala Powder may be given as well to concentrate on the spleen deficiency, both in pill form.

There are many prepared medicines of plant origin designed to help people control depression that are sold commercially in China:

Pinyin	English Name	Chinese Name
Shū Gān Wán	Liver-soothing Pill	舒肝丸
Ān Shén Yǎng Xīn Wán	Spirit-calming Heart-supporting Pill	安神养心丸
Zhū Shā Ān Shén Wán	Cinnabar Spirit-calming Pill	朱砂安神丸
Xiāo Yáo Wán	Free Wanderer Powder	逍遥丸
Guī Pí Wán	Spleen-restoring Pill	归脾丸
Yǎng Xuè Ān Shén Piàn	Blood-Nourishing Spirit-calming Tablet	养血安神片
Qīng Nǎo Fù Shén Yè	Brain-clearing Spirit-restoring Oral Liquid	清脑复神液
Wǔ Wèi Zǐ Táng Jiāng	Schisandra Syrup	五味子糖浆

Pinyin	English Name	Chinese Name
Shēn Qí Piàn	Shen Qi Tablet	参芪片
Chái Hú Shū Gān Wán	Chai Hu Liver-dredging Pill	柴胡疏肝丸
Mù Xiāng Shùn Qì Wán	Costus Root Qi-balancing Pill	木香顺气丸
Ān Shén Wán	Spirit-calming Pill	安神丸
Niú Huáng Qīng Xīn Piàn	Bovine Bezoar Heart-clearing Tablet	牛黄清心片
Shēng Mài Yǐn	Pulse-engendering Beverage	生脉饮
Qī Yè Shén Ān Piàn	Qi Ye Spirit-calming Tablet	七叶神安片

These formulas contain many different combinations of medicinals, but since they are all designed specifically for depression management, they have much in common. Since the most common presentation of patterns in a depression patient is qi stagnation and *shén* disturbance, most of these products contain medicinals that regulate *shén* and qi movement. Also, since internal heat, stagnation, qi and blood deficiency and spleen, heart, and kidney weakness are also common, many of these patterns are addressed. Since each prepared medicine is slightly different, a trained professional will need to help you choose the best one.

> Granules

Chinese medicinals in granule form is a modern creation and represents a middle path between decoctions and prepared medicines. Granules of medicinals have been in use for the past 20 years and are a popular choice in today's busy world. To make granules, individual medicinals or whole formulas are cooked down until a concentrated powder remains. These are packaged and can be combined to fit the patient's exact pattern. Unlike preparing a decoction, the patient just takes the granule packets, empties them into a cup or container, pours hot water over the mixture, stirs to dissolve, and drinks.

This eliminates the need to prepare the medicinals at home, allows a more convenient preparation and individualized formula design, and still holds much of the original decoction's potency. However, it is generally thought that taking medicinals in granule form is slightly less effective than decoctions. Despite this, granules have become popular with many patients and practitioners in recent years due to their ease of preparation.

> External application

Chinese medicinals are sometimes prepared so that they may be applied directly to the skin to be absorbed superficially. External applications are usually used for problems of the skin and superficial channels. They are used often in dermatology, but are also often used to treat pain, numbness, and injury of a local area. Application of medicinals to acupoints aim to regulate the channels, yin-yang, and qi and blood for preventing and treating diseases by exerting influences on the flow of qi. Zhu Xiu-ping[64] treated 80 cases of deficient and cold pattern in the spleen and stomach by external application of medicinal paste on acupoints, the results showed remarkable effect in 52 cases, improvement in 24 cases, failure in 4 cases, and the total effective rate was 95.0%, indicating remarkable therapeutic effects were achieved with the external application of medicinal paste on acupoints in this case.

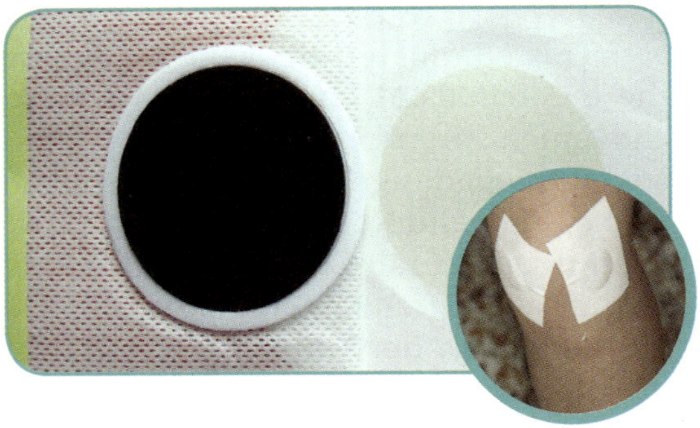

The simplest way to make an external application is to boil medicinals like you would cook a decoction, and apply the cooled liquid to the skin. This can then be wrapped in gauze for better effect. External applications do not need to be as specific as decoctions that are taken internally. For this reason, many practitioners use some kind of prepared medicine, usually as an alcohol extract, an oil, a cream, or sometimes a plaster that will stick to the body.

> Foot fumigation or foot bath

Foot fumigation or foot bath refers to therapies that use a warm medicinal decoction to bathe or fumigate the feet. It is used to prevent or treat peripheral vascular complications. The warmth combined with the medicinals act on the feet to benefit the flow of qi and blood. The ingredients in the decoction should be given by your practitioner based on your specific pattern identification. Medicinals that can move blood and remove stasis are often used to promote local circulation and metabolism. In addition, medicinals that supplement qi and open the channels are often used to treat the root condition. A lot of research showing the effectiveness of medicinal foot baths has been done.

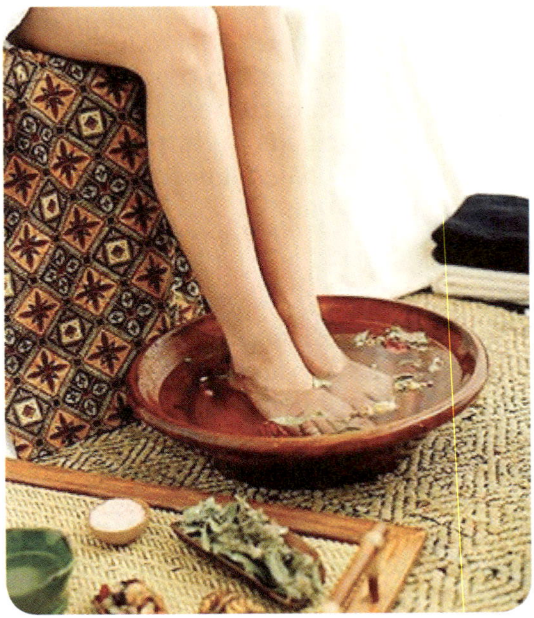

Warning!

The information in this section is not meant to be a cookbook for you to choose from. It is presented in order to help you understand more about Chinese medicine. The selection of medicinals must be done by a trained Chinese medical practitioner. If Chinese medicinals are used improperly, those drugs may also cause side effects, trigger allergic reactions, or interact with other medicinals or biomedicine. Always let your Chinese medical practitioner know about any allergies or medication use before using any Chinese therapies.

3. Research and References

➡ **Wang YT** et al.[62] investigated the therapeutic effects of *Sì Nì Săn* on laboratory animals of the chronic restraint stress (CRS) model. *Sì Nì Săn* was administered in the animal's drinking water at a concentration of 100mg/kg for 21 days (7 days pre-CRS and 14 days during the CRS). Spatial learning and memory were measured 24 hours after the CRS procedures using the Morris Water Maze (MWM). Aggressive behavior and body weight were determined as well. The *Sì Nì Săn* treatment decreased aggressive behaviors and reversed CRS-induced impairment of spatial learning and memory as well as decreased rate of growth. This study concluded that *Sì Nì Săn* does exert measurable therapeutic effects in an experimental chronic stress model.

➡ **Wu LK** et al.[63] observed the effects of Ping Yu capsule on such important regulatory factors as cAMP, PKA, and PKC of the signal transduction in rats with chronic stress-induced depression. Wistar male rats were randomly divided into control group, model group, paroxetine group, and Ping Yu capsule low, middle, and high doses groups; rats in all groups but the control group were fed in a single cage for 21 days and were given such irritations as electric shock to the pelma, ice water swimming, pyretic fumigation, and tail clipping during this period; lobe cortex and hippocampus of all rats were taken out for detection of the cAMP content by means of radioactive immunization, PKA and PKC content by Elisa, and the PKA and PKC activity by radioactive isotope. Content of cAMP in lobe cortex and hippocampus, content and activity of PKA in the hippocampus, and content of PKC in lobe cortex of rats in the model group were lower than those in the normal group. Ping Yu capsule and paroxetine can increase those numbers. It concluded the anti-depression effect of Ping Yu capsule may be related to its function of adjusting the signal transduction of cAMP-PKA.

➡ **Mao QQ** et al.[64] conducted a study of the antidepressant-like effects of total glycosides of peony (TGP). The antidepressant-like effects of TGP was determined by using animal models of depression including forced swimming and tail suspension tests. The acting mechanism was explored by determining the effect of TGP on the activities of monoamine oxidases. Results revealed that intragastric administration of TGP at 80 and 160 mg/kg for seven days caused a significant reduction in immobility time in both forced swimming and tail suspension tests, yet TGP did not stimulate locomotor activity in the open-field test. In addition, TGP treatment antagonized reserpine-induced ptosis and inhibited the activities of monoamine oxidases in mouse cerebrum. These results suggested that the antidepressive effects of TGP are mediated, at least in part, by the inhibition of monoamine oxidases.

➡ **Wei XH** et al.[65] conducted a study to evaluate the antidepressant activity of Yue Ju Wan (YJ) ethanol extract (YJ-E) and its four different fractions, the petroleum ether fraction (YJ-EA), ethyl acetate fraction (YJ-EB), n-butanol fraction (YJ-EC) and final aqueous fraction (YJ-ED). Two experimental despair animal models: the mice tail suspension test (TST) and the mice forced swimming test (FST) were used to evaluate the antidepressant activity of YJ-E and its fractions. These extracts or fractions were administered orally for 7 days, while the parallel positive control was given at the same time using fluoxetine hydrochloride (FLU) in TST and imipramine hydrochloride (IMI) in FST respectively. Results showed that YJ-E high dose (YJ-E2), YJ-EA, YJ-EC, and the positive control groups could decrease the duration of immobility in the TST and FST and have no significant changes in locomotor activity. YJ-E low dose (YJ-E1), YJ-EB, YJ-ED, and the vehicle solvent (VEH) control group have no obvious effect on these same tests. This study concluded that in these despair animal models, YJ ethanol extract, the petroleum ether fraction and n-butanol fraction showed potent antidepressant effects. The petroleum ether fraction and n-butanol fraction appeared to be the active fractions of YJ-E.

➡ **He Q** et al.[66] performed a study to evaluate the therapeutic effect and safety of acupuncture plus TCM medication for treatment of mental depression. Sixty-one cases of mental depression were randomly divided into a treatment group of 30 cases and a control group of 31 cases. The former group was treated by acupuncture plus TCM medication, and the latter with TCM medication alone. The Hamilton Mental Depression (HAMD) scoring system was adopted to evaluate the therapeutic effects, and the Treatment Emergent Symptom Scale (TESS) was used to evaluate the adverse reactions. RESULTS: The treatment group was superior to the control group in the total effective effect (*P*<0.05), with a significant difference in the HAMD score before and after treatment between the 2 groups (*P*<0.01). There were marked differences in the reducing rate of the HAMD score at the end of the second and sixth week of the treatment between the 2 groups (*P*<0.05) and the difference was very obvious at the end of the fourth week (*P*<0.01). No remarkable difference was found in adverse reactions between the 2 groups (*P*>0.05). This study concluded that acupuncture plus TCM medication showed satisfactory results for mental depression, indicating that a synergic action may exist between acupuncture and TCM medication.

➡ **Mao QQ** et al.[67] reviewed the reports concerning the mechanisms of traditional Chinese medicine in treating depression in recent years, combined with the research achievements of the authors, and summarized the research progress on the therapeutic mechanism of depression treated by traditional Chinese medicine. Previous research proved that traditional Chinese medicine played an antidepressant role by affecting the monoamine neurotransmitters, excitotoxicity, hypothalamus-pituitary-adrenal axis, hippocampal neurons, and neurotrophic factors. This study stated that depression treated by traditional Chinese medicine can be achieved through a lot of channels, target spots, and levels.

➡ **Chen JX** et al.[68] examined the effects of the *Xiāo Yáo Săn* (XYS) decoction, a Chinese traditional prescription containing eight commonly used medicinals, on tail suspension behavior and the levels of brain-derived neurotrophic factor (BDNF), tyroxine hydroxylase (TrkB), and neurotrophin 3 (NT-3) in the frontal cortex and hippocampus. Rats subjected to chronic immobilization stress (CIS) exhibited decreases in weight-gain, food intake, and ambulation in the open field test; they also showed an increase in immobility in the tail suspension test. These were all attenuated by the XYS decoction. Biochemically, the XYS decoction also reversed CIS-induced decreases in BDNF and increases in TrkB and NT-3 in the frontal cortex and the hippocampal CA(1) subregion. The behavioral effects of the XYS were correlated to the biochemical actions. These results suggested that the XYS decoction produces an antidepressant-like effect, which appears to be involved by BDNF in the brain.

➡ **Li YJ** et al.[69] investigated the effect of *Dān Zhī Xiāo Yáo* Powder (DXP) on neuro-immuno-endocrine systems in patients with depression. A randomized double-blinded and controlled study was conducted in 63 cases of depression. They were assigned to the DXP group (32 cases, treated with DXP) and the control group

(31 cases, treated with maprotiline). The curative effect was evaluated with Hamilton's depressive scale (HAMD) before and at the end of the 2nd, 4th, and 6th week of treatment. Serum levels of serotonin (5-HT), norepinephrine (NE), brain derived neurotrophic factor (BDNF), cortisol (CORT), interleukin-6 (IL-6), and interleukin-1beta (IL-1beta) were detected before, and at the 6th week of treatment. Results revealed that after 2 weeks of treatment, the total score of HAMD decreased remarkably in both groups ($P<0.01$), and the total score, as well as the scores of the three factors, i.e. anxiety/somatization, cognitive impairment, and feeling of despair, were lower in the DXP group than that in the control group, respectively ($P<0.05$ or $P<0.01$). After 4 and 6 weeks of treatment the total score and score of the three factors all reduced significantly in both groups ($P<0.01$), with insignificant difference between the groups. After 6 weeks of treatment, the serum levels of 5-HT and BDNF increased ($P<0.01$), and the serum IL-6 level decreased in both groups ($P<0.05$ or $P<0.01$). The serum CORT level reduced in the DXP group ($P<0.01$), while the serum NE level elevated in the control group ($P<0.01$). This study concluded that DXP is effective in improving symptoms of depression by regulating the levels of 5-HT, BDNF, CORT, and IL-6.

➡ **Ushiroyama T** et al.[70] performed a study to compare the effects of *chái hú guì zhī gān jiāng tāng*, a formula used in improving depressed mood, on plasma interleukin-6 (IL-6) and soluble interleukin-6 receptor (sIL-6R) concentrations as compared with those of anti-depressants in peri- and post-menopausal women. Ninety patients complaining of menopausal symptoms including insomnia who were diagnosed with mood disorder based on DSM-IV were recruited and separated into two groups (*chái hú guì zhī gān jiāng tāng* group was selected on the basis of SHO for 42 cases, while antidepressants were used for 48 cases), and plasma IL-6 and sIL-6R concentrations were determined three months before and after the treatment. There were no significant differences in the decrease in both climacteric and Hamilton depression score after treatment between the two groups. Plasma IL-6 and sIL-6R concentrations were significantly lower in the *chái hú guì zhī gān jiāng tāng* group (-34.8±15.5% and -22.4±14.6%, respectively) than in the antidepressant group (7.5±4.8% and 2.4 ± 3.8%, respectively) after 3 months of treatment. Correlations between rate of decrease in climacteric score and plasma IL-6 (R=0.498, $P=0.0056$) and sIL-6R (R=0.512, $P=0.0045$) concentrations were observed. *Chái hú guì zhī gān jiāng tāng* reduced plasma IL-6 and sIL-6R concentrations in relation to improvement of depressed mood during treatment. The findings of this study suggested that *chái hú guì zhī gān jiāng tāng* has the potential to decrease morbidity by alleviation of stress reactions in peri- and post-menopausal women.

Tui Na (Massage)

1. What Is Tui Na?

In ancient China, medical therapy was often divided into external and internal treatments. As one of the external methods, tui na has been used extensively in China for over 2,000 years and is a form of Chinese manipulative therapy often used in combination with Chinese medicinal, acupuncture, moxibustion, cupping, tai ji, and qi gong. In the *Sui* and *Tang* dynasties, Chinese medicine witnessed geat development and tui na developed into an independent discipline. At the beginning of the Ming Dynasty, it was classified as one of the 13 medical disciplines by the imperial hospital, with the specialized discipline of pediatric massage coming into being. During the process of development, diverse schools of tui na took shape gradually thanks to various academy sources and different masters. Generally, most Chinese medicine hospitals in China have a massage department.

Developed over 2,000 years ago, tui na, literally "pushing and grasping", but usually simply translated as massage, is a hands-on-body practice of manipulating and acupressuring the body performed by highly-skilled practitioners with the purpose of bringing the body into balance. Tui na works with the qi system in the body, which flows through channels. By stimulating the specific areas (acupoints or channels) with well-honed techniques, the channels can be opened, the flow of qi and blood will be promoted and regulated, and the balance will be restored. The body's qi will be strengthened and so will its resistance to disease. Tui na is an important element of Chinese medicine and is effective for musculoskeletal pain, headaches, stress, fatigue, anxiety, depression, insomnia, weakened immune systems, digestive problems, female problems, and stroke patients. It is popular with everyday people as it is simple, convenient, effective, and cheap.

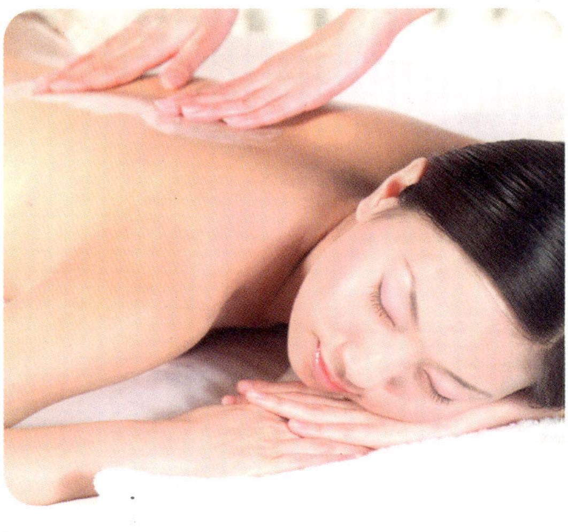

Tui na is often called "acupuncture without needles" and is irreplaceable as a natural kind of physical therapy. You may have already tried other kinds of massage, but tui na is unique because it is deeply rooted in Chinese medical theory. Diagnosis and treatment are based on the same theories as acupuncture, but tui na is a system of hands-on treatment with specific massage techniques to remove blockages to the flow of vital substances which would otherwise cause pain, edema, dark thoughts and other problems. According to the theory of Chinese medicine, pain is either due to stagnation or deficiency, and local stagnation of the flow of qi and blood is the most common cause. Tui na can relieve this kind of pain by applying forceful, smooth, and penetrating manipulations in order to remove stagnation and promote the flow of qi and blood. Pain with a different diagnosis would be managed differently, in accordance to the theory. As in all aspects of Chinese medicine, applying individualized treatment is of primary importance. Discovering the unique pattern of disharmony in each patient is vital in order to apply the correct treatment methods.

In the treatment of depression, tui na is effective, though it often plays a supplementary role. Manual stimulus on acupoints (acupressure) will also produce effects similar to acupuncture according to the theory of Chinese medicine. In general, tui na restores the balance of yin and yang, regulates the *zang-fu* organs, unblocks the channels, and enhances the flow of qi and blood. And as a holistic treatment, tui na treats the mind and the body as a whole, letting people feel deep relaxation, physically and mentally, thus increasing vitality and overall wellbeing. Tui na is more convenient and also may sound safer if you are afraid of needles, since the physician lets their hands and fingers work on your body usually through clothes instead of needles. If applied regularly, tui na can not only relieve your symptoms, but can also make you feel relaxed and refreshed every time you leave the clinic. You will know how well tui na works once you try it.

Tui na has fewer side effects than other medical therapies when being performed properly. It has been used to treat or complement the treatment of many medical conditions. The practitioner may adopt various manipulative techniques to get the energy moving, then use range of motion and traction to strech the muscles and channels, with the stimulation of acupressure points. As an integral part of Chinese medicine, tui na is taught in Chinese medicine universities and colleges as part of formal training in China. Many martial arts practitioners also learn tui na for the treatment of injury and pain caused by training.

2. What Can I Expect?

After inquiring about your condition and performing a detailed examination,

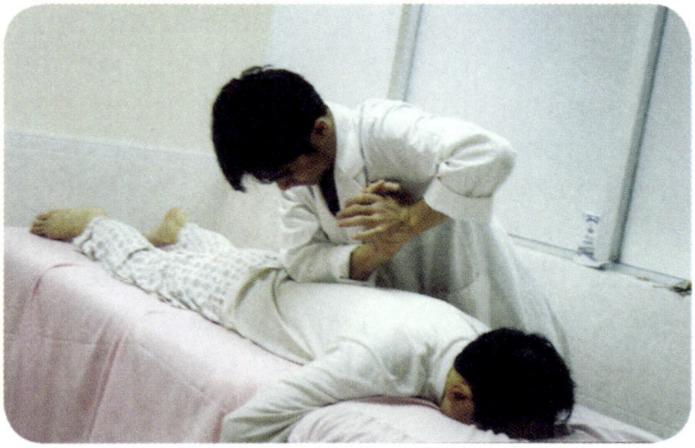

the practitioner will decide on a tui na procedure based on the pattern identification presented. Since tui na is a direct, manual therapy, treatment can take place almost anywhere and in many positions, but most often the patients will be asked to lie on their back or stomach. Sometimes the massage will be done in the sitting position. If necessary, the position may be changed during the treatment.

A pair of trained hands is all that is necessary for a tui na treatment to be performed. Other parts of the practitioner's body might also be used, such as elbows and arms. The manipulations are called "*shŏu fă*" (hand techniques) in Chinese, such as one-finger-pushing manipulation, ligation, rolling manipulation, ointment rubbing, kneading manipulation, rubbing manipulation, scrubbing manipulation, pushing manipulation, palm-pushing manipulation, foulage manipulation, shaking manipulation, pressing manipulation, point-pricking method, pinching manipulation, pinching along spine, grasping manipulation, treading manipulation, tapping manipulation, patting-striking manipulation, flicking manipulation, foulage and rolling for relaxing tendons, rotating manipulation, back-carrying manipulation, pulling manipulation, backward stretching-pulling manipulation, and oblique pulling manipulation. Those different manipulation methods emphasize particular aspects of therapeutic effects. Occasionally, a practitioner might use some kind of massage tool.

Special oil or medicinal paste may sometimes be used to lubricate and protect the skin and for their own therapeutic effects. The most common ingredients are common oily substances like lanolin or beeswax mixed with medicinals that invigorate qi and blood. In ancient China, such lubricants as onion juice solution, ginger juice solution, sesame oil, and Chinese holly oil, were used. If you are allergic to certain substances, please inform the practitioner before treatment begins. Sometimes medicinal pastes are specially made to manage certain conditions. For example, one kind of paste for deficiency pain, another for stagnation pain; one kind for the upper body and a different type for the lower half.

3. At-home Massage

You should know that tui na manipulation is not as simple as it looks, even though many of the procedures are simple actions performed every day such as pushing, grasping, pressing, and kneading. It is actually a set of highly-skilled techniques and expert movements that are performed according to Chinese medical theory. It uses the same system of channels and collaterals and acupoints as those in acupuncture, but the hands and fingers take the place of needles. The manipulation must be performed by trained practitioners to promote internal self-adjustment of the channel system without harming the local tissues of the body. The effect of tui na depends more on the skill with which the manipulations are performed rather on the sheer force of the pressure. Force, even a small amount, applied improperly can be harmful to the body. Sometimes patients come to the clinic who have been given tui na therapy by a non-professional practitioner showing bruises or other injuries. It is not suggested to perform or receive tui na treatments that you have observed in the clinic on or by your friends or family members without the presence of an instructor.

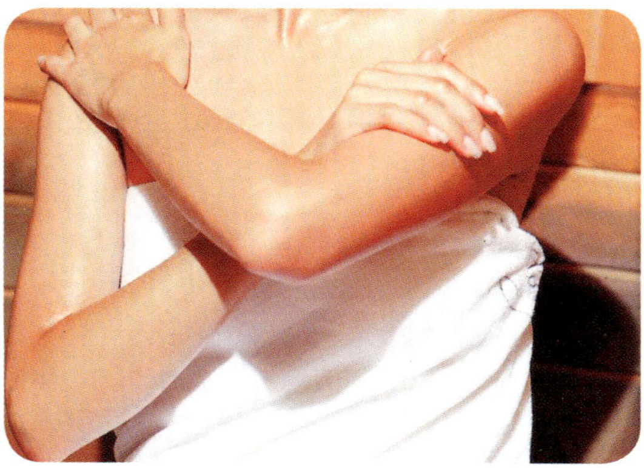

Nonetheless, there are some self-massage techniques that are safe, simple, convenient, and designed for patients with depression to soothe their body and mind, regulate organ function, and serve as a supplement to the medical treatment of depression. Self-massage is a method that uses a variety of techniques to stimulate the flow of qi in the channels and acupoints, to releases blockages in these vital substances, and to balance vital substances and the internal organs. This is also a process of active exercise.

Simple massage routines can be done at home either alone or with the help of a friend or family member. It can be done in a sitting, standing, or lying position as whatever you like and makes you comfortable. When you perform it, please be calm and attentive, and breathe normally. The manipulation, force, mental activities, and the flow of qi in your body are expected to be well-coordinated. During the process of massage, special attention should be paid to the force you use and the reaction of the skin. It is usually performed twice a day, once in the morning and once at night, 20-30 minutes each time.

Please note that there are numerous tui na routines and self-massage protocols recommended for patients. The most important thing is to find something that helps you and feels good.

Self-massage on the Head

Below are simple and effective self-massage techniques for the head that you can perform at home.[71] All of them are helpful for strengthening the brain, enhancing intelligence, tranquilizing the mind, and eliminating spiritual disturbance. They are valuable for the prevention and treatment of such ailments as headache, insomnia, dizziness, or mental disturbance.

> Pushing the forehead on either side simultaneously

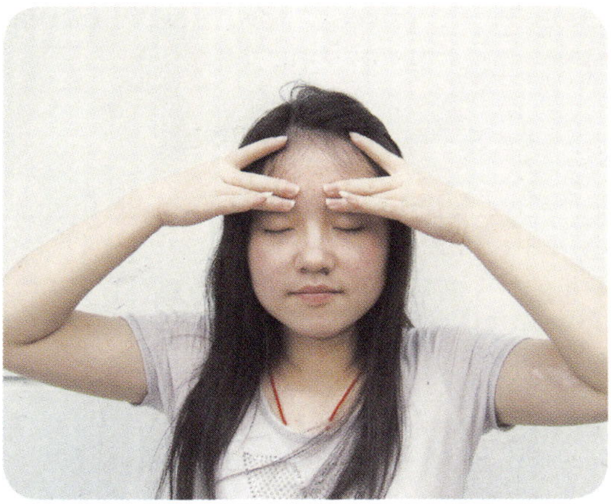

Start from the midline of the forehead, conduct top-down push with the radial side of the second knuckle of the bent index fingers towards SJ 23 (*sī zhú kōng*), *tài yáng*, and ST 8 (*tóu wéi*) bilaterally 30-50 times.

> Pressing the temples

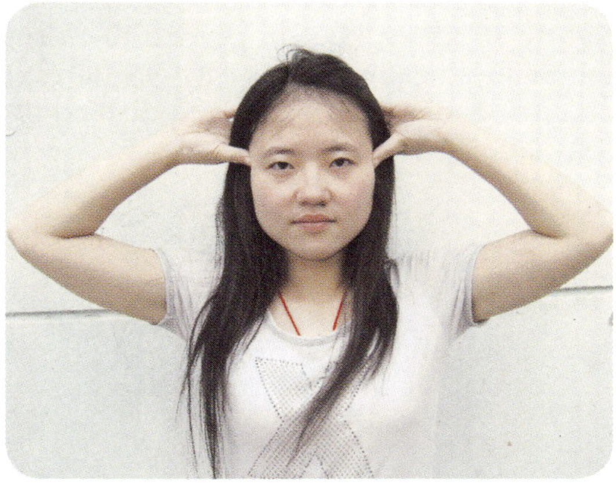

Press the temples forcefully with the thumbprint surface of the thumb. Push forward and backward about 30 times until a sore and distending feeling is obtained.

> Pressing and kneading the back of the head

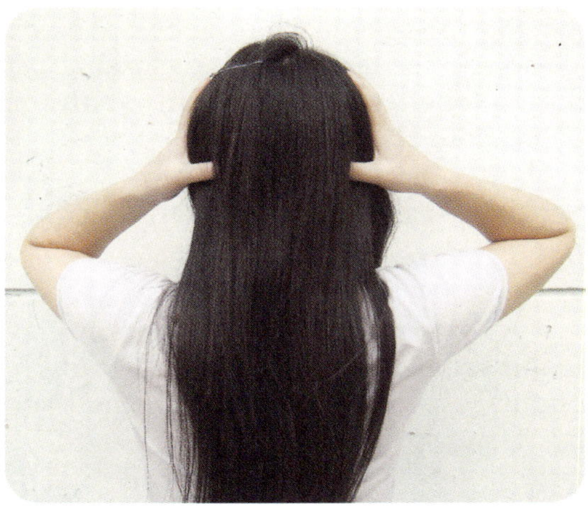

Press GB 20 (*fēng chí*) with the thumbprint surface or the tip of the thumbs tightly 10 times, kneading-press them rotationally, kneading-press *nǎo kōng* (GB 19) about 80 times until a sore and distending sensation is achieved.

> Patting-striking the vertex

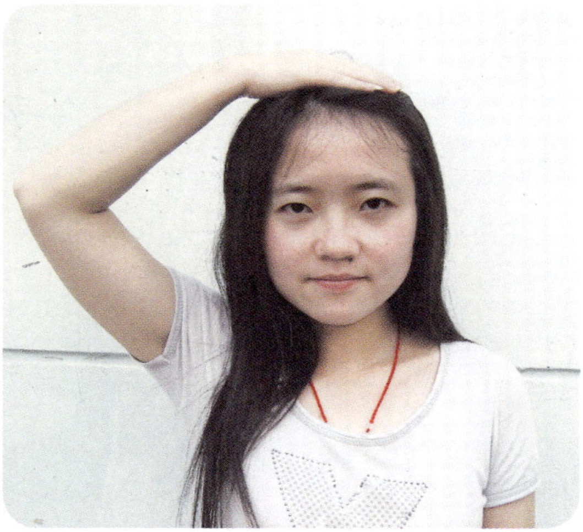

Sit up straight with the eyes looking ahead and the teeth clenched, striking-pat the fontanel area rhythmically with the palm about 10 times.

Self-Massage for Regulation of *Zang-fu* Organs

As you may know, depression may result from the disturbance of *zang-fu* organs, especially disorders of the liver, heart, and spleen.

> Rubbing the lower abdomen

Sit up straight or lay on your back, put the two hands below the hypochondriac regions, push and rub obliquely through the lower abdomen to the pubis back and forth 20 times. This plays a role of soothing the liver and regulating the flow of qi.

> Stirring the tongue within the mouth

Rotate the tongue outside the upper and lower gums in the oral cavity first from left to right, then from right to left about 10 times. Swallow the saliva generated by the motion of tongue in three portions. This is effective for relieving mental stress and tranquilizing the mind.

> Pressing ST 36 (*zú sān lǐ*)

Overlap the index and middle fingers of both hands, press and knead ST 36 (*zú sān lǐ*) on both sides respectively 50 times. This method acts upon the spleen and stomach.

> Rubbing DU 14 (*dà zhuī*)

Sit up straight, put the palm horizontally on DU 14 (*dà zhuī*, below the spinous process of the 7th cervical vertebra), rub it back and forth with the major thenar eminence and the index and the middle finger until it becomes hot. It is used for activating the lung and regulating qi.

> Rubbing KI 1 (*yǒng quán*)

Put one palm horizontally on KI 1 (*yǒng quán*) (at the anterior 1/3 point of the sole and in the depression appearing on the sole when the foot is in plantar flexion), rub it to and fro about 50 times. Repeat this to the other side. This is applicable in reinforcing the kidney essence and relieving mental disturbance.

> Sighing method

Relax the whole body, inhale deeply, exhale as much as possible, make a sound of "*xu*"※ when exhaling, and open your eyes wide. Repeat this process 10 times. This method is believed to eliminate liver qi stagnation.

Self-Massage with Music

Massage is very soothing and invigorating. It also incorporates the therapeutic effects of touch. Music's ability to "heal the soul" is the stuff of legend in every culture.[72]

➡ Turn on your music.

➡ Start with your head and work your way down to your toes.

➡ Pour some massage oil onto your palms, and using flat hands, rub it vigorously into your hair and scalp.

➡ Use your fingertips to cover your head with small circular movements.

➡ Gently massage your face and ears, and then your neck.

➡ Knead your shoulders and vigorously massage your arms, with up-and-down motions. Use circular movements on your elbows and knead your hands and fingers.

➡ Massage your chest and stomach using large gentle circular motions. Massage your sides and back if you can reach it without straining.

➡ Use vigorous up-and-down motions on your legs, with circular movement at your knees and ankles.

➡ Massage your feet-tops and bottoms and use your fingers to massage your toes.

When you are done, take a warm shower and use a mild soap to wash off the excess oil. The oil that has penetrated or remains on the surface of the skin conditions the skin and helps keep your body warm.

※ [Note: the pronunciation of "xu" is halfway between "s" and "sh" in English. It is similar, but unvoiced, to the "su" in the word "usual."]

Foot Spa

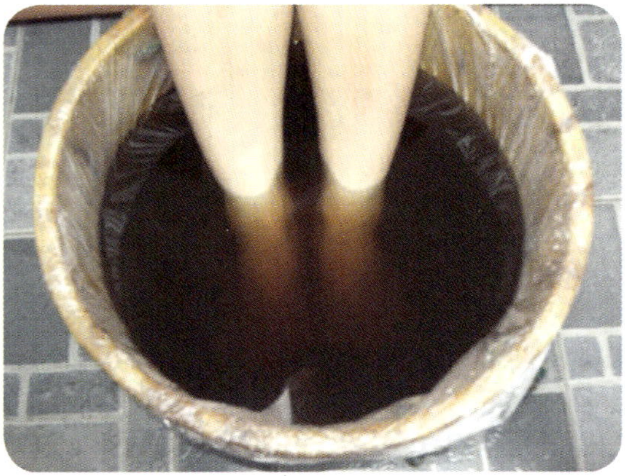

Washing your feet with warm water is the most convenient way to keep healthy. It is one of the most common methods for health preservation. Soaking your feet in warm water before sleeping can not only relieve fatigue but also improve the quality of sleep.[73]

Firstly, the foot is averse to cool and cold, so attention should be paid to keeping your feet warm. Do not become addicted to cold in summer, please keep warm in winter by forming the daily habit of bathing your feet in warm water.

Secondly, kneading the sole of the foot is helpful. Every night sit on the bed after having a foot spa and bending your left leg, hold the left foot with the left hand, rub the left sole with the left palm up and down 50 times; then bend the right leg, hold the right foot with the right hand, rub the right sole with the right palm up and down 50 times. This movement has the effects of promoting heart-kidney interaction, nourishing qi and blood, clearing the liver and gallbladder, lowering blood pressure, nourishing the heart, and tranquilizing the spirit. It should be practiced with proper force and perseverance, so as to strengthen the body.

Thirdly, the effect of health preservation is much better when adding some natural ingredients such as milk, red wine, or tea into the basin, the specialized essential oil or Chinese medicinals are preferred.

Additionally, you may soak your feet in cold water no longer than 2 minutes, and then knead and rub them forcefully until your feet become red. It can promote blood circulation.

Hand, Ear, and Foot Self-massage

All of these therapies are based on the holistic view of Chinese medicine, together with channel theory and modern holographic theory. Holographic therapies on the hands and feet are commonly known as reflexology. These techniques work on the idea that the larger image (macrocosm) of the body is reflected on smaller images (microcosms) like the hands, feet, or ears. Treatment on the microcosm can be therapeutic for the larger body (macrocosm).

The basic theory of reflexology states there are reflex points (or areas) on the foot related to various areas of the body, such as the feet, hands, ears, etc. If the function of an organ in the body becomes abnormal, there will also be abnormal signs which can be detected on the corresponding reflex area. In turn, working on the reflex point (area) can also help to adjust the function of the related organ and the body as a whole to put it back to balance.

By stimulating the reflex points on the hands, ears, or feet, the internal organs can be stimulated and regulated. Gentle self-massage of the hands, ears, and feet can be done by people of all ages and conditions - children, adults, the elderly, the sick - anywhere, and with or without lotion. Calming music may be used during the massage. With just a five-to-ten-minute massage you can feel relaxed and relieved. You can follow the procedure recommended here, or one recommended by your practitioner. You can do this at home by yourself or with the help of a friend or family member.

Wash your hands, face, and feet with warm water. Play music lightly in the background if you like. Sit comfortably. Relax yourself and empty your mind. You can also use lotion on your hands, especially if your skin is dry.

➡ Rub your hands gently as if you are washing them.

➡ Open the palm of your hand with the other one, gently pressing the palm and stretching the muscles of the hand.

➡ Massage the muscles and tendons between the bones of the hand.

➡ Use your wrist to massage the opposite palm.

➡ Massage each finger and pull the fingers visualizing the tension pouring out of the fingertips.

➡ Massage your face with your fingertips from jaw to cheeks using gentle, circular motions. Widen the circle to touch the ears.

➡ Massage your ears all over and warm them with your hands.

➡ Rest for a few minutes if you are feeling tired.

➡ Adjust your position to make yourself comfortable. Prop one foot in your lap and let the other extend in front of you. Massage one foot and when finished, change position and do the other.

➡ Put one hand on top of the foot and the other closer to your toes, then stroke smoothly from your toes to your ankles.

➡ Glide your hands to the sole of your foot and massage any sensitive point on the sole.

➡ Massage the whole foot and pull the

toes gently visualizing the tension pulling out the tip of the toes.

➡ Press the arch of the foot with your wrist.

➡ Again put one hand on top of the foot and the other closer to your toes, then stroke smoothly from your toes to your ankles.

You can do the above procedure every other day or twice a week. In a month you will feel better. Continue to massage yourself regularly to ensure a lasting effect.

4. Research and References

➡ **Field TM**[74] stated that massage therapy is older than recorded time, and rubbing was the primary form of medicine until the pharmaceutical revolution of the 1940s. Popularized again as part of the alternative medicine movement, massage therapy has recently received empirical support for facilitating growth, reducing pain, increasing alertness, diminishing depression, and enhancing immune function. In this article studies are reviewed that document these effects, and models are proposed for potential underlying mechanisms.

➡ **Field T** et al.[75] randomly assigned 47 prenatally depressed women into the group that received massage twice weekly from their partners from 20 weeks gestation until the end of pregnancy, and the control group, and found that self-reported leg pain, back pain, depression, anxiety, and anger decreased more for the massaged pregnant women than for the control group women; the partners who massaged the pregnant women versus the control group partners reported less depressed mood, anxiety, and anger across the course of the massage therapy period; scores on a relationship questionnaire improved more for both the women and the partners in the massage group. This data suggests that not only mood states but also relationships improve when depressed pregnant women are massaged by their partners.

➡ **Lee YM**[76] conducted a study on 46 middle-aged women (40-64 years) who were recruited from the Community Health Center in Busan City to identify the effects of a self-foot reflexology massage on depression, stress responses and functions of the immune system of middle-aged women. This study was a one group pre-test/post-test experimental design and the data was collected from August 1st, 2004 to May 31st, 2005. Those women were trained in self foot reflexology massage for two weeks, and then they practiced daily foot massage for six weeks (two days at the research center, five days at home). The outcome variables were measured 4 times, at baseline, pre-training, post-training, and after the intervention. The collected data was analyzed by repeated measure ANOVA by the SPSS/WIN program. The results revealed a statistically significant difference in depression, perceived stress, systolic blood pressure, natural-killer cells, and Ig G, indicating that self-foot reflexology massage could be utilized as an effective nursing intervention to reduce depression and stress responses, and to strengthen immune systems in middle-aged women.

➡ **Song RH**[77] investigated the effects of foot reflexology massage on sleep disturbance, depression disorder, and the physiological index of the elderly in nursing homes. The research design was a non-equivalent control group pre-test/post-test quasi-experimental study. The subjects were 50 elderly people who resided in two different nursing homes in the same region. An experimental group and a control group were organized with 25 subjects respectively, and foot reflexion massage was provided for 12 sessions, 30 minutes per session. The selected dependent variables were sleep disturbance, depression disorder, and physiological indices (blood plasma serotonin, serum cortisol), which were all measured before and after foot reflexology massage was offered. Data analysis included "chi2-test," "t-test," paired "t-test," and ANCOVA, using the SPSS program package. The results demonstrated that the experimental group improved sleep quality more than the control group; the experimental group had less depression disorder than the control group; the experimental group had higher serotonin levels than the control group, suggesting it is necessary to give foot reflexology massage as a successful nursing intervention to elderly who undergo a change in sleep, and suffer from a depression disorder due to a deterioration in sleep.

➡ **Field T** et al.[78] recruited 84 depressed pregnant women during the second trimester of pregnancy and randomly assigned them to a massage therapy group, a progressive muscle relaxation group or a control group that received standard prenatal care alone. These groups were compared to each other and to a non-depressed group at the end of pregnancy. The massage therapy group participants received two 20-minute therapy sessions by their significant others each week for 16 weeks of the pregnancy, starting during the second trimester. The relaxation group provided themselves with progressive muscle relaxation sessions on the same time schedule. Immediately after the massage therapy sessions on the first and last days of the 16-week period the women reported lower levels of anxiety, depression and less leg and back pain. By the end of the study the massage group had higher dopamine and serotonin levels and lower levels of cortisol and norepinephrine. These changes may have contributed to the reduced fetal activity and the better neonatal outcome for the massage group (i.e. lesser incidence of prematurity and low birthweight), as well as their better performance on the Brazelton Neonatal Behavior Assessment. The data suggests that depressed pregnant women and their offspring can benefit from massage therapy.

➡ **Jones NA**[79] assessed the effects of massage therapy and music therapy on frontal EEG asymmetry in depressed adolescents. Thirty adolescents with greater relative right frontal EEG activation and symptoms of depression were given either massage therapy (n=14) or music therapy (n=16). An EEG was recorded for three-minute periods before, during, and after therapy. Frontal EEG asymmetry was significantly attenuated during and after the massage and music sessions.

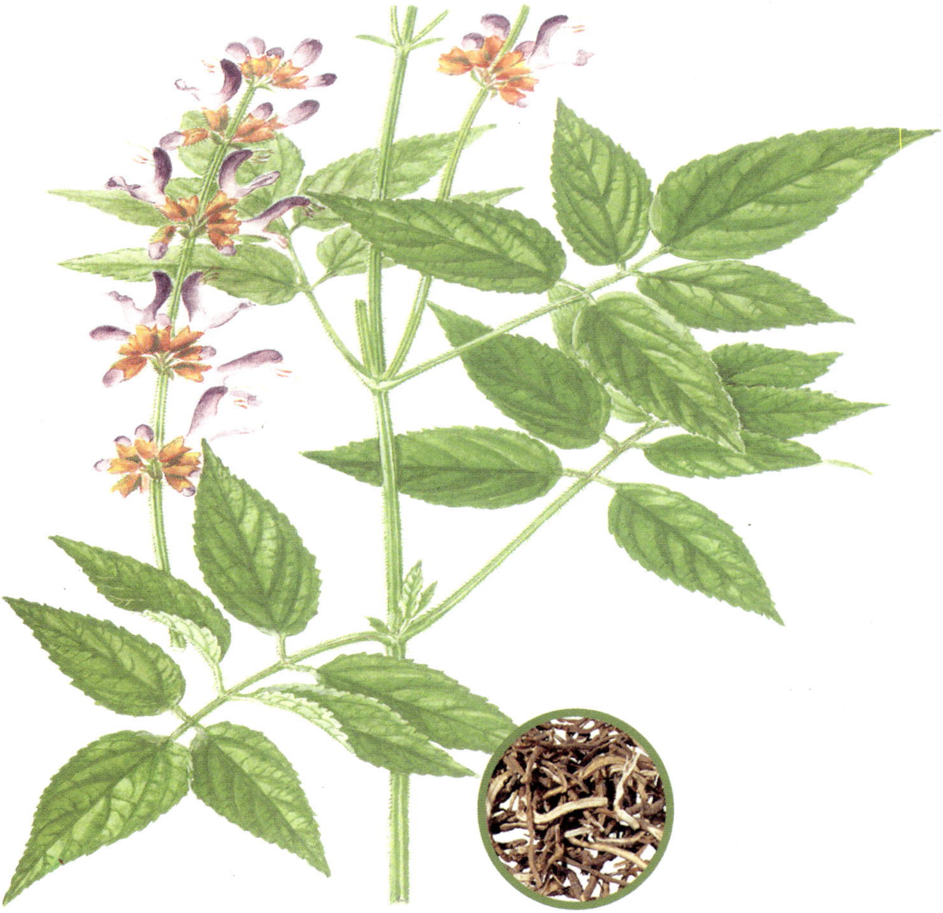

Salvia

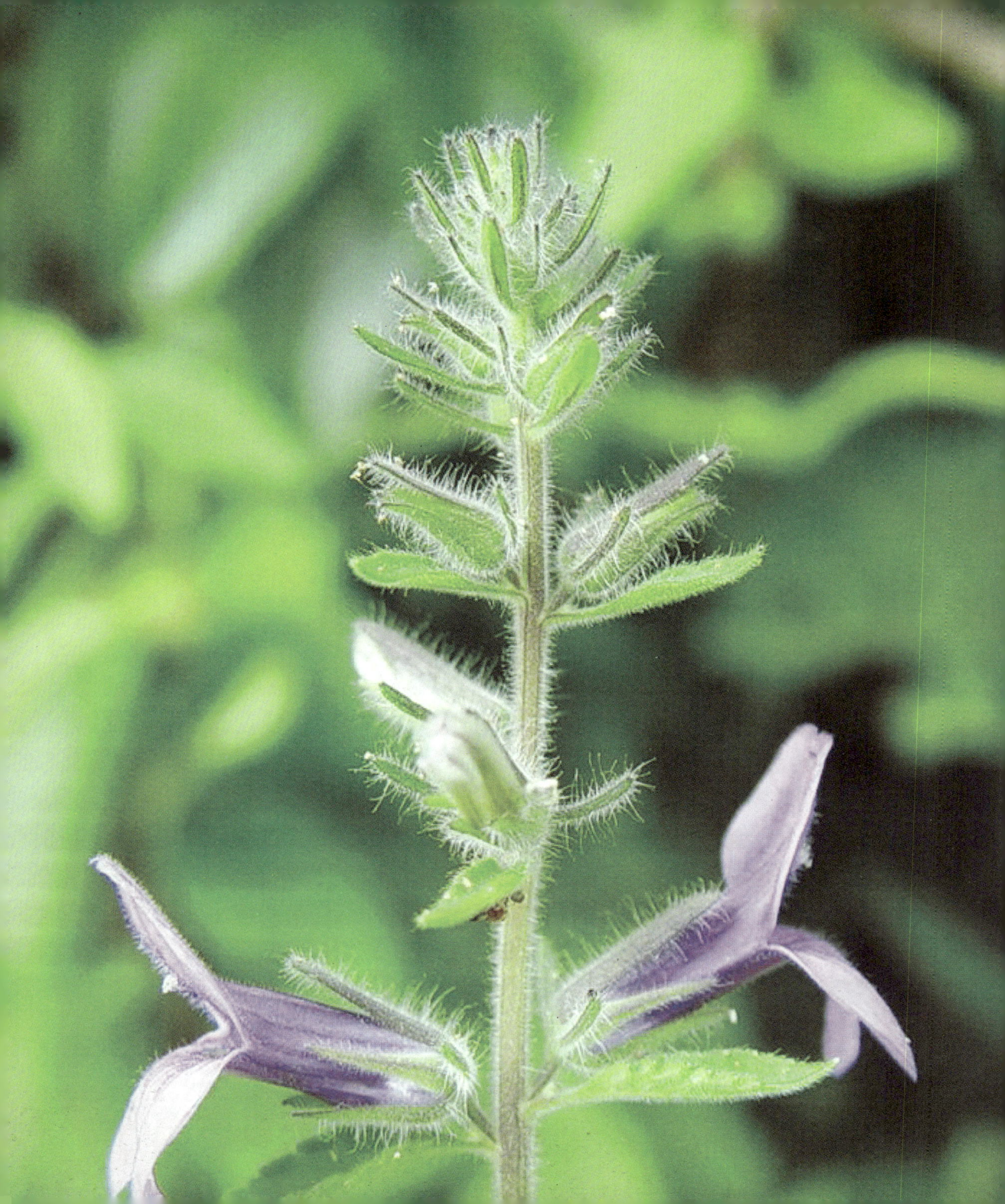

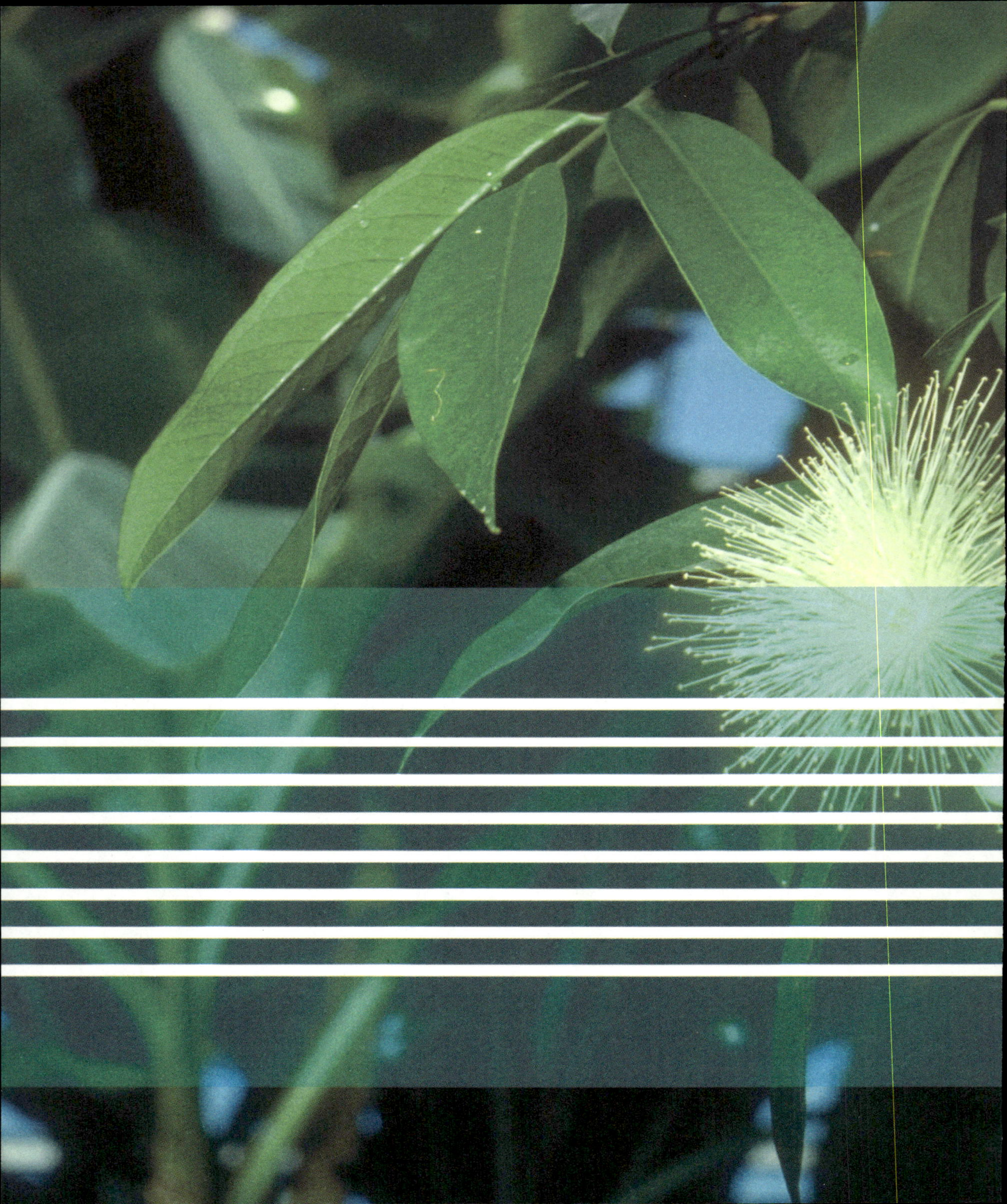

Chapter 5

Case Studies

This final chapter includes case histories from real patients who are trying to manage their depression. They represent the standard of care with Chinese medicine. As you have seen above, depression treatment has been rigorously studied both in the clinic and the laboratory. These cases are to show you that by using this knowledge, real people have been able to bring their problems under control and lead healthy lives. You may notice that nearly all the case histories in this book involve treatment with medicinals, usually prescribed to be taken as a decoction every day for a number of weeks or months. For those who were initially attracted to treatment with Chinese medicine because of what they heard about acupuncture, we encourage you to also give medicinals a fair trial. It is the most effective, safest, and fastest way to health with Chinese medicine.

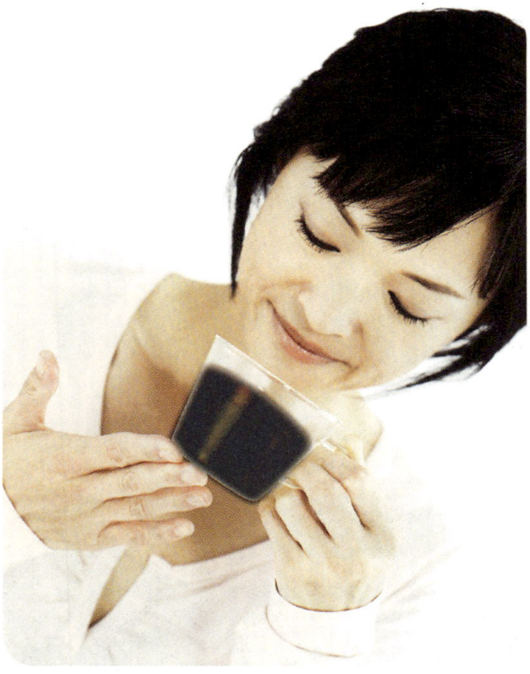

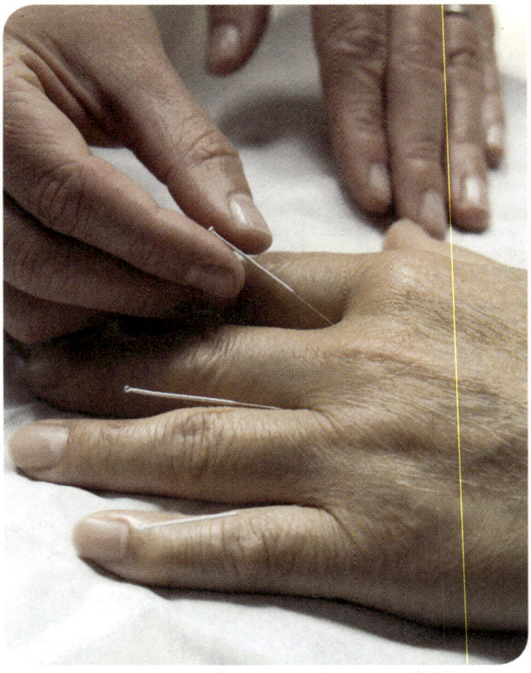

Case One

A 38-year-old female patient with depression for six months[80]

At the very first beginning, she had quarrels with her neighbor and felt depressed. Gradually, she had chest stuffiness, distension and fullness of the hypochondrium, belching, poor appetite, a haggard face, lassitude, slight edema of the lower limbs, insomnia, thin and white tongue coating, and wiry pulses. Her condition was on a seesaw, up and down. Upper gastrointestinal barium meal type-B ultrasonic examination showed a negative result.

The pattern differentiated was liver qi stagnation, and the corresponding therapeutic principles were to soothe the liver, regulate qi circulation, relieve depression, and revive the spleen. A medicinal prescription based on *Chái Hú Shū Gān Săn* (Bupleurum Liver-Soothing Powder) was given, including *chái hú, zhĭ qiào*, and *xiāng fù* to soothe the liver, regulate qi circulation, and relieve depression; *chuān xiōng, chì sháo*, and *zhì gān căo* to promote blood circulation, relieve blood stagnation, and kill pain; and *chén pí* and *fú líng* to revive the spleen and relieve dampness.

Chinese Name	Pinyin	Dose	Latin Name
柴胡	*chái hú*	9 g	Radix Bupleuri
赤芍	*chì sháo*	9 g	Radix Paeoniae Rubra
枳壳	*zhĭ qiào*	9 g	Fructus Aurantii
香附	*xiāng fù*	9 g	Rhizoma Cyperi
川芎	*chuān xiōng*	12 g	Rhizoma Chuanxiong
陈皮	*chén pí*	12 g	Pericarpium Citri Reticulatae
茯苓	*fú líng*	15 g	Poria
炙甘草	*zhì gān căo*	3 g	Radix et Rhizoma Glycyrrhizae Praeparata cum Melle

The patient was asked to drink the warm decoction of medicinals twice a day, one dose per day. She felt much better after taking three doses, and she got complete relief from depression after continuing to take the same formula for another six doses. In order to consolidate the therapeutic effect, she took *Shū Gān Jiàn Pí Wèi Wán* for one week. After six months, the condition had still not returned.

Case Two

A 48-year-old female patient, long-term depression[81]

During the past ten years, her bad relationship with her family caused her to suffer from long-standing depression, restlessness, and weeping. She had recently gotten divorced, which, in turn, made her more depressed, with the manifestation of distension and fullness of the sternocostal region, insomnia, bad memory, no desire for life, suicide attempts, thin and white tongue coating, as well as wiry and thin pulses.

The pattern was differentiated as qi stagnation and the corresponding therapeutic principles were to resuscitate *shén*, soothe the liver, and relieve depression. The selected acupoints were PC 6 (*nèi guān*), DU 26 (*shuǐ gōu*), SP 6 (*sān yīn jiāo*), DU 23 (*shàng xīng*), *yìn táng*, DU 20 (*bǎi huì*), *sì shén cōng*, ear *shén mén*, and RN 17 (*dàn zhōng*). After two acupuncture treatments she felt better; and after another five treatments, her symptoms were improved to a large degree, with a relatively good mental attitude and no thoughts of suicide. But sometimes the distension and fullness of chest still bothered her, so the treatment was continued for another 8 treatments to consolidate the therapeutic effect. After that, her emotions were stable and her symptoms were completely relieved.

Case Three

A 20-year-old female patient with depression for two years[82]

She did not respond to previous biomedicine treatments. During her first visit to the clinic, she showed the signs and symptoms of depression, dull expression, anxiety, oversensitivity, chest stuffiness, frequent sighing, muttering, insomnia, poor appetite, normal urine and stool, a reddish tongue with a thin, white, and greasy tongue coating, as well as wiry and slippery pulses.

The pattern was diagnosed as stagnation of phlegm and qi, and the corresponding therapeutic principles were to soothe the liver, regulate qi circulation, remove depression, and relieve phlegm. Acupoints RN 15 (*jiū wěi*), RN 13 (*shàng wǎn*), LV14 (*qī mén*), LV 3 (*tài chōng*), and ST 40 (*fēng lóng*) were selected to soothe the liver, regulate qi, control depression, and relieve phlegm; RN 12 (*zhōng wǎn*) and ST 36 (*zú sān lǐ*) to tonify the spleen and stomach; and HT 7 (*shén mén*), PC 6 (*nèi guān*), and DU 20 (*bǎ i huì*) to resuscitate. A mild reinforcing-reducing method was adopted to manipulate, the needle was retained for two hours after the patient got needling sensation, once a day. A modified formula was prescribed for her with the purpose of tranquilizing the mind through soothing the liver, relieving depression, strengthening the spleen, and removing phlegm, one dose per day. She got better and seemed to be normal three weeks after receiving the combined treatment of acupuncture and medicinals. One year later, she received the same treatment for one week to consolidate the therapeutic effects. Thereafter, no relapse was observed over a two-year follow-up period.

Chinese Name	Pinyin	Dose	Latin Name
柴胡	*chái hú*	15 g	Radix Bupleuri
枳壳	*zhǐ qiào*	15 g	Fructus Aurantii
姜半夏	*jiāng bàn xià*	15 g	Rhizoma Pinelliae Praeparatum
陈皮	*chén pí*	20 g	Pericarpium Citri Reticulatae
厚朴	*hòu pò*	20 g	Cortex Magnoliae Officinalis
郁金	*yù jīn*	20 g	Radix Curcumae
合欢皮	*hé huān pí*	20 g	Cortex Albiziae
白术	*bái zhú*	20 g	Rhizoma Atractylodis Macrocephalae
炒酸枣仁	*chǎo suān zǎo rén*	25 g	Semen Ziziphi Spinosae
远志	*yuǎn zhì*	20 g	Radix Polygalae
琥珀	*hǔ pò*	30 g	Succinum

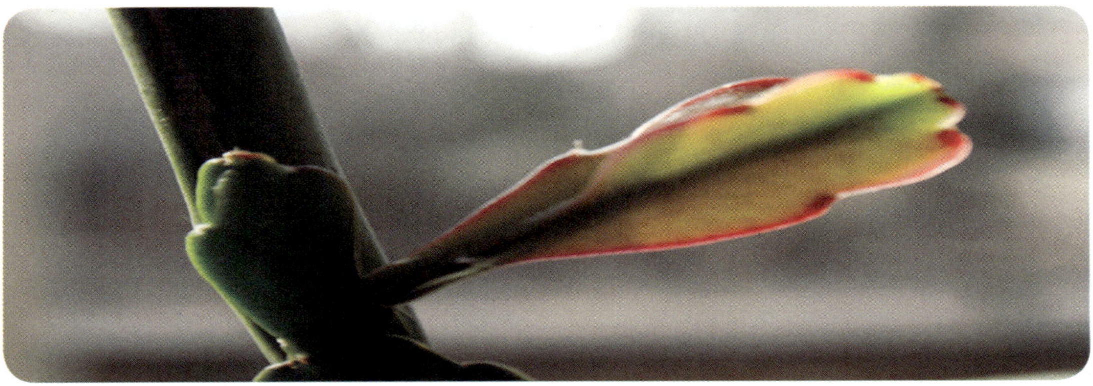

Conclusion

To manage and overcome depression is sometimes a very challenging process. The first step is to admit that you are depressed and not to be ashamed of it, then it will take time, patience, love, and understanding no matter what type of medicine you choose to follow.

Chinese medicine is a safe and effective way to deal with depression. It has been used in China for over 2,000 years, but only made its debut on the international stage in the last few decades. It includes a wide range of traditional medical practices, such as medicinals, acupuncture, dietary therapy, tui na, medical massage, and tai ji, all of which are effective to some extent and leave no worry about associated side effects and possible withdrawal symptoms. It will absolutely give you more options to help in relieving your depression.

Chinese medicine is not a magic pill, nor is biomedicine. Each system studies the amazing human body in its own way, with its own philosophy. Biomedicine sees the human body as a machine and analyzes each part in fantastic detail. Its strength is its precision and accuracy. Eventually, it will have the entire human body mapped out in the greatest detail. A doctor's job is to nail down the exact part that is broken down and fix it. The question for a doctor is: "What is wrong?" As a patient, it is difficult to understand much about your treatments as biomedicine is extremely technical and there are so many details.

Meanwhile, Chinese medicine sketches a figure that is inseparable from his complex surroundings. In Chinese medicine, a human is neither a jigsaw puzzle nor a machine, but like a tree growing in soil, a fish swimming in water, or a bird flying in the sky. When it comes to accuracy and precision, Chinese medicine may never compare to biomedicine. Its strength is seeing the big picture. A practitioner's job is to evaluate the patient's general condition and find where the imbalances lie. As a patient, you may not have the training to evaluate your own imbalances of yin, yang, qi, and blood, but you have the ability to understand what is wrong, and more importantly, how you can act to restore your health.

We sincerely hope this book has given you another option when it comes to managing your health.

Appendix

1. Basic Depression Information (Biomedicine)

Introduction

According to the World Health Organization, depression is defined as a common mental disorder that presents a depressed mood, loss of interest or pleasure, feelings of guilt or low self-worth, disturbed sleep or appetite, low energy, and poor concentration. These problems can become chronic or recurrent and lead to substantial impairments in an individual's ability to take care of his or her everyday responsibilities.

There are several different types of depression, such as major depressive disorder (also known as major depression or clinical depression), dysthymic disorder (also referred to as dysthymia), manic depression (now known as bipolar disorder), post partum depression, seasonal affective disorder (SAD). They are distinguished from each other in terms of prevalent features, duration and severity of symptoms.

The reasons why there are so many victims of depression are varied and complicated. You are more likely to be attacked by depression due to one or the combination of the following environmental and biological variables:

➡ Chemical imbalance in the brain, involving the neurotransmitters dopamine, norepinephrine, and serotonin, has been regarded as the root cause of depression, since the neurotransmitter is responsible for controlling the important physiological aspects of the body. And the decrease of these brain chemicals can inhibit the normal brain transmission of signals by the nerve cells, exerting an influence on every aspect of the body.

➡ Poor physical condition, especially chronically and refractory ailments, AIDS, endocrine disorders such as hypothyroidism and diabetes, neurological disorders, multiple sclerosis, etc. are not uncommon for the onset or aggravation of depression. These disorders plus depression make people more and more debilitated.

➡ Other psychological diseases such as anxiety disorder, schizophrenia, and substance abuse.

➡ Family history research shows evidence that the biological element of genetics may play an important role in depression, and blood relatives of people with depressive disorders were found to be more vulnerable to depression in comparison to members of the general population.

➡ A trigger such as a trauma or a stressful event. Financial problems, breaking up with someone you love, loss of one's job, death of a loved one, stressful but hopeless career, etc. may result in an episode of depression.

➡ Sudden changes in your life. Starting a new job, living in a new country or new place, graduating from school, getting married or divorced, getting a promotion with a heavy workload, etc. may cause you to be depressed.

➡ Pessimistic personality in combination with low self-esteem. It seems like people with a pessimistic personality are more likely to be hit by depression than others when facing the same environmental factors.

➡ Medications or withdraw from them.

(Adopted from http://www.depression.com/causes_of_depression.html)

Measurement

The ICD-10 Classification of Mental and Behavioural Disorders by the World Health Organization, Geneva, 1992.

According to DSM-IV, the diagnostic manual from American Psychiatric Association, criteria used by mental health professionals, you have Major Depressive Disorder if you: have had an episode of depression lasting at least two weeks with at least five of the following symptoms:

➡ You are depressed, sad, blue, or tearful.

➡ You have lost interest or pleasure in things you previously liked to do.

➡ Your appetite is much less or much greater than usual and you have lost or gained weight.

➡ You have a lot of trouble sleeping or sleep too much.

➡ You are so agitated, restless, or slowed down that others have begun to notice.

➡ You are tired and have no energy.

➡ You feel worthless or excessively guilty about things you have done or not done.

➡ You have trouble concentrating, thinking clearly, or making decisions.

➡ You feel you would be better off dead or have thoughts about killing yourself.

These symptoms are severe enough to upset your daily routine, or to seriously impair your work, or to interfere with your relationships. The depression does not have a specific cause like alcohol, drugs, medication side effect, or physical illness. Your depression is not just a normal reaction to the death of a loved one.

(Adopted from http://www.holisticonline.com/Remedies/Depression/dep_diagnosis_1.htm)

Signs and Symptoms

➡ Feeling worthless, helpless, or hopeless

➡ Sleeping more or less than usual

➡ Eating more or less than usual

➡ Having difficulty concentrating or making decisions

➡ Loss of interest in taking part in activities

➡ Decreased sex drive

➡ Avoiding other people

➡ Overwhelming feelings of sadness or grief

➡ Feeling unreasonably guilty

➡ Loss of energy, feeling very tired

➡ Thoughts of death or suicide

(Adopted from http://www.cmha.calgary.ab.ca/mentalhealth/Types_of_Mental_Illness/Depression1.aspx)

Treatments

➡ With appropriate treatment, more than 80% of people with depression get full relief from their symptoms or at least substantial improvements.

➡ Most people respond to a combination of medication and psychotherapy.

➡ In some cases, electroconvulsive therapy (ECT) may be helpful.

➡ People with mild or moderate depression may benefit from medicinal extracts of St. John's Wort (hypericum perforatum).

➡ Light therapy can benefit people with seasonal affective disorder ("winter depression").

➡ Regular exercise and a healthy diet can help lessen overall symptoms.

➡ Spiritual faith or practice can give hope.

➡ People with mild depression may benefit from accenting the positive and increasing pleasurable activities.

(Adopted from http://www.kwantlen.ca/__shared/assets/Wellness_InFocus_-_Depression7838.pdf)

2. Global / National Statistics

Depression is one of the greatest problems and killers of our times. Here is the latest depression statistics, revealing surprising facts.

➡ In 2002, depression accounted for 4.5% of the worldwide total burden attributable to non-fatal health outcomes, accounting for almost 12% of total years lived with disability worldwide.

➡ Number of people worldwide suffering from depression: 121,000,000; the 4th leading cause, worldwide, of life years lost due to disability: depressive disorders (behind infectious diseases, heart disease and respiratory infections, and before HIV/AIDS); depressive disorders is the ailment expected to rank 2nd in global diseases, after heart disease, by 2020; depression is the mental disorder most commonly leading to suicide.

➡ Depression is the leading cause of disability as measured by YLDs and the 4th leading contributor to the global burden of disease (DALYs) in 2000. By the year 2020, depression is projected to reach 2nd place of the ranking of DALYs calcuated for all ages and both sexes. Today, depression is already the 2nd cause of DALYs in the age category 15-44 years for both sexes combined.

➡ Major depression affects approximately 15 million American adults or about 8% of the U.S. population age 18 and older in a given year; bipolar disorder (manic depression) affects approximately 6 million American adults or about 3% of the population in a given year; women experience depression about twice as often as men, over their lifetime about 12% of women will have clinical depression; approximately 80% of people experiencing depression are not currently receiving treatment; 80-90% of people who live with a serious mental illness are unemployed; more than 90% of persons who die by suicide have a diagnosable mental illness, commonly a depressive disorder; approximately 4% of adolescents develop serious depression each year, suicide is the third leading cause of death for ages of 10 to 24; depression is also known to weaken the immune system, making the body more susceptible to other medical illnesses; by the year 2020, depression will be the 2nd most common health problem in the world; and depression is one of the most treatable illnesses: 80-90% find relief.

➡ In any two-week period, 5.4% of Americans 12 years of age and older experienced depression, rates were higher in 40-59 year olds, women, and non-Hispanic black persons than in other demographic groups; rates of depression were higher among poor persons than among those with higher incomes; approximately 80% of persons with depression reported some level of functional impairment because of their depression, and 27% reported serious difficulties in work and home life; and only 29% of all persons with depression reported contacting a mental health professional in the past year, and among the subset with severe depression, only 39% reported contact.

➡ Mixed anxiety and depression is the most common mental disorder in Britain;

1/4 of the people will experience some kind of mental health problem in the course of a year; women are more likely to have been treated for a mental health problem than men; about 10% of children have a mental health problem at any one time; British men are three times as likely as British women to die by suicide; the UK has one of the highest rates of self harm in Europe, at 400 per 100,000 population; only one in 10 prisoners has no mental disorder.

(Adopted from:
http://www.heretohelp.bc.ca/publications/fact-sheets/depression#stats
http://www.who.int/mental_health/management/depression/definition/en/
http://www.pbs.org/wgbh/takeonestep/depression/pdf/dep_stats.pdf
http://www.mentalhealth.org.uk/information/mental-health-overview/statistics/)

3. Depression Survey – Are You Depressed?

The following are depression indicators. This is not a scientific tool but rather a way for you to identify contributing conditions in your life. We have listed two types of indicators: yellow indicators, which signal caution and should be monitored, and red indicators, which signal identified symptoms of depression. Red indicators are certainly important for you to be aware of, but don't overlook the yellow indicators. Yellows tend to turn to reds over time if not addressed. Yellow indicators can include conditions that have been present in your life for a long time, even a number of years. Red indicators come from the established criteria for clinical depression and, because of their severity can have a much shorter duration.

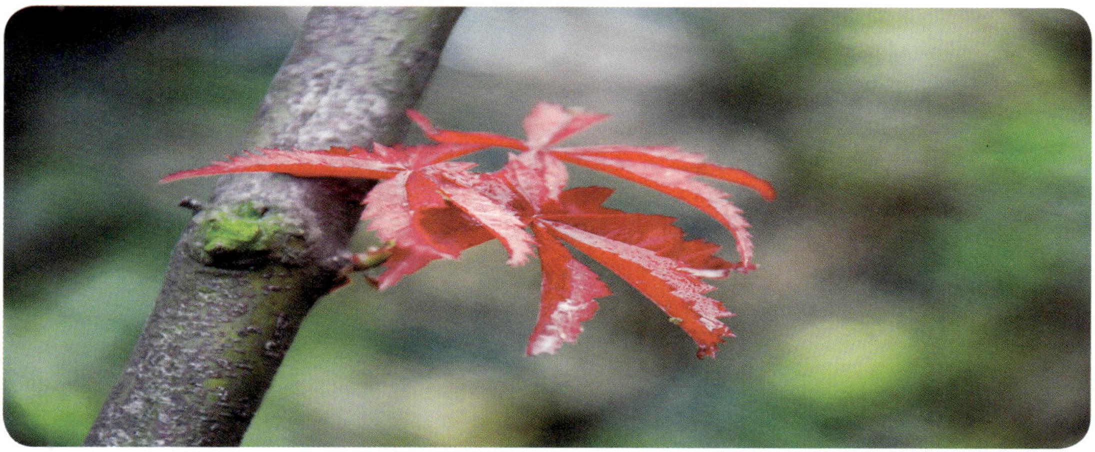

Check the indicators that you are experiencing:

Yellow Indicators

1	Loss of enjoyment in established activities
2	Restlessness, fatigue, or a lack of motivation at work
3	An increase in irritability or impatience
4	A sense of being either wound up or weighed down
5	A sense of being overburdened with life and its activities
6	A lack of spiritual peace or wellbeing
7	Relief fueled by controlling aspects of your personal behavior, including consuming liquids or food
8	A fear of expressing strong emotions
9	Constant anxiety or a vague fear about the future
10	A sense of being unappreciated by others
11	Feelings of martyrdom, as if you are constantly asked to do others' work
12	A pattern of impulsive thinking or rash judgments
13	Sexual difficulties or a loss of interest in sexual activities
14	Enjoyment in seeing others' discomfort
15	Anger at God for how you feel
16	A recurrent pattern of headaches, muscle aches, body pains
17	Social isolation and distance from family or friends
18	A sense of being trapped by the day's activities
19	A pattern of pessimistic or critical comments and/or behaviors
20	The belief that your best days are behind you and the future holds little promise
21	A sense of being left out of life
22	A binge on high-calorie foods to feel better
23	Upon waking, apathy about how the day will turn out
24	A preference just to do things yourself instead of working with others
25	Recurring gastrointestinal difficulties
26	A sense of being trapped inside your body
27	Dread of family get-togethers or social gatherings
28	The self-perception of being overweight, unattractive, or unlovable
29	A sense of being old, discarded, without value
30	No motivation to try new activities, contemplate new ideas, or enter into new relationships

Red Indicators

1	A significant change in appetite, lasting longer than two weeks, resulting in either marked weight loss (if not dieting) or weight gain
2	Recurring disturbances in sleep patterns for longer than two weeks, resulting in difficulty falling and staying asleep or sleeping too much
3	Increased agitation or inability to relax for an extended period of time (more than two weeks)
4	Fatigue, lethargy, or loss of energy for an extended period of time (more than two weeks)
5	Sadness, despondency, despair, loneliness, or feelings of worthlessness for an extended period of time (more than two weeks)
6	Inability to concentrate, focus, or make decisions, recurring over a period of time (more than two weeks)
7	Recurring thoughts of death or suicide
8	Plans for a suicide or an attempt at suicide

(Adopted from http://www.aplaceofhope.com/depressionsurvey.html)

4. Additional Reading Material

Chinese Medicine

Xu Yi-bing. *An Illustrated Guide to Chinese Medicine*. Beijing: People's Medical Publishing House; 2007

Paul Pritchford. *Healing With Whole Foods: Asian Traditions and Modern Nutrition*. Berkeley: North Atlantic Books; 2003

Harriet Beinfield, Efrem Korngold. *Between Heaven and Earth*. New York: Random House; 1991

Tom Williams. *Complete Illustrated Guide to Chinese Medicine*. New York: Barnes and Noble Inc.; 1996

Yang Jia-san. *The Way to Locate Acupoints*. Beijing: Foreign Language Press; 1982

Li De-yin. *Taiji Quan*. Beijing: Foreign Language Press; 2004

Cai Jing-feng. *Eating Your Way to Health – Diet Therapy in Traditional Chinese Medicine*. Beijing: Foreign Language Press; 1996

http://www.acupuncture.com/education/tcmbasics/index.htm
http://www.acupuncturetoday.com/abc/

http://www.healthy.net/
http://nccam.nih.gov/health/
http://www.tcmstudent.com/
http://www.nlm.nih.gov/hmd/chinese/chinesehome.html
http://qi-journal.com/
http://www.medicalacupuncture.org/
http://nccam.nih.gov/
http://www.medicinalnet.com/
http://www.medical-acupuncture.co.uk/
http://www.acupuncture.com/referrals/can.htm
http://www.who.int/mental_health/en/

Depression Treatment

Liu Zheng-cai. *The Mystery of Longevity*. Beijing: Foreign Language Press; 1990

Xu Jin-shui, Cheng Li-hong. *Chinese-English Edition of Acupuncture Treatment for Depression*. Shanghai: Shanghai Scientific and Technical Publishers; 2007

http://www.yinyanghouse.com/treatments/chinesemedicine_depression_treatment
http://chinese-medicine.suite101.com/article.cfm/chinese_medicine_helps_depression

5. Finding a Practitioner of Chinese Medicine

Finding a practitioner of Chinese medicine is often as easy as looking in your local phone book. Most cities now have an "Acupuncture" heading in the yellow pages. Since acupuncture is the best-known modality of Chinese medicine in Western countries, those that practice Chinese medicine will often also be listed in this section. In many places, there will probably not be a practitioner who specializes in treating depression, but you may be able to find someone in the larger cities if you call around.

Most countries have established educational and licensure standards. A practitioner should be able to verify that these standards have been met.

The web can offer many ways to find a practitioner. Just searching for "acupuncture" and your town/area's name will probably locate something. The following internet resources should help you find a practitioner in your local area:

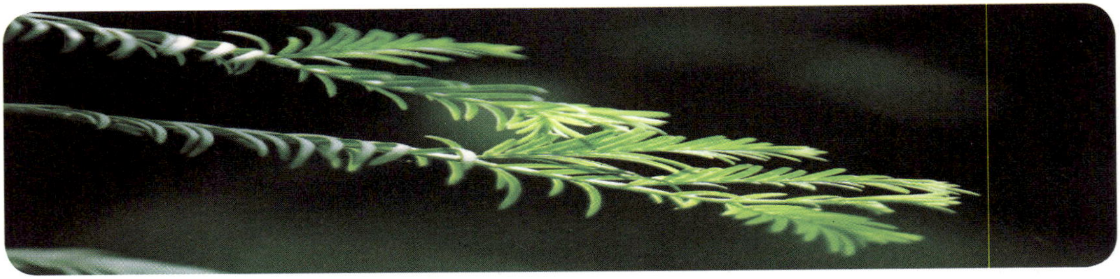

International Acupuncture Referral	http://www.acufinder.com http://www.gancao.net
Australia	Australian Acupuncture and Chinese Medicine Association http://www.acupuncture.org.au/
Canada	Traditional Chinese Medicine Association of British Columbia http://tcmabc.org/ Ordre des Acupuncteurs, Quebec http://www.ordredesacupuncteurs.qc.ca/
New Zealand	New Zealand Registrar of Acupuncture http://acupuncture.org.nz/
United Kingdom	Register of Chinese Medicinals http://www.rchm.cwww.acupuncture.org.uk/ The British Medical Acupuncture Society http://www.medical-acupuncture.co.uk/
United States of America	National Certification Commission for Acupuncture and Oriental Medicine http://nccaom.org/ Council of Colleges of Acupuncture and Oriental Medicine http://www.ccaom.org/
Tai Ji - Qi Gong Information	http://www.worldtaichiday.org http://www.qi.org

References

1. *Traditional Chinese Medicine Acknowledged by World,* http://english.peopledaily.com.cn/english/200004/24/eng20000424_39547.html.

2. National Institute of Health. *Estimates of Funding for Various Diseases, Conditions, Research Areas.* http://www.nih.gov/news/fundingresearchareas.htm, 2007.

3. CDC: *Antidepressants Most Prescribed Drugs in U.S.,* http://edition.cnn.com/2007/HEALTH/07/09/antidepressants/index.html.

4. Thomas J. Moore. *Prescription for Disaster: The Hidden Dangers in Your Medicine Cabinet,* New York: Simon and Schuster, 1998.

5. Anahad O'Conner. *"Has the Romance Gone? Was It the Drug?"* New York Times, May 4, 2004. Also available online: http://www.nytimes.com/2004/05/04/health/has-the-romance-gone-was-it-the-drug.html.

6. *Five-Medicinal Combo Can Control Eczema, Study Says,* http://chinesemedicinenews.com/2007/08/03/5-medicinal-combo-can-control-eczema-study-says/.

7. Peter Sherwood. *Healing*. Australian College of Natural Medicine, 2006.

8. Zhen Cheng. *The Pandemic of Influenza Eighty Years Ago.* Chinese Journal of Medical History. No. 4, 1998.

9. The Times. *Olympic Athletes Queue to Try Old Chinese Remedies,* http://www.timesonline.co.uk/tol/sport/olympics/article4510344.ece.

10. Hao Wang-shan. *The Therapeutic Effect of Modified Chai Gui Wen Dang Ding Zhi Tang on Depression.* Journal of Beijing University of Traditional Chinese Medicine, 1997, 20(3) :64.

11. Jin Guang-liang. *Study on the Seasonal Pathogenesis of Depression.* Journal of Beijing University of Traditional Chinese Medicine, 1997, 20(1) :151.

12. Zheng Yi-lun. *Discussion on the diagnosis and treatment principle of depression from the perspective of brain spirit and the theory of five-zang organs and spirit.* Research of Traditional Chinese Medicine, 1998, 14 (2): 31.

13. Zhang Jian and Li Fu-ren. *Experience of Treating Senile Depression.* Journal of Traditional Chinese Medicine, 2000, 41 (4): 208.

14. Wang Yong-yan. *Depression*: Internal Medicine of Traditional Chinese Medi-

cine, First Edition. Shanghai Scientific and Technical Publishers, 1997.

15. *Psycho-Emotional Practice: PNE Balancing Therapy*, http://www.acupuncturetoday.com/mpacms/at/article.php?id=29058.

16. *Emotional Wellbeing through Chinese Medicine*, http://www.fivepetalshealth.com/Emotional.

17. Zhang Guo-xi. *Zhang Guoxi's Experience on Health-preservation of Chinese Medicine.* http://lz.book.sohu.com/chapter-9964-1-7.html.

18. Jin Hong-zhu and Yang Hong-ying. *Chinese Tui Na (Massage)*. Publishing House of Shanghai University of Traditional Chinese Medicine, First edition, 2002.

19. Zhang En-qin. *Chinese Medicated Diet.* Publishing House of Shanghai University of Traditional Chinese Medicine, First edition, 1996.6 14.

20. Brosse AL, Sheets ES, Lett HS, et al. *Exercise and the Treatment of Clinical Depression in Adults: Recent Findings and Future Directions.* Sports Medicine, 2002;32(12):741-760.

21. Luan Jia-qin. *Wisdom of Keeping Healthy.* Jiangsu Arts and Literature Publishing House. http://read.dangdang.com/content_567144.

22. Lee MS, Shin BC, Jeong DM. *An Exploratory Study of the Relationship between the Midday-midnight Law and Electrical Conduction Properties of Corresponding Acupuncture Points.* Acupuncture and Electro-therapy Research, 2005; 30 (3-4): 201-206.

23. Irwin MR, Olmstead R, and Motivala SJ. *Improving Sleep Quality in Older Adults with Moderate Sleep Complaints: A randomized Controlled Trial of Tai Chi Chih.* Sleep, 2008 Jul 1; 31(7):1001-1008.

24. Kerr CE, Shaw JR, Wasserman RH, Chen VW, Kanojia A, Bayer T, and Kelley JM. *Tactile Acuity in Experienced Tai Chi Practitioners: Evidence for use Dependent Plasticity as an Effect of Sensory-attentional Training.* Experimental Brain Research. 2008, 188 (2):317-322.

25. Mustian KM, Palesh OG, Flecksteiner SA. *Tai Chi Chuan for Breast Cancer Survivors.* Medicine and Sports Science. 2008; 52:209–217.

26. Wang Y. *Tai Chi Exercise and the Improvement of Mental and Physical Health among College Students.* Medicine and Sports Science. 2008; 52:135–45.

27. Tsang HW, Fung KM. *A Review on Neurobiological and Psychological Mechanisms Underlying the Anti-depressive Effect of Qi Gong Exercise.* Journal of Health Psychology, 2008, 13 (7):857-863.

28. Kim SD, Kim HS. *Effects of a Relaxation*

Breathing Exercise on Anxiety, Depression, and Leukocyte in Hemopoietic Stem Cell Transplantation Patients. Cancer Nursing. 2005, 28(1):79-83.

29. *Acupunture.* http://www.mamashealth.com/massage/acupuncture.asp.

30. *Chinese Medicine.* http://www.health.com/health/library/topic/0, aa140227spec_tp 21268, 00. html.

31. *Acupuncture: An Introduction.* http://nccam.nih.gov/health/acupuncture/introduction.htm.

32. TCM. http://www.drdonfan.ca/tcm.html.

33. *Questions and Answers about Acupuncture,* http://www.medem.com/medlib/article/ZZZ8QS2P9CF.

34. *About Acupuncture.* http://www.healthynj.org/health-wellness/acupuncture/main.htm.

35. *The World Health Organization Viewpoint on Acupuncture.* http://www.roseacupuncture.com/conditions_treated.php#WHO.

36. Jennifer Dubowsky. L.Ac., M.S.O.M., Dipl.Ac. *Acupuncture and Depression: An Old Answer to an Old Problem.* http://www.acufinder.com/Acupuncture+Information/Detail/Acupuncture+and+Depression+An+Old+Answer+to+an+Old+Problem.

37. Xu Jin-shui, Cheng Li-hong. *Chinese-English Edition of Acupuncture Treatment for Depression.* Shanghai Scientific and Technical Publishers. 2007.

38. Wang Yu-ying. *Application of Electro-acupuncture in the Treatment of Depression.* Foreign Medical Sciences (Traditional Chinese Medicine), 1994, 16(2): 50.

39. Ye Guo-chuan. *Treatment of 36 Cases of Depression by Acupuncture.* Shanghai Journal of Acupuncture and Moxibustion, 2000, 19 (6):30.

40. Lin Hong. *Treatment of 53 cases of Postpartum Depression by Acupuncture.* Tianjin Journal of Traditional Chinese Medicine, 1996, 13 (3) :11-12.

41. Jiang Feng-lian. *Treatment of Senile Depression by Acupuncture.* Henan Traditional Chinese Medicine, 1997, 17 (6):373.

42. Kang Bo, Zhang Ping-gen, Xiong Sheng-cai, et al. *Comparison of Electro-acupuncture and Amitriptyline in the Treatment of Depressive States.* Chinese Acupuncture and Moxibustion, 2002, 22 (6) :383–384.

43. Luo He-chun, Hou Dong-fen. *Clinical Observation on the Treatment of 30 Cases with Post Stroke Depression by Electro-acupuncturing Yin Tang.* Chinese Acupuncture and Moxibustion, 1996, 8:23–24.

44. Dong Zi-ping. *Treatment of 101 Cases with Depression by Electro-acupuncture.* Chi-

nese Acupuncture and Moxibustion, 2001, 2 (1): 6.

45. He Ling, Liu Zhi-bin. *Treatment of 32 Cases with Hot Sensation and Profuse Sweating Caused by Menopause by Pressing Earpoints.* Shaanxi Journal of Traditional Chinese Medicine, 2002, 23 (11):1022–1023.

46. Ren Jian-ning. *Treatment of 50 Cases of Depression by Ear Acupuncture.* Henan Traditional Chinese Medicine, 2005, 25 (2):75.

47. Song Yin, Liang Hao-rong. *Clinical Observation on the Treatment of Post Stroke Depression by Scalp Acupuncture.* Shanghai Journal of Acupuncture and Moxibustion, 1999, 18 (1):8.

48. Li Han-jun. *Treatment of 75 Cases with Neurasthenia by Acupuncturing Baihui towards Si Shen Cong.* Heilongjiang Journal of Traditional Chinese Medicine, 1997, 1:45.

49. Zhao Xiu-min, Ji Peng-wen, Chen Feng-kuan, et al. *Treatment of Depression by Combining Acupuncture Point Injection of Back-shu Points and with Acupunture.* Chinese Journal of Information on Traditional Chinese Medicine, 2001, 8 (12):78279.

50. Qian Jie, Zhang Jie, Pei Yin. *Treatment of Depression by Cupping Therapy.* Beijing Journal of Traditional Chinese Medicine, 2003, 22 (5) :15-16.

51. Wang Wei-hong, Yi Fang-hong. *Treatment of 35 Cases with Menopause Depression by Acupuncture and Cupping.* Shanghai Journal of Acupuncture and Moxibustion, 2005, 24 (5) :8.

52. Zhong ZG, Cai H, Li XL, et al. *Effect of Acupuncture Combined with Massage of Sole on Sleeping Quality of the Patient with Insomnia.* Chinese Acupuncture and Moxibustion. 2008 Jun; 28(6): 411–413.

53. Wang H, Qi H, Wang BS, et al. *Is Acupuncture Beneficial in Depression: a Meta-analysis of 8 Randomized Controlled Trials?* Journal of Affective Disorders. 2008 Dec;111(2-3):125-134.

54. Li SJ, Liu T. *Clinical Observation on Treatment of Melancholia by Acupuncture following Principle of Relieving Depression and Regulating Mentality.* Chinese Journal of Integrative Medicine, 2007 Feb; 27(2):155–7.

55. Zhang C. *The Brain-resuscitation Acupuncture Method for Treatment of Post Wind-stroke Mental Depression-A Report of 45 Cases.* Journal of Traditional Chinese Medicine, 2005 ,25(4):243-246.

56. Han C, Li X, Luo H, et al. *Clinical Study on Electro-acupuncture Treatment for 30 Cases of Mental Depression.* Journal of Traditional Chinese Medicine, 2004, 24 (3):172-6.

57. Tsay SL, Cho YC, Chen ML. *Acupressure and Transcutaneous Electrical Acupoint Stimulation in Improving Fatigue, Sleep Quality, and Depression in Hemodialysis Pa-*

tients. American Journal of Chinese Medicine, 2004; 32 (3): 407-16.

58. Lei Zai-quan. *Science of Chinese Materia Medica, First Edition.* Shanghai Scientific and Technical Publishers, 1995.

59. Chen Shi-hong. *Common Medicinal Groups Used in the Treatment of Depression.* Journal of Practical Traditional Chinese Internal Medicine, 2005, 19 (4): 382.

60. Wang Li-ren. *Formula Analysis Commonly Used in the Treatment of Depression.* Guangming Journal of Chinese Medicine, 2000, 15 (88):7-8.

61. Wang Yong-yan. *Depression: Internal Medicine of Traditional Chinese Medicine, First Edition.* Shanghai Scientific and Technical Publishers, 1997.

62. Wang YT, Tan QR, Sun LL, et al. *Possible Therapeutic Effect of a Traditional Chinese Medicine, Sinisan, on Chronic Restraint Stress Related Disorders.* Neuroscience Letters. 2009, Jan 16; 449 (3): 215–219.

63. Wu LK, Zhang JJ, Wang JX, et al. *Effects of Pingyu Capsule on Signal Transduction of Rats with Chronic Stress-induced Depression.* China Journal of Chinese Materia Medica, 2008, Jul; 33 (14):1743-1746.

64. Mao QQ, Ip SP, Tsai SH, et al. *Antidepressant-like Effect of Peony Glycosides in Mice.* Journal of Ethnopharmacology. 2008, Sep 26; 119 (2): 272-275.

65. Wei XH, Cheng XM, Shen JS, Wang ZT. *Antidepressant Effect of Yueju-Wan Ethanol Extract and its Fractions in Mice Models of Despair.* Journal of Ethnopharmacology, May 8, 2008; 117 (2):339-344.

66. He Q, Zhang J, Tang Y. *A Controlled Study on Treatment of Mental Depression by Acupuncture plus TCM Medication.* Journal of Traditional Chinese Medicine. 2007, 27(3): 166-169.

67. Mao QQ, Huang Z. *Research Progress on Therapeutic Mechanism of Depression Treated by Traditional Chinese Medicine.* China Journal of Chinese Materia Medica. 2007 May; 32 (10): 877–80.

68. Chen JX, Li W, Zhao X, et al. *Effects of the Chinese traditional prescription Xiaoyao-san decoction on chronic immobilization stress-induced changes in behavior and brain BDNF, TrkB, and NT-3 in rats.* Cellular and Molecular Neurobiology. 2008, 28(5):745-755.

69. Li YJ, Luo HC, Qian RQ. *Effect of Danzhi Xiaoyao Powder on Neuro-immuno-endocrine System in Patients with Depression.* Chinese Journal of Integrative Medicine. 2007, 27(3):197–200.

70. Ushiroyama T, Ikeda A, Sakuma K, Ueki M. *Chai-hu-gui-zhi-gan-jiang-tang Regulates Plasma Interleukin-6 and Soluble Interleukin-6 Receptor Concentrations and Improves Depressed Mood in Climacteric Women with Insomnia.* American Journal of Chinese Medicine. 2005; 33(5): 703-711.

71. Jin Hong-zhu, Yang Hong-ying. *Chinese Tui Na (Massage).* Publishing House of Shanghai University of Traditional Chinese Medicine. First edition, 2002.

72. *Self Massage for Depression,* http://www.holisticonline.com/remedies/Depression/dep_massage.htm.

73. Zhang Guo-xi. Zhang Guo-xi's Experience on the Health-preservation of Chinese Medicine. http://vip.book.sina.com.cn/book/chapter_61377_39538.html.

74. Field TM. *Massage Therapy Effects.* American Psychology. 1998 Dec;53(12):1270-81.

75. Field T, Figueiredo B, Hernandez-Reif M, Diego M, Deeds O, Ascencio A. *Massage Therapy Reduces Pain in Pregnant Women, Alleviates Prenatal Depression in Both Parents and Improves their Relationships.* Journal of Bodywork and Movement Therapies. 2008 Apr; 12 (2):146-150.

76. Lee YM. *Effect of Self-foot Reflexology Massage on Depression, Stress Responses and Immune Functions of Middle Aged Women.* Taehan Kanho Hakhoe Chi Journal. 2006, 36(1):179-188.

77. Song RH, Kim DH. *The Effects of Foot Reflexion Massage on Sleep Disturbance, Depression Disorder, and the Physiological Index of the Elderly.* Taehan Kanho Hakhoe Chi Journal. 2006, 36 (1):15-24.

78. Field T, Diego MA, Hernandez-Reif M, Schanberg S, Kuhn C. *Massage Therapy Effects on Depressed Pregnant Women.* Journal of Psychosomatic Obstetrics and Gynecology. 2004, 25(2):115-122.

79. Jones NA, Field T. *Massage and Music Therapies Attenuate Frontal EEG Asymmetry in Depressed Adolescents.* Journal of Adolescence. 1999, 34 (135): 529-534.

80. Hua Gang. *Treatment of 46 Cases with Depression by the Modification of Chai Hu Shu Gan San.* Shaanxi Journal of Traditional Chinese Medicine, 2003, 24 (6): 539-554.

81. Zhang Chun-hong, Li Jin-bo, Wang Shu. *Observation on Therapeutic Effect of Activating Brain and Opening Orifice on Depression in Germany.* Journal of Clinical Acupuncture and Moxibustion, 2002, 18 (8): 6-7.

82. Yang Wen-bin, Chen Shu-jiang, Wang Xin. *Case Report of Treating Depression and Mania by Acupuncture and Medicinals.* Liaoning Journal of Traditional Chinese Medicine, 2003, 12 (30): 1003.

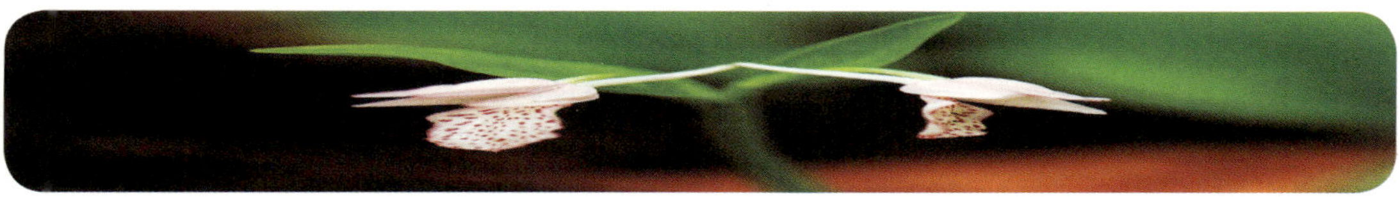

Index

A

B

C

D

E

F

G

H

I

J

K

L

M

N

O

P

Q

R

S

W

X

Y

Z

图书在版编目（CIP）数据

中医科普系列—抑郁症（英文）/陈云慧等主编.
—北京：人民卫生出版社，2009.10
ISBN 978-7-117-11472-1
Ⅰ.中… Ⅱ.陈… Ⅲ.R473.6 Ⅳ.R473.6

中国版本图书馆CIP数据核字（2009）第104649号

中医科普系列—抑郁症

（英文）

主　　编：陈云慧　卡尔·斯蒂姆森
出版发行：人民卫生出版社（中继线＋8610－6761－6688）
地　　址：中国北京市丰台区方庄芳群园三区3号楼
邮　　编：100078
E－mail：pmph@pmph.com
发　　行：pmphsales@gmail.com
购书热线：＋8610-6769-1034（电话及传真）
开　　本：850×1168　1/24
版　　次：2009年10月第1版　2009年10月第1版第1次印刷
标准书号：ISBN 978-7-117-11472-1/R·11473